Essential Operational Components for High-Performing Healthcare Enterprises

ACHE Management Series

Essential Operational Components for High-Performing Healthcare Enterprises

Jon Burroughs, Editor

Foreword by David B. Nash

ACHE Management Series

Your board, staff, or clients may also benefit from this book's insight. For more information on quantity discounts, contact the Health Administration Press Marketing Manager at (312) 424-9450.

23   22   21   20   19   5   4   3   2

Library of Congress Cataloging-in-Publication Data
Names: Burroughs, Jonathan H., editor.
Title: Essential operational components for high-performing healthcare
   enterprises / edited by Jon Burroughs.
Description: Chicago, IL : Health Administration Press, [2018] | Series:
   HAP/ACHE management series | Includes bibliographical references. |
   Identifiers: LCCN 2018023024 (print) | LCCN 2018031220 (ebook) | ISBN
   9781640550025 (xml) | ISBN 9781640550032 (epub) | ISBN 9781640550049
   (mobi) | ISBN 9781640550001 | ISBN 9781640550001q(alk. paper)
Subjects: LCSH: Health services administration.
Classification: LCC RA971 (ebook) | LCC RA971 .E88 2018 (print) | DDC
   362.1068--dc23
LC record available at https://lccn.loc.gov/2018023024

Acquisitions editor: Jennette McClain; Cover designer: Brad Norr; Layout: PerfecType

Found an error or a typo? We want to know! Please e-mail it to hapbooks@ache.org, mentioning the book's title and putting "Book Error" in the subject line.

For photocopying and copyright information, please contact Copyright Clearance Center at www.copyright.com or at (978) 750-8400.

Health Administration Press
A division of the Foundation of the American
   College of Healthcare Executives
300 S. Riverside Plaza, Suite 1900
Chicago, IL 60606–6698
(312) 424-2800

This book is dedicated to my daughter Serena, my son Seth,
my daughter-in-law Elli, and my grandson Aristides,
that they may inherit and support an even better
healthcare system for the generations that will follow.

Contents

Foreword

David B. Nash, MD
Jefferson College of Population Health
Thomas Jefferson University

IN MY TRAVELS across the country, I see healthcare-related organizations that are talking the talk but seem unable to walk the talk in our national transition from traditional fee-for-service reimbursement to value-based care. This shift is a dangerous journey through unchartered waters. It's a journey that calls for a modern-day guide, a Sherpa who knows every risk and can lead us through perilous, unknown terrain. Jon Burroughs is this Sherpa, perfectly situated for this hazardous journey!

In *Essential Operational Components for High-Performing Healthcare Enterprises*, I believe Jon has encapsulated the challenge in his pithy phrase "eliminating non-value-added clinical and business outcome variation," which constitutes a central theme and directional beacon for the journey. The book is built on the four Cs of communication, collaboration, continued learning, and caring about communities.

Jon has assembled a well-known group of contributors, almost all of whom I count as my professional friends. Among my favorite chapters is James E. Orlikoff's "Governing the Future of Healthcare Systems." Governance responsibilities, in the contemporary era, transcend a singular focus on finance and strategic planning and now encompass the entire healthcare journey: prevention, wellness, and care coordination in every setting.

Given my role as the dean of the nation's first college of population health, I was also drawn to chapters on information technology that support population health. As a result, chapters 8 and 11 resonated with me particularly.

I was happily surprised to read chapter 9 on managing actuarial risks. Actuarial expertise is my own personal litmus test for leaders of integrated systems; that is, if a leader doesn't have actuaries on staff, I am prone to dismiss his plans outright. The lack of such individuals is testimony to the leader's failure to understand the core transition of the system.

I also admire the way Jon weaves in some of the industry's best contemporary learnings from foremost scholars such as Atul Gawande and Clay Christensen. Jon does not pay homage to these individuals but rather cleverly distills their main messages in a way that supports his own, as well as the clarity of his own prose.

At its essence, this book attempts to transfer a skill set historically identified with the for-profit managed care industry—for-profit leaders have already been practicing a form of population-based care and have attempted to drive the adoption of value-based purchasing. Say what you will about the for-profit managed care industry—it has been at the forefront of this movement and, as a result, has been a target of the traditional hospital and provider community.

I would bet we have not heard the last from Jon, but this book will be an outstanding guide for leaders who want to seriously walk the talk on the journey toward reducing unexplained variation—those who seek to move our broken system from a "the more we do, the more we get paid" approach to an approach focused on asking the far more difficult question, "Why are we doing these things in the first place, and what value do they add?"

Sign me up for the journey, as long as I have Jon Burroughs at my side leading the way! I'm confident that the reader will readily recognize Jon's navigational skills, and those who spend the time with this book will be richly rewarded when they reach the final destination before most of their competitors.

Acknowledgments

THIS BOOK IS the result of three years of research, travel, on-site visits, consulting engagements, communications, and reflection. The exhilarating part of synthesizing new knowledge is that there are few established references. The healthcare industry is evolving rapidly and, contrary to popular belief, that change is less the result of a federal mandate than a bottom-up reaction to intransigent economic pressures that require and even demand transformation.

I would like to first thank several organizations that were the original inspiration for this book through their extraordinarily innovative and imaginative work in clinical integration. They are the following:

- Intermountain Healthcare, Salt Lake City, Utah
- St. Luke's Health System, Boise, Idaho
- Baylor Scott & White Health, Dallas, Texas
- Memorial Hermann Health System, Houston, Texas

These organizations have been blessed with gifted and visionary healthcare leaders whom I both respect and consider personal and professional friends. They include Brent James, MD, former chief quality officer, Intermountain Healthcare; Susan Dubois, assistant vice president, Intermountain Healthcare and past president, National Association Medical Staff Services; David Pate, MD, JD, president and CEO, St. Luke's Health System; Joel Allison, past president and CEO, Baylor Scott & White Health; Paul Convery, past system CMO, Baylor Scott & White Health; Carl Couch, MD, past senior vice president and chief innovation officer, Baylor Scott & White Health; and Keith Fernandez, MD, past chair of the board, past president and CEO, the Memorial Hermann Physician Network.

To create a text with the latest best practices in clinical integration, I had the privilege of recruiting some of the most outstanding healthcare thought leaders in our country. They have all contributed significantly to the value of this book through their individual groundbreaking work in our field. I count many among my personal and professional friends. They include the following:

- Tom Atchison, EdD, president and founder, Atchison Consulting LLC
- Mary A. Baker, DHA, CPCS, CPMSM, president, Medical Staff Plus Consulting LLC
- Kathleen Bartholomew, RN, MSN
- Steve Berger, FACHE, FHFMA, CPA, president, Berger Healthcare Executive Training and Consulting, LLC
- Brian C. Betner, Esq., shareholder, Hall, Render, Killian, Heath, and Lyman, PC
- Carl Couch, MD, MMM
- Daron Cowley, senior director of corporate communications, Intermountain Healthcare
- Dan Grauman, MBA, CPA, managing director and CEO, Veralon
- Michael R. Greer, Esq., Hall, Render, Killian, Heath, and Lyman, PC
- Mike Harmer, enterprise analytics lead, Intermountain Healthcare
- John Harris, MBA, director, Veralon
- Brent Heaton, data governance manager, Intermountain Healthcare
- Steven P. Johnson, PhD, president and CEO, Health First

- Naveen Maram, MD, MSHI, MPH, partner, care transformation, Intermountain Healthcare
- John J. Nance, JD
- David Nash, MD, MBA, founding dean, Jefferson School of Population Health
- Lonny Northrup, medical informaticist, Intermountain Healthcare
- Jamie Orlikoff, president, Orlikoff and Associates, Inc.
- Lee Pierce, MIS, chief data officer, Intermountain Healthcare
- Jake Poore, founder, president, and CEO, Integrated Loyalty Systems
- Sidney Thornton, PhD, partner, care transformation, Intermountain Healthcare
- Bill Vanaskie, FACHE

Healthcare Administration Press provided a top-notch team to oversee the editorial process necessary to support a book of this complexity. Jennette McClain served as the acquisitions editor and oversaw the entire project. Nancy Vitucci and Lauren Wilk built HAP's marketing campaign.

Finally, I would like to thank my wife, Anita, who has served as my psychological and emotional anchor throughout the three-year project. She is my partner in business and in life, and without her, I could not explore the far reaches of our field. I give her my love and gratitude for this and more.

Introduction

Jon Burroughs

THE UNITED STATES is committed to moving its healthcare system from a volume-based reimbursement method to one centered on value. By 2018, the Centers for Medicare & Medicaid Services (CMS) will have shifted 50 percent of its payment methodologies to "pay for value," with 90 percent of its payment programs tied to some form of quality measures. Commercial payers are following CMS's lead. Amy Oldenburg, vice president of network and product strategy accountable care solutions at Aetna, estimates that 75 percent of Aetna's spending will be absorbed by some form of value-based payment by 2020 (Gruessner 2016).

Thus, time is short as healthcare organizations transform their care and business models in an effort to provide value-based services that can meet key benchmarks for clinical and business outcomes (particularly concerning cost of care). But what will get us there? Certainly not the traditional twentieth-century models. Their stand-alone hospitals providing primary and secondary service areas with both employed and self-employed physicians (who work through productivity-based contracts) are on the decline.

The stand-alone hospital must evolve into a coordinated and integrated delivery system that can leverage the facility as a cost center intended to treat the seriously ill and injured. Organizations must build a new ambulatory infrastructure whose purpose is to prevent patients from resorting to the hospital, emergency department, and physician's office. Doctors must be fully aligned and integrated with large healthcare systems so that they can work in collaboration with management and other healthcare facilities, working toward common clinical and business goals. Hospitals will be part of clinically integrated delivery systems that include patients and their families in their homes, schools, home health agencies, health clubs, freestanding imaging centers, inpatient and outpatient rehabilitation facilities, nursing homes and other long-term care facilities, post-acute care facilities, and more. This spectrum of facilities will be tied in with health information exchanges, employers, Medicaid and other state-supported programs, and the federal government (CMS); they will require the support of clinical and business analytics with access to a data warehouse covering the whole enterprise. With these elements in place, healthcare systems can work with large payers toward mutual, value-based goals and objectives.

Contracts with all parties will need to be dynamic, transparent, and shared. These measures will ensure that all parties are working together to achieve the objective of better health outcomes at a reduced cost.

This book describes the fundamental operational components that all healthcare organizations must share to achieve success in this rapidly emerging world. The specific structure of each organization will differ based on local market and payer conditions and the availability of resources across widely diverse geographic, political, and economic regions. Each chapter describes a component or building block integral to the rapid transformation of a volume-based "sickness" industry into a value-based "health" industry. The following are short descriptions of the chapters.

CHAPTER 1: A HEALTHCARE VISION FOR THE NEXT-LEVEL HEALTHCARE ENTERPRISE (JON BURROUGHS, FACHE)

This chapter articulates the compelling economic, clinical, and political mandate to redesign the healthcare enterprise and describes the new models necessary to move the traditional model toward prevention and population health.

CHAPTER 2: SUSTAINABLE CHANGE IN HEALTHCARE: LEADERSHIP FOR THE TWENTY-FIRST CENTURY (TOM ATCHISON)

Forging ahead in a radically altered business model requires new leadership and management skills. The top-down style of the twentieth century will be replaced by collaborative executives able to guide change in a complex matrix management configuration. Such leaders bring stakeholders together, helping them to envision collaboration and supporting overarching strategies that benefit broader constituencies. Hospital executives will evolve into *healthcare* executives who oversee clinically integrated networks of largely ambulatory facilities and resources. The personal traits of such leaders must evolve as well; with direct control replaced by influence, vision, and collaboration. This chapter examines the characteristics of effective contemporary leaders and the leadership skills that are essential in the twenty-first century.

CHAPTER 3: GOVERNING THE FUTURE OF HEALTHCARE SYSTEMS (JAMES E. ORLIKOFF)

Governance models for integrated systems are significantly different from those for stand-alone hospitals. As healthcare enterprises become increasingly complex and interconnected, novel governance competencies will be in high demand. Governing members are required to have greater skill, commitment, and knowledge of the healthcare sector. These advantages will enable them to partner effectively with management and medical staff, improving quality and financial outcomes. This chapter covers emerging governance models and analyzes the fundamental competencies required to govern effectively in the twenty-first century.

CHAPTER 4: THE EVOLVING ROLE OF THE PHYSICIAN, NURSE, MEDICAL STAFF SERVICES PROFESSIONAL, AND ORGANIZED MEDICAL STAFF (JON BURROUGHS, FACHE; KATHLEEN BARTHOLOMEW; AND MARY A. BAKER)

As healthcare becomes more patient centered, lower-cost providers will be patients' primary contact point with their healthcare systems. Physicians will take on coordination and oversight roles, delegating responsibility for direct, routine services and documentation to others while overseeing the management of larger populations for whom they will be held accountable according to specific, measurable outcomes. The boundaries between physician, nurse, medical staff services professional, and healthcare executive will blur as clinical professionals gain increasing operational and financial experience and assume greater management responsibilities. The organized medical staff will shift from being an entity that once functioned like a protective professional guild to more dynamic units capable of moving with management through ever-accelerating change in an agile and collaborative way.

CHAPTER 5: STRATEGIC PLANNING FOR THE FUTURE HEALTHCARE ENTERPRISE (JOHN M. HARRIS AND DAN GRAUMAN)

As strategic, operating, and business plans become more adaptable to accommodate unforeseeable change, the ability to plan will require different skills. Analytics shared among healthcare enterprises, payers, regulators, and patients will alter the dynamic of healthcare planning, which will evolve to include the integration and alignment of key stakeholders. This chapter looks at the new ways in which healthcare organizations will plan for an increasingly transformed future.

CHAPTER 6: MODELS AND COMPETENCIES FOR CLINICAL INTEGRATION (JON BURROUGHS, FACHE; AND CARL COUCH)

Clinically integrated networks (CINs) take many forms, ranging from accountable care organizations to acute care episode–bundled-payment projects. This chapter explores the various models of clinical integration and the fundamental operational components and competencies necessary for any successful CIN, regardless of its structure. It will also discuss the Baylor Scott & White Quality Alliance, one of largest and most successful ACOs in the United States, as an example of the complexities of a well-designed, clinically integrated enterprise.

CHAPTER 7: TAKING THE SERVICE LINE TO THE NEXT LEVEL IN THE TWENTY-FIRST CENTURY (WILLIAM VANASKIE, FACHE)

One of the fundamental building blocks of any clinically integrated network is the service line, or horizontally integrated clinical institute. These units involve multiple clinical disciplines coming together, through aligned contracts, to develop evidence-based approaches to managing high-volume or variable-risk conditions. Service lines are often governed and managed collaboratively through dyad or triad models of physician–nurse–executive oversight to manage overarching organizational initiatives. This chapter explores the success factors for service lines, regardless of operational structures, and how they can support more consistent clinical and business outcomes.

CHAPTER 8: HEALTH INFORMATION MANAGEMENT FOR THE TWENTY-FIRST-CENTURY HEALTHCARE ENTERPRISE (LEE PIERCE, MIKE HARMER, BRENT HEATON, LONNY NORTHRUP, NAVEEN MARAM, AND SID THORNTON)

Like finance industries, population health requires the seamless transmission of information throughout the world—from the patient to all key healthcare personnel and institutions. This seamlessness requires a series of tools within, between, and beyond clinical enterprises, including

- electronic medical records (internal and interorganizational),
- multi-institutional health information exchanges,
- customized patient portals,
- clinical and business analytics with decision alerts to key stakeholders, and
- enterprise data warehousing.

These elements must be connected via global systems that readily interface and provide superb interconnectivity. Intermountain Healthcare has one of the largest and most sophisticated health information management systems in the world, and this chapter summarizes the fundamental components necessary for sharing and transmitting information throughout any clinically integrated delivery system.

CHAPTER 9: MANAGING ACTUARIAL RISK (STEVEN JOHNSON)

Clinical and business analytics provide real-time, predictive, actionable information that enables healthcare enterprises to optimize value by managing clinical outcomes while minimizing costs. One of the overarching purposes of predictive analytics is to manage actuarial risk for defined populations of covered lives. The question of using internal versus outsourced talent is of less importance than the skill with which an organization can implement this component of its model. Steven Johnson, who oversees a sophisticated health plan, discusses how to manage actuarial risk generically and how to apply these skills to manage insurance products that will be an essential part of any effective healthcare system of the future.

CHAPTER 10: BEST-PRACTICE EVIDENCE-BASED MANAGEMENT THAT MINIMIZES COSTS AND OPTIMIZES OUTCOMES (JON BURROUGHS, FACHE; AND STEVE BERGER, FACHE)

One of healthcare's contemporary strategies is to employ evidence-based management of labor and supply chains for higher-quality healthcare at a fraction of the cost. This goal requires the adoption of clinical and business analytics that use real-time and predictive information, enabling a smaller number of managers to gain greater control over operational processes. This chapter examines healthcare organizations' best practices, used to achieve significantly lower costs while optimizing quality and safety.

CHAPTER 11: OPERATIONAL BUILDING BLOCKS AND SUCCESS FACTORS FOR POPULATION HEALTH (JON BURROUGHS, FACHE)

Population health represents the rationalization of healthcare resources for risk-stratified subpopulations of covered lives. Operational elements of population health include the following:

- Palliative care for patients with life-threatening conditions
- Disease management for patients with complex, chronic conditions
- Post-acute care and ambulatory disease management following discharge for acute care services
- Retail medicine for healthy individuals with minor, acute, episodic problems
- Ongoing access to e-health platforms and customized healthcare management systems and solutions for the healthy majority

This chapter covers the key operational elements of each of these services, describes their contributions to the well-being of defined subpopulations, and discusses the ways in which they will optimize healthcare outcomes and minimize costs.

CHAPTER 12: CREATING A HIGH-RELIABILITY ORGANIZATION FOR THE TWENTY-FIRST CENTURY (KATHLEEN BARTHOLOMEW; JOHN NANCE; AND JON BURROUGHS, FACHE)

High reliability, along with the elimination of non-value-added variation, is essential to optimal outcomes and constitutes a fundamental public expectation of all healthcare organizations. Sustaining a culture of safety is even more challenging in a clinically integrated network, in which traditional hospital strategies are implemented throughout the network. Contractual performance expectations for all collaborative partners and care providers add a layer of complexity. This chapter discusses the approach that organizations must take to link all venues of care while keeping in sight goals such as excellent outcomes and the elimination of preventable harm.

CHAPTER 13: BUILDING A CULTURE OF SERVICE EXCELLENCE FOR THE TWENTY-FIRST CENTURY (JAKE POORE)

As healthcare continues to become standardized and commoditized, service will be the great differentiator between competent and outstanding healthcare organizations. It is currently a leading indicator of optimized clinical and financial performance. Traditional, hospital-based tactics will no longer be enough—clinically integrated networks span the entire continuum of care from home health care to community-based ambulatory settings to long-term care facilities. To optimize service delivery for all populations throughout the enterprise, collaborative at-risk contracts will include the expectation of systemwide best practices for service.

CHAPTER 14: LEGAL CHALLENGES FOR CLINICALLY INTEGRATED NETWORKS (BRIAN BETNER AND MICHAEL GREER)

Innovative healthcare models will create new and unique legal, regulatory, and accreditation challenges as care shifts from inpatient settings to accommodate more complex and innovative integrated structures. Chapter 14 discusses these developments, along with the traditional issues surrounding price fixing, antitrust regulations, civil monetary penalties law, the Health Insurance Portability and Accountability Act, the corporate practice of medicine, state requirements, insurance regulations, the Stark law, the antikickback statute, fraud and abuse, and the False Claims Act. As healthcare becomes increasingly regulated and managed by international, federal, state, and accreditation organizations, legal challenges will become more pressing for leaders.

CHAPTER 15: INTERMOUNTAIN HEALTHCARE: AN EVOLVING INTEGRATED DELIVERY SYSTEM (JON BURROUGHS, FACHE)

This chapter chronicles and celebrates an innovative organization willing to pioneer new models for clinical integration in order to provide cost-effective healthcare to defined populations. Intermountain Healthcare is one of several organizations that has chosen to become a positive outlier by forging unique links between its clinical and business enterprises. We look at this organization in greater detail and explore some of the factors that define its status as a leader in innovative, clinically integrated models.

CONCLUSION (JON BURROUGHS, FACHE)

This postscript sums up the key learnings from *Essential Operational Components for High-Performing Healthcare Enterprises* that will enable all healthcare organizations to pursue an up-to-date model to catalyze success in the new pay-for-value world.

REFERENCE

Gruessner, V. 2016. "Private Payers Follow CMS Lead, Adopt Value-Based Payment." Health Payer Intelligence. Published October 17. https://healthpayerintelligence.com/news/private-payers -follow-cms-lead-adopt-value-based-care-payment.

CHAPTER 1

A Healthcare Vision for the Next-Level Healthcare Enterprise

Jon Burroughs

THE HEALTHCARE INDUSTRY is experiencing a seismic shift greater in scope and magnitude than ever before. One hundred years ago, healthcare evolved from a disorganized industry to an organized industry; today, it is even more rapidly evolving from an organized industry to a transformed industry. Soon, it will be standardized, commoditized, digitized, and globalized. This chapter provides a brief history of healthcare's evolution and discusses the extraordinary shifts that twenty-first-century healthcare requires.

EARLY TWENTIETH CENTURY: FROM A DISORGANIZED INDUSTRY TO AN ORGANIZED INDUSTRY

The late nineteenth-century US healthcare system was characterized by largely rural practitioners using traditional remedies passed down from physician to apprentice despite the rapid growth of scientific medicine in Europe. Physicians had no standards of practice, and they determined treatment modalities based on experience and heuristic trial and error. Hospitals existed to care for seriously ill, injured, or infirm people and served to protect communities from communicable diseases that were typically the most common cause of death.

By 1900, the United States began to more widely adopt the germ theory of antisepsis and other, more scientific approaches advocated in European centers. Morbidity and mortality rates began to improve. As a result, there was greater interest in incorporating European methods, and in 1910 the Carnegie Foundation recruited Abraham Flexner to create a blueprint for how the European approach to healthcare could be adapted to the frontier and rural environments of the United States and Canada.

The Flexner Report encouraged universal standards for medical education, resulting in the closure of more than half the existing schools. It also encouraged two years of basic science education, two years of clinical preparation, and one year of internship prior to clinical practice. Hospitals affiliated with these new programs implemented a more scientific method, and professors were encouraged to engage in basic scientific research to promulgate new knowledge and approaches. Laboratories and sterile operating facilities became an integral part of the new centers of healing. These more complex medical institutions required professional management and coincided with the first business schools established to train business leaders in healthcare and other industries.

To encourage physicians to work together for the betterment of clinical quality, the American Surgical Society (now the American College of Surgeons) created the notion of an organized medical staff in 1919 as part of its first Minimum Standards for Hospitals. Similarly, in 1933, the American College of Hospital Administrators (later the American College of Healthcare Executives) was founded to encourage healthcare leaders to share information and to improve their professional skills and knowledge.

The adoption of a distinctly American version of the European model brought rich dividends, with the rapid growth of Western scientific discoveries leading to the development of commercial antibiotics, sophisticated technology, and sterile equipment, as well as the rapid development of new vaccines. Healthcare organizations and physicians could now offer life-saving treatments more reliably; thus, the field rose in stature and skill.

The twentieth century saw many other great advances in healthcare. For example, anesthetic agents made better surgical outcomes routine, and improvements in water and food sanitation reduced communicable diseases. The introduction of the birth control pill gave women greater control over their reproductive lives, and advances in obstetric care made childbirth safer. Cardiac care improved, creating a significant reduction in morbidity and mortality. The advancement of radiologic imaging (including the introduction of computed tomography [CT] scans in the 1970s) obviated the need for most exploratory surgeries. Organ transplantation enabled those with failing organs to gain years of productive life.

Healthcare financing changed radically in the twentieth century, progressing from a cash-based system to an insurance-based system. This was in part the result of the influenza pandemic of 1918, which afflicted 25 percent of the US population and killed 675,000 Americans (many of whom were young and able-bodied), as well as 100 million people worldwide (Knobler, Mack, and Mahmoud 2005). To protect their pool of workers, great industrialists such as Henry Ford, John D. Rockefeller, and Andrew Carnegie pressured the federal government to support the introduction of third-party payment for healthcare. Many methods of health insurance coverage arose over the century. Employer-based healthcare coverage emerged in the mid-1930s following a spike in deaths during the Great Depression as a result of malnutrition and suicide. The Health Care Financing Administration, the precursor to the Centers for Medicare & Medicaid Services (CMS), was established in 1965. By the end of the twentieth century, approximately 40 million Americans (slightly more than 15 percent of US citizens) were left without any healthcare insurance coverage (Kaiser Family Foundation 2017).

The two major healthcare business models of the twentieth century became the physician's office and the hospital. At the physician's office, patients could receive care for routine or minor conditions, or they could obtain ongoing evaluation and treatment of major chronic conditions. At the hospital, patients with acute or significant medical and surgical conditions could be diagnosed, initially treated, and stabilized. In the late twentieth century, the emergency department (ED) became the after-hours physician's office and hospital gateway, treating both minor and major conditions and providing safety-net care for people without health insurance.

As a result of rapid biomedical advances, previously life-threatening conditions such as tuberculosis, HIV, and heart disease became chronic conditions that many patients could manage throughout their lives. Unfortunately, traditional reimbursement methodologies did not evolve with this trend, and many with chronic diseases went untreated or minimally treated through lack of incentives for hospitals, physicians, and patients.

The twentieth century saw tremendous growth in the number of physicians in the United States—from 131,640 in 1900 to almost 800,000 in 2000. There was also significant growth in the number of specialties and subspecialties—the American Board of Medical Specialties and the Accreditation Council for Graduate Medical Education now list almost 50 major medical/surgical specialties and more than 60 subspecialties. The number of hospitals grew as well, from just more than 200 in 1900 to more than 5,000 today.

A close working relationship evolved between the healthcare sector and corporate suppliers who contributed to and profited from the development of new technology. These advances added both value and cost to the system. By the conclusion of the century, healthcare made up 14 percent of the US gross domestic product, and observers began to use the term *medical–industrial complex* to characterize this phenomenon (first used by Ehrenreich and Ehrenreich in 1969).

THE CHALLENGES OF TWENTIETH-CENTURY HEALTHCARE

The great healthcare advances of the twentieth century resulted in greater medical access for at least 85 percent of US citizens and a 67 percent reduction in mortality rates (from 1 in 42 deaths in 1900 to 1 in 125 in 1998) (Francis 2018). However, a number of challenges emerged that must be addressed to create a sustainable twenty-first-century healthcare model.

Challenge: Unaligned Payment Methodologies and Revenue Cycles

With rare exceptions, the predominant healthcare payment methodology in the United States is a discounted and politicized fee-for-service system. This methodology creates significant incentives for healthcare organizations and physicians to "follow the money"—prescribing high-margin procedures, tests, and treatment modalities.

The system arose because suppliers support politicians through political action committees. These politicians oversee the funding for CMS, which in turn influences the Medicare Payment Advisory Commission's establishment of conversion-factor rates for Medicare reimbursement through work relative value units (wRVUs). The commission's payment methodology is emulated by most commercial payers and ultimately results in significant differentials in payment for various treatment modalities. For instance, the two most important causes of premature heart disease are smoking and obesity. However, the two highest reimbursement rates for the treatment of heart disease involve placement of cardiac stents and performance of coronary artery bypass grafts. Although effective for late-stage coronary artery disease, these do little to prevent heart disease in its earliest stages.

This payment methodology is based on a return on investment for suppliers and has less impact on long-term clinical outcomes, though the latter ought to be the major concern of a rational reimbursement methodology. To complicate matters, most payers will not disclose in advance the amount they are willing to contribute. Because of the lack of transparency over third-party reimbursement, healthcare organizations have had to create a fictional category called *gross revenues* or *gross charges* to overestimate likely payment, so that no money is left on the table, and then call the difference between the overestimation of reimbursement and actual payment *deductions from revenue* or *contractual allowances*. Worse, critical-access hospitals must provide Medicare cost reports based on historical, fictional costs recorded on their chargemaster (historic gross charges) to justify cost plus payments (101 percent of Medicare costs), which further distorts financial accounting. In short, the lack of appropriate incentives to bolster health and prevent disease, along with a lack of transparency for both costs and quality outcomes, has created perverse incentives that do not reward healthcare organizations or physicians for providing the best possible care to achieve optimal clinical and business outcomes.

Challenge: Non-Value-Added Clinical and Business Outcome Variation

Healthcare was originally established as a cottage industry that permitted each physician to determine the appropriate approach with each patient. This culture created enormous variation in the way physicians treated identical conditions. Similarly, healthcare leaders and executives, lacking real-time information or standards, followed an individualized trial-and-error, or heuristic, approach to management decisions using retrospective data. These approaches have created a significant range of outcomes, eloquently described by Atul Gawande (2004) in his landmark article "The Bell Curve." He recounts variations in survival and life expectancy for individuals with cystic fibrosis, each treated by different physicians and organizations in their own way; these discrepancies in survival could be more than 25 years. Another example of the healthcare field's scattershot approach is found in organizations that are able to perform true cost accounting and measure the direct variable costs of treatment ordered by individual physicians for the care of patients with identical diagnosis-related groups (DRGs). The variation in cost can be as great as 1,000 percent, with those who spend less driving superior outcomes.

In 2013, the Advisory Board announced that preventable medical errors were the third leading cause of death in the United States, with 220,000 to 440,000 fatalities per year resulting from non-value-added variation. In fact, the Rand Corporation has asserted that appropriate care is administered only 45 percent of the time (National Center for Health Statistics 2018). Other manifestations of non-value-added variation include the following:

- Too much care rendered (e.g., excessive testing and procedures, inappropriate use of antibiotics)
- Too little care rendered (e.g., non- or undertreatment of hypertension while billions are spent on treatment of resultant strokes)
- Wrong care rendered (e.g., misdiagnosis, failure to diagnose, delay in diagnosis)

The challenge for all healthcare professionals is to reduce both clinical and managerial variation by eliminating non-value-added variation that places individuals and the organization at risk for both inferior outcomes and management waste. At the same time, we must preserve value-added variation that optimizes both clinical and business outcomes.

Challenge: High Costs

The United States currently spends $3.3 trillion on healthcare per year—almost 18 percent of the country's total gross domestic product

(CMS 2018b). This figure amounts to an almost 28 percent increase in healthcare expenditures for large employers and 25 percent of disposable income expenditures for the average American family over the past five years. Healthcare is the leading cause of personal bankruptcy among working Americans as a result of high-deductible policies, lack of insurance, and high out-of-pocket expenses for life-threatening chronic diseases. The average American family has approximately 90 days' cash on hand, including its total assets (e.g., home equity, retirement funds), and according to David Himmelstein and colleagues (2018), may be "only one serious illness away from bankruptcy."

As a result of the unfunded liabilities of the Medicare and Medicaid programs, the US healthcare system is the second leading cause of federal debt. According to the US Government Accountability Office (GAO 2018), our national debt is currently $21.3 trillion, with a virtual (unreported) deficit of $80 to $100 trillion. These figures are based on unfunded liabilities pertaining to Social Security (24 percent), interest on the national debt (16 percent; predicted to be the largest percentage in ten years), Medicare (14 percent), and Medicaid (9 percent). According to the GAO, to balance the federal budget by 2040, federal spending would have to be cut by 60 percent or taxes would have to be raised by 250 percent—neither of which is politically feasible (Chernew, Baicker, and Hsu 2010).

In 2000, large employers and purchasers founded the Leapfrog Group to exert political pressure on Washington to reform the US healthcare system. The Leapfrog Group now also provides safety ratings (from A to F) on more than 1,800 hospitals and healthcare organizations nationally. It is important to note that large employers are driving the national initiative to decrease the costs and improve the quality of healthcare through transformational projects.

Challenge: Fragmentation and Lack of Access

Healthcare transformation is an economic issue in the guise of a political conflict. Access is a major problem for people who are uninsured or underinsured, live in regions with physician shortages, cannot afford out-of-pocket costs, or live in low-income areas that cannot support qualified clinicians. These individuals may present to EDs well after they are in need of care or are dying and have nowhere to go. This backward approach drives up the cost of care for everyone (through risk sharing and undiluted high-risk pools) and increases both bad debt and charity care, placing healthcare organizations and patients at significant financial risk.

According to the American Hospital Association, almost one-third of hospitals reported negative operating margins in 2016 and are in danger of poor financial performance in the future. Moreover, according to the Association of American Medical Colleges (Kirsch and Petelle 2017), there are many geographic regions that have significant physician and practitioner shortages. Some areas, such as Boston, are rich in specialty and subspecialty physicians (because of the many academic medical centers in the area) but have such primary care shortages that average wait times may exceed two months.

Even with reasonable access, our healthcare system is fragmented. Imagine a woman who discovers a lump in her breast. Is it cancer? The following represents a typical scenario for her treatment:

1. Sees her primary care physician for an examination. He confirms a lump and refers her to an imaging center for mammography (fee-for-service unit charge).
2. Undergoes a mammography (unit charges for imaging center and radiologist).
3. Sees her primary care physician. He informs her of a suspicious lesion and refers her to a surgeon for a breast biopsy (unit charge).

4. Undergoes a biopsy by a surgeon in an ambulatory surgery center (ASC). Biopsy result is read by a clinical pathologist (unit charges for surgeon, ASC, pathologist, and laboratory).
5. Sees her primary care physician. He informs her of the preliminary diagnosis of adenocarcinoma of the breast and refers her to an oncologic surgeon for staging procedure and evaluation (unit charges for surgeon and ASC).
6. Surgeon performs sentinel node biopsy (which is sent to a pathologist), and radiologist performs a positron emission tomography scan and relevant magnetic resonance imaging and CT scans to determine staging (unit charges for surgeon, radiologist, pathologist, ASC, imaging center, and laboratory).
7. Sees her primary care physician. He informs her that she has stage 2 adenocarcinoma and refers her for oncologic evaluation (unit charge).
8. Oncologist performs an evaluation, places her on chemotherapy, and refers her to a radiation oncologist, who starts radiation treatments (unit charges for oncologist, radiation oncologist, oncology facility, radiation center, pharmacist, oncology nurse who administers treatments, and infusion center).
9. Follows up with her primary care physician for ongoing surveillance and healthcare maintenance (unit charge).

This process typically takes between one and three months and involves physicians who do not work together, share an integrated electronic information system, or function in an economically or clinically aligned manner. In addition, the number of handoffs creates a high probability of error and, most important, a delay in the diagnosis and treatment of a potentially life-threatening condition. Our current healthcare system does not make it easy, convenient, or cost-effective for people to seek evaluation and treatment for complex, life-threatening conditions.

Challenge: Lack of Alignment and Engagement

Alignment has many meanings. In healthcare, alignment means that all stakeholders' self-interests coincide with optimized clinical and business outcomes. When all parties—patients, physicians, healthcare leaders, payers, regulators, and accreditors—are working toward the same fundamental goals and objectives, the system is aligned.

The definition of *engagement* is this context is closely related. When a stakeholder has a sense of "ownership" that results from alignment, that person or organization may be thought of as fully engaged. Unfortunately, most participants in healthcare are neither aligned nor engaged.

For instance, consider the financial motivations of the current healthcare system. Hospitals (despite the 3 percent Medicare penalty for readmissions) and physicians earn more with higher bed days, higher wRVU volume, more complex care, and more expensive procedures and tests. Payers earn more by denying benefits, denying access, paying physicians and healthcare systems less, and covering low-risk pools of healthy people. Patients save by purchasing high-deductible policies, not paying the balance of their bills, claiming disability, or divesting assets to access public benefits. This dynamic leads to what economists might call a *tragedy of the commons*, in which self-interest differs from the greater community interest and everyone loses over time. In healthcare, everyone must be engaged and aligned to produce optimal outcomes at low cost. This goal requires the input of all parties to create a system that works for everyone.

Challenge: Lack of Real-Time Information

As a result of its complexity, healthcare is the last sector to become fully digitized. The aim is real-time and predictive analytics that enable all parties to manage both clinical and business risks effectively. However, what we have is an expensive, complex, and dysfunctional amalgam of paper and digital technologies that may not be compatible, interconnected, or functionally interoperable.

We have additional problems. The technology sector is evolving so rapidly that the latest application is often partially obsolete the day it is installed, and without a functional and international health information exchange (HIE), protected health information cannot seamlessly travel around the globe and be accessed on demand. Finally, most healthcare systems do not have access to a robust enterprise data warehouse (EDW) to convert data into role-based analytics that produce actionable information that each healthcare professional needs in real time to do her job effectively. Such analyses can provide highly selective, aggregated, actionable information concurrently so that both patients and enterprises can be managed optimally and effectively at any point and time of care.

POTENTIAL SOLUTIONS

The following represent potential solutions, many with proven value, that healthcare organizations currently pursue to address these contemporary challenges. They are potential because, like most new initiatives, unanticipated consequences may arise that must be addressed through rapid-cycle adjustments and improvements. However, organizations that react quickly are able to adapt to an evolving economic environment and write some of their own rules as they go.

Potential Solution: Aligned Payment Methodologies

The most important and fundamental change that must occur is the move from a volume-based (fee-for-service) reimbursement system to a value-based (at-risk global or capitated) healthcare payment model. The latter properly incentivizes providers and systems so that they work to keep people healthy instead of profit when people are sick or injured. Much has been written about the perverse incentives of fee-for-service, but Elizabeth McGlynn and colleagues (2003) have provided the simplest explanation: Most people receive approximately 50 percent of the healthcare they should, either because the appropriate healthcare (e.g., preventive healthcare services) has little, if any, reimbursement attached to it or because the incentive to offer unnecessary services and procedures is so great.

Thus, the business model of healthcare must optimize cost-effective healthcare outcomes and not reward complications, waste, and unnecessary services. Many organizations are voluntarily moving toward a form of risk-based reimbursement by pursuing varied solutions (e.g., pay for performance, shared savings, bundled payment, global payment, capitated reimbursement). States such as California and Maryland are also moving in this direction—California through pursuit of reference-based capitated payments, and Maryland through global budgets for episodes of care and treatment.

Through the CMS Innovation Center, Medicare currently uses almost a hundred reimbursement methodologies (e.g., shared savings, bundled payments) that are often customized for organizations willing to take on risk and potentially improve the cost-to-outcome ratio for both CMS and Medicare beneficiaries. The center works with healthcare organizations to develop innovation models organized into the following categories:

- Accountable care organizations (ACOs) and shared savings programs to reduce costs and optimize quality
- Episode-based payment initiatives with cost and quality parameters for defined healthcare events, such as a hospitalization or elective procedure (e.g., joint replacement)
- Primary care transformation that provides incentives for adopting advanced primary care models (e.g., the patient-centered medical home, which combines preventive

care services, information technology and analytics, care coordination, and shared decision-making).
- Initiatives focused on Medicaid populations and the Children's Health Insurance Program, which include innovative programs such as Oregon's Coordinated Care Organization, Colorado's Regional Care Collaborative Organization, and Minnesota's Integrated Health Partnerships. (These are all ACOs for the Medicaid population, which have saved millions of dollars and improved care for high-risk populations.)
- Initiatives focused on the high-risk pool of dual-eligible Medicare and Medicaid beneficiaries who make up a disproportionate percentage of Medicare costs (because they require a systematic disease management or palliative care program and represent the greatest potential for cost savings and quality improvement)
- Experiments to accelerate the development and testing of new payment and service delivery models (e.g., through collaboration with the CMS Innovation Center to develop new ideas for reimbursement methodologies)— an opportunity for forward-thinking leaders who seek to develop more effective clinical and business models
- Initiatives to speed the adoption of best practices (e.g., coalitions of healthcare organizations, payers, health plans, providers, federal agencies, professional societies, and experts to promulgate best practices, speed the diffusion of innovations, and ensure the widespread availability of up-to-date treatments [CMS 2018a])

Organizations such as Intermountain Healthcare, St. Luke's Health System (Boise, Idaho), Baylor Healthcare System, Memorial Hermann Health System, Advocate Health Care, and Geisinger Health have developed three- to five-year strategic plans to manage the period of transition from fee-for-service to multiple at-risk payment systems). This change requires shifts in both the business model and the care-delivery model; as readmissions, ED use, elective procedures, ancillary revenue, and office visits drop, the organization will be rewarded and not penalized for improving health and reducing both volume and capacity.

Any such fundamental changes to an organizational paradigm constitute a complex process, because most organizations require a capital reserve to compensate for a short-term loss of operating margin before they can invest in a population health infrastructure. Chapter 10 covers the operational and collaborative elements required to support these new care and payment models and describes a method to stage this difficult financial transition using the various operational components of population health.

Multiple payment methods are currently available to consider as transition models, enabling organizations to acquire the clinical, operational, information technology, and financial competencies necessary to make the full transition. Each model has its pros and cons. Consider exhibit 1.1.

Healthcare leaders may feel overwhelmed by the complexity and disruptive nature of these changes and may be tempted to resist the shift to these new models. Unfortunately, successfully fulfilling the new payment methodologies requires time and planning, but once a critical mass of payers (including CMS and commercial payers) adopts value-based payments, organizations that resist change will find themselves at a significant disadvantage. Fortunately, a growing number of financial accounting simulators or "gameification" programs can now run the numbers prior to such strategic discussions to determine which payment methodologies are appropriate for a given organization and market.

Potential Solution: Elimination of Non-Value-Added Clinical and Business Outcome Variation

Many organizations have begun the arduous process of eliminating non-value-added variation on both the clinical side and the

Exhibit 1.1: Possible Payment Methodology Models

Model	Benefits	Risks
Discounted fee-for-service	First step on the road to transformation	• Continuously decreasing payments • Necessity to exit as population health initiatives become more robust
Care coordination payments	Opportunities to employ nurse navigators and patient registries	Start-up and overhead costs
Pay for performance (P4P)	• Begins to focus delivery on specific outcomes • Begins process of physician alignment	Subsidization of ninetieth-percentile performers at the cost of lowest-decile performers
Bundled payments (most common DRGs, with payment for acute and post-acute care)	Gainsharing opportunities to align physicians and reduce operating costs	• Volume incentivized • Potential losses if cost reductions are not realized
Shared savings	• Begins to focus on lower cost of care; opportunities for shared-savings gains • Focus on agreed-on quality measures	• Possibility of shared losses or no gains • Diminishing returns over time • Significant start-up and overhead costs
Risk-based global or capitated payments	Focus on prevention, disease management, palliative care, and wellness with aligned incentives and metrics	Inappropriate withholding of essential services if appropriate risk-based incentives are not incorporated

management side. This process is challenging because it involves changing the fundamental culture of both clinicians and leaders, both of whom value independence and the autonomy to make decisions in a customized and personalized way. The key to shifting the culture is to reassure everyone that value-added variation—customization and personalization that add value to cost-effective care—will always be supported. Only the adverse part of professional autonomy (that which inadvertently harms people and adds waste) must be eliminated.

The Memorial Hermann Physician Network (formerly the Memorial Hermann Health Network Providers and Memorial Hermann Physician Clinically Integrated Network) began this process when it was founded in 1982. Its evolution accelerated around 2008 when, under the former president Dr. Keith Fernandez (2013), the physicians began to standardize their work. They formed more than 200 clinical program committees, which evaluated the top 20 DRGs of their respective specialties and developed a single evidence-based approach to each diagnostic entity, consulting available scientific literature, clinical guidelines, and the clinical judgment of group members. They agreed that, when encountering a patient with an uncomplicated DRG, they would follow the clinical guidelines they established, but they gave each practitioner the right to divert from the guidelines with the understanding that each exception would be peer audited within 24 hours. They also decided that whenever any new or significant information emerged, the group would meet to decide whether to incorporate it into the existing standard. For instance, when it was discovered that prostate-specific antigen studies had a higher-than-predicted rate of false positives, the urologists modified the pathway for the evaluation of prostate cancer to rely more heavily on other clinical findings. They also would occasionally use exceptions to modify the pathway itself in the event that the customization worked better than the standardized approach.

Based on its innovative committee system, Memorial Hermann was able to accomplish improvements relative to many other healthcare organizations. Memorial Hermann achieved a 5 percent reduction in length of stay, a 91 percent reduction in hospital-acquired infections, a 66 percent reduction in general complications, a 43 percent reduction in 30-day readmissions, and a 23 percent reduction in mortality rate (Fernandez 2013).

Payers took note. Aetna immediately offered the physician group a new contract with premium payment—a move eventually duplicated by United and Blue Cross Blue Shield, the other major payers in the region. Aetna further incentivized participation by offering significant bonuses, to both physicians and management, for every 10 percent increase in payer network membership. In addition to this new pay-for-performance premium (paid on the backs of performers in the lowest tenth percentile), the group was able to save the system more than $500 million in costs over the first three years (2008–2011) by eliminating the majority of vendor groups and simplifying its supply chain.

Memorial Hermann's results are impressive, but achieving them does not mean abandoning physician autonomy. In his book *The Checklist Manifesto*, Atul Gawande (2009) emphasizes that the purpose of standardization is not to diminish the essential role of the professional clinical or business leader but rather to reduce complexity to a manageable level so that critical executive decisions can be made in a more accurate, effective, and timely way.

Most healthcare systems are just beginning the journey toward greater efficiency. Their tool kits contain new models of clinical integration and alignment that allow them to manage both clinical and business variation in real time. Chapters 4, 6, and 10 cover these topics in more detail.

Potential Solution: Elimination of Cost-Prohibitive Systems

When it comes to driving down costs, large employers in the United States are pushing the hardest. Their influence over politicians trickles down to the US Department of Health and Human Services, which, in turn, oversees CMS, the agency that sets Medicare rates.

Large employers seek to change policy because healthcare expenses pose a real threat to their ability to compete in a global market. For example, Ford Motor Company now spends more on healthcare than it does on raw materials for its auto assembly process. This situation has created a tremendous competitive disadvantage for US companies in global markets.

In 1975, sociologist Samuel Preston mapped out the comparative relationship between per capita healthcare spending and life expectancy, called the *Preston curve* (Organization for Economic Cooperation and Development [OECD] 2018). Exhibit 1.2 shows a 2011 Preston curve for countries around the world. Not only do Americans spend almost twice as much on healthcare as people do in other industrialized nations, they also live shorter lives. The US healthcare system emphasizes expensive tests and procedures to treat the later stages of disease while shortchanging prevention and early treatment, which are far more cost-effective.

Large employers do the following to lower the cost of healthcare:

- Transfer risk to employees (beneficiaries) through defined contributions to tax-deferred health savings accounts, which enable workers to self-insure over time as they put money aside for their future healthcare needs.
- Provide incentives to employees who use employer-created, narrow, tiered networks, and choose practitioners and organizations that demonstrate high quality and low cost through the creation of private exchanges (marketplaces); these exchanges consist of healthcare organizations and providers who offer a bundled-payment contract with guaranteed contractual outcomes.
- Employ disease management programs to standardize care for high-cost, high-risk illnesses and other causes of absenteeism and presenteeism (employees who come to work unable to perform their jobs fully).
- Use navigators (often advanced-practice nurses with public health backgrounds who understand the entire

Exhibit 1.2: International Preston Curve, 2011

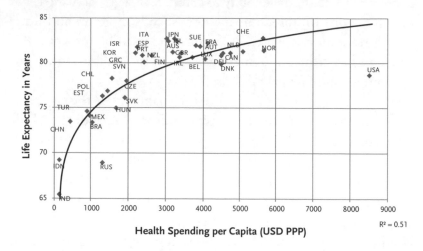

X-axis: Health Spending per Capita (USD PPP)

Y-axis: Life Expectancy in Years

$R^2 = 0.51$

Source: Adapted from OECD (2018).
Note: USD PPP = US dollars purchasing power parity

health ecosystem, including relevant payer contracts), and establish registries (databases that use predictive analytics to identify at-risk employees).

- Contract directly with healthcare organizations throughout the country to provide high-cost services to employees at a discount.

For example, Walmart contracts with Cleveland Clinic, Mayo Clinic, Geisinger Medical Center, Scripps Health, Scott & White Memorial Hospital, Virginia Mason Medical Center, and Mercy Hospital to provide bundled-payment agreements that guarantee quality outcomes. If a covered procedure must be redone, the follow-up care is performed at no cost to Walmart. The company is able to pay for all travel and living expenses for its employees and their family members who seek care at designated centers of excellence and still reap significant savings (estimated to be hundreds of millions of dollars annually). In 2016, Walmart announced that any surgery performed outside its centers of excellence network would be paid at 50 percent of the rate for in-network care (Emerick 2016).

US citizens adapt this idea on a global level to pursue high-value, low-cost care through international medical tourism. In 2017, approximately 2 million Americans sought healthcare abroad to save up to 95 percent on costs, often for life-threatening conditions. For those with chronic illnesses such as cancer or hepatitis C, for which out-of-pocket expenses may exceed $100,000 annually in the United States, their travel may be the difference between solvency and bankruptcy. Medical tourism is now a $246 billion sector, growing at a rate of approximately 15–25 percent annually throughout the world. Relative to the US market, estimated savings from medical tourism range from 20 percent (Brazil) to 95 percent (India) (Woodman 2015).

How can healthcare organizations lower their cost structures significantly? The traditional wisdom was to use techniques such as Lean or Six Sigma to both simplify and standardize processes, eliminating waste and lowering costs by 10–15 percent. However, to compete with health systems internationally, both business and care models must restructure to lower costs by 50–60 percent or more. Then Americans with disposable income will be able to stay in the United States for care, with patients from other nations coming to take advantage of more sophisticated American technology at costs equivalent to those abroad.

Thus, the following must occur:

- *Reduction of labor costs.* Providers should be able to perform all healthcare activities at the top of their license. Organizations will monitor labor costs through real-time and predictive labor analytics (see detailed discussion in chapter 10).
- *Reduction of supply chain costs.* Healthcare entities can simplify and modernize the supply chain through the use of value analysis, computerized and automated supply

chain tracking systems, and supply chain analytics (see chapter 10).

- *Development of new business and clinical models.* More cost-effective approaches to risk-stratifying subpopulations include addressing the socioeconomic (nonclinical) determinants of health (this issue will be discussed at length in chapter 11).
- *Construction of a retail medicine infrastructure.* The US healthcare system must be able to provide acute care services (outside of the ED and urgent care) to those who have minor conditions or economic challenges but are otherwise healthy (chapter 11 focuses on this issue).
- *Creation of an e-health infrastructure.* We can provide ongoing healthcare services to healthy people with minor acute problems and those with stable chronic diseases through a far more cost-effective e-health approach (see chapter 11).
- *Cooperation with national and state agencies.* Many patients with terminal conditions receive futile care that is responsible for almost $1 trillion in healthcare expenditures annually but that adds few, if any, years of quality health. Healthcare organizations should team up with governments to develop national and regional approaches to easing this problem (this issue is discussed at length in chapter 11).

Potential Solution: New Models for Unified and Accessible Care

Several new models of healthcare delivery have been described to address issues of healthcare access and fragmentation, most prominently in the groundbreaking book *The Innovator's Prescription* (Christensen, Grossman, and Hwang 2009). The three models include *solution shops* for complex undifferentiated problems;

value-added processes for significant, serious, or potentially life-threatening conditions; and *facilitated networks* for chronic conditions that add significant costs to our system.

Solution Shops

Remember the example given earlier of the woman with a lump in her breast who goes through a lengthy ordeal to receive breast cancer treatment? What if this process could be done more efficiently?

In an alternate vision, this woman could see a team made up of all the specialists and subspecialists she visited along her journey as well as a care coordinator, a social services specialist, and a pharmacist. Instead of seeing independent, unaffiliated practitioners, she could see physicians organized into a service line of like-minded professionals willing to develop best-practice, evidence-based approaches to the diagnosis and treatment of breast conditions. In place of a fragmented process with multiple handoffs that cause information to fall through the cracks, there could be one standardized, seamless process that eliminates delays in this potentially life-threatening situation.

The woman could dispense with the long process of visiting providers in disparate or unaffiliated organizations. Instead, she could see practitioners who use a completely integrated health information management (HIM) system to acquire and share information in real time. Rather than a fee-for-service, per-unit reimbursement approach, the physicians, practitioners, and facilities could be paid with either a bundled fee or a global services fee that incentivizes all to arrive at a cost-effective and timely solution to this patient's complex and potentially life-threatening problem.

The Mayo Clinic does this process as well as any organization in the United States, but it still has some distance to go. It accomplishes its greater alignment through an employment model (although any alignment model is sufficient) that emphasizes the cooperation of physicians and leaders, all of whom work together to create standardized processes.

The Innovator's Prescription describes Mayo's process. Jerome Grossman, MD, one of the three authors, died of renal cell carcinoma with metastasis to the heart shortly before the book's publication. He had sought a diagnosis from some of the finest specialists in the world—in vain—and finally went to the Mayo Clinic. There, his problem was identified by a team that included a nephrologist who suggested this rare disease. On his return from the Mayo Clinic, Dr. Grossman reportedly said, "They have a process! It's not a one-size-fits-all process. Every patient has a different disease, but they have a practiced way to treat every patient uniquely" (Christensen, Grossman, and Hwang 2009).

Obviously, most people do not have access to care at the Mayo Clinic. Nor is the organization designed to cost-effectively diagnose all clinical problems or large enough to accommodate even a fraction of them. However, Mayo represents a model we should be moving toward for people with complex, undiagnosed, and potentially serious conditions.

To reach this goal, healthcare organizations must be willing to

- align with all relevant practitioners through some form of at-risk contracts;
- create service line or clinical institute (horizontally integrated service lines) structures to reorganize and standardize care for defined conditions (see chapter 7);
- build an integrated HIE supported by clinical and business analytics to provide information in real-time decision supports, such as those provided by IBM Watson, or proactively through predictive analytics (this will be discussed in greater detail in chapters 8 and 11); and
- create at-risk bundled- or global payment contracts with payers and large employers to incentivize such optimized care.

This model, referred to as a *solution shop*, should be consistent with local cultures and sensibilities but focus on developing solutions to complex and potentially life-threatening clinical problems in a timely and cost-effective manner.

Value-Added Processes

It is now well established that healthcare services that are complex, high-risk, and high-cost should be regionalized so that a smaller number of organizations can improve outcomes and lower costs. Hundreds of studies now confirm the benefits of evidence-based referrals. Many healthcare leaders throughout the country are committed to advocating for the needs of patients first by establishing new policies to triage, guide, and manage high-risk care.

These aims require new ideas. In a *New England Journal of Medicine* article, David Urbach (2015) describes the volume pledge taken by physician and administrative leadership at several prominent medical centers. In an effort to ensure patient safety and secure optimum healthcare outcomes, they commit to disallowing certain predefined, high-risk procedures by low-volume surgeons or facilities.

Despite 36 years of "exhaustive" research in this area, financial incentives (for both surgeons and hospitals) still reward low-volume facilities for taking on high-risk cases, though counter to the best interests of the patient, surgeon, and organization (Urbach 2015). This issue is highly controversial because many organizations cannot (or feel they cannot) give up these services in a fee-for-service environment that rewards organizations that provide this level of high-margin care.

To address this dilemma, Clayton Christensen, Jerome Grossman, and Jason Hwang (2009) advocate for a value-added process—more commonly known as a *focused factory*—that includes the following components:

- Singular focus with a standardized approach, culture, and service
- World-class quality, cost-effectiveness, and service
- Team-based approach that allows practitioners to adapt and standardize processes based on the latest available evidence
- Reimbursement model based on bundled payments or global payments for outcomes

- Strong regional and worldwide brand

A well-known example of this approach is the Shouldice Hernia Centre in Thornhill, Ontario, Canada. The center was founded in 1945 by a surgeon frustrated by the number of surgical failures in what ought to be a straightforward procedure—the repair of commonly occurring hernias. He standardized a surgical repair process, taught other surgeons how to apply this approach, and began performing large numbers of hernia operations with outstanding outcomes at low costs. Today, Shouldice performs more than 7,500 hernia repairs annually in five operating rooms. Each of its surgeons performs at least 700 procedures per year and enjoys a 99.5 percent success rate after more than 300,000 repairs. Similar examples include the Heart Center at the Cleveland Clinic and the central line–focused factory at the Cedars-Sinai Medical Center, which takes a standardized, evidence-based approach to the insertion of all peripherally inserted catheter and arterial lines.

Facilitated Networks

As the authors of *The Innovator's Prescription* point out, the vast majority of day-to-day decisions about medications, diet, exercise level, lifestyle, and attitudes are made by patients themselves, based on their own personal values and beliefs, nonclinical determinants of care (e.g., socioeconomic, genetic, and environmental factors), and peers who experience the same clinical conditions. Alcoholics learn from alcoholics, people with diabetes from other people with diabetes, and schizophrenics from schizophrenics. Thus, physicians' attempts to enforce dependence on medical advice may be neither productive nor effective. Enabling patients to have access to supportive peer groups—and good medical advice when needed—is an important role for any healthcare system.

The role of these *facilitated networks* is to support self-empowered care, not deliver it. Examples include Alcoholics Anonymous, d-Life (for people with diabetes), and the Restless Legs Syndrome Foundation. Physicians and healthcare organizations have a role to play in coordinating, guiding, and facilitating the care of patients with chronic diseases, and a viable business model for this approach emphasizes a capitated or global services fee for supporting these facilitated network groups and facilitating access.

Potential Solution: True Patient and Stakeholder Alignment and Engagement

Most industries are going through a new form of consumer empowerment, in which consumers are no longer dependent on others for services, knowledge, or even guidance. For instance, most people plan their own travel without a travel agent, bank on demand without a banker, and purchase clothing online without a salesperson. It should not come as any surprise that the same changes are coming to healthcare. To provide a sense of empowerment to individuals and stakeholders, a healthcare organization must make a deliberate attempt to align its interests with those of all stakeholders, including physicians, consumers, payers, accreditors, and community agencies. The key is that alignment must be compelling enough to convince people to sacrifice some of their independence to contribute to the greater good and more cost-effective outcomes.

Health insurance is a case in point. When all people participate (particularly low-cost, healthy ones), the insurance is more affordable for everyone, particularly those with the greatest need (and cost). Similarly, if a patient is willing to sacrifice some of her personal choice by conforming to evidence-based recommendations and treatments, the cost for everyone's care drops as a result of a dilution of the high-risk pool by optimizing clinical outcomes.

More and more state governments, such as those of Minnesota and Oregon, are implementing Medicaid managed care programs in which Medicaid beneficiaries partner with healthcare providers and systems to lower the overall cost of care while improving outcomes. Medicare managed care programs use private-sector coverage to provide incentives for patients who seek to receive radiologic and laboratory testing or ambulatory surgery at lower-cost venues in their state. For instance, Anthem Blue Cross Blue Shield in New Hampshire noted that the difference in cost for an abdominal CT scan at various facilities ranged from $750 to $2,850. On the other hand, if the beneficiary is willing to drive to the lower-cost venue, the insurance carrier will pay $150. However, if the beneficiary chooses a higher-cost venue, the higher cost will come out of the person's deductible. Although traditional Medicare and Medicaid programs cannot, under federal law, penalize beneficiaries for making unwise healthcare decisions, they can legally incentivize patients to make decisions that will ultimately lower costs and improve outcomes.

These trends are leading toward a transparent healthcare market in which all quality, safety, service, and cost data are publicly shared, enabling patients, payers, physicians, and leaders to make good choices based on consumer knowledge of both quality and cost. Increasingly, healthcare systems and payers are negotiating dynamic pay-for-value contracts with transparent metrics that permit parties to share information and understand key variables (e.g., cost, quality), enabling the agreements to modulate over time based on changing conditions. These instruments are discussed in chapter 11.

One of the greatest opportunities for engagement and alignment is between and among payers, healthcare systems, and both employed and self-employed physicians through at-risk arrangements. Chapter 4 provides more detail on this rapidly growing phenomenon.

Potential Solution: Real-Time Information for All Stakeholders

A common question from healthcare consultants is, "What is the lag time between the provision of care and accurate information on how well you did or how much it cost?" With rare exceptions, the typical answer is one to three months. Virtually every other industry has reached a point where information can not only be gleaned in real time but also anticipated with relative accuracy through predictive analytics. Healthcare is embarking on a transformation that the banking industry began in 1969, when the first ATM was introduced in the United States. Banking can now be performed around the clock almost anywhere in the world through a computer, smartphone, or tablet using encrypted information and secure firewalls. To provide comprehensive services, the healthcare sector must support the same.

To achieve this, the following fundamental building blocks must be assembled:

- All healthcare-related information (e.g., clinical, financial, demographic) must be digitized to enable the seamless transmission of cloud-based information throughout the internet.
- All healthcare entities and stakeholders must be connected through an HIE so that all participants in any healthcare system can access real-time information from participating systems anywhere in the world.
- Via an EDW, data must be converted into role-based clinical and business analytics that give every participant in the system the information needed to fully and optimally participate (see chapters 8 and 11 for a more detailed discussion of this process).
- Every organization must have some form of data governance to organize how data and analytics are created, used, shared, and managed, both within and beyond the system's boundaries, to ensure their credibility, integrity, and security.
- Both national and international standards must be created to ensure that data and analytics systems are compatible and interoperable and that they meet minimum standards for accuracy and privacy.
- Small healthcare organizations and practices must be able to connect with a larger system to access contemporary infrastructures and tools.

Potential Solution: Disruptive Innovation

Contrary to popular opinion, the notion of disruptive innovation, as popularized in *The Innovator's Dilemma* (Christensen 2011) and *The Innovator's Solution* (Christensen and Raynor 2013), does not encompass unusual or innovative ideas that suddenly emerge to disrupt and supplant an existing industry. It represents an exit, by the industry itself, of its own "low" end, to permit new entrants to arrive, gain a foothold, and work their way upstream.

How does this phenomenon work from a pragmatic perspective? As healthcare reimbursement declines, both physicians and healthcare leaders are forced to focus on increasingly profitable procedures and services to maintain a sustainable margin—so they advertently (or inadvertently) abandon such basic services as preventive medicine, mental and behavioral health care, and wellness initiatives. This gap provides an opportunity for new entrants—such as Walgreens, CVS, and Walmart—to bring an entirely different business model to bear on these low-end demands. For instance, the retail pharmacy industry brings a much lower cost structure to the creation of retail medicine units, which can be housed in a structure already devoted to diverse sales models. In addition, these businesses can offer attractive customer-based benefits and services such as short-notice appointments, decision support tools, customized health maintenance plans, integration with payers, and pharmacy benefits management to create a seamless solution for consumers frustrated by the lack of easy access to basic medical services.

Another significant disruptive innovation is the development of e-health platforms and solutions that enable immediate access to qualified physicians worldwide for a relatively low cost and with excellent, reproducible results for high-volume, low-risk conditions. Many otherwise healthy patients are not interested in a traditional and personal relationship with a physician but rather want on-demand, convenient appointments with a qualified physician for the management of minor medical/surgical conditions.

This innovation is not surprising, as it has already occurred in many other fields. All business sectors are rapidly moving to a completely digitized, convenient model that can be accessed on any smartphone. In the medical field, this additional resource can function as a supplement to the relatively expensive and inconvenient traditional healthcare delivery process, which lacks a consumer-focused approach. People with unique, complex, difficult-to-diagnose, or tough-to-manage clinical conditions always require a more customized and individualized model of care that includes a team-based approach. Most individuals, however, can be cared for with less in-depth attention. Think of the traditional model of physician, hospital, and ED as the Ritz-Carlton and other disruptive models as less expensive, though "good enough," lodgings that may be lower quality but serve their purpose in a far more pragmatic and cost-effective way. The healthy majority will be served, and likely satisfied, with lower-cost options, while the sickest (or wealthiest) will require or demand a higher level of service.

PUTTING IT ALL TOGETHER

The challenge with twentieth-century healthcare was that it had two predominant business models—the physician's office and the hospital—both of which provided care for everyone whether they were sick or well. Too much care was provided to the healthy majority, and too little was given to the unhealthy minority with serious and often complex conditions.

This imbalance has led to the need for population healthcare models in which groups of covered lives (e.g., Medicare recipients, commercial payers) are risk stratified through predictive analytics. These groups are then sorted into subpopulations by cost and risk so that healthcare resources can be rationalized into a more sustainable and cost-effective model. The redistribution of resources makes sense because the so-called vital few, who require the greatest resources, shift costs onto the healthy many, affecting the cost of care for all. In short, overall care must be system based and risk stratified to ensure a more sustainable and pragmatic availability of resources.

Managing actuarial risk (covered in chapter 9) is essentially the ability to stratify covered lives by risk and, within a defined global budget, to manage each subpopulation—all while optimizing outcomes and working within a defined medical loss ratio (percentage of the premium dollar used for the direct care of beneficiaries). This approach is now a fundamental competency of any healthcare system meeting the expectations of pay-for-value contracts.

There will always be people who choose or can afford more personalized services (think a private investment adviser, banker, cook, lawyer), per the primary business model in the twentieth century. However, the majority of people will choose services that are quick, easy to access, available around the clock, reliable, transparent, and affordable. Offering this type of healthcare requires a more commoditized, automated, and standardized approach, particularly for the high-volume, low-risk services that make up the majority of healthcare encounters. This type of care can be easily provided through e-health services, retail clinics, home health services, advanced primary care models, and interactions with navigators and care coordinators (all discussed in chapter 11).

There will be a need to identify, through predictive analytics, patients who make up the vital few and require more specialized, in-depth, timely, and multidisciplinary services led by physicians and executed by care coordinators. These people may require palliative care (intensive disease management) for life-threatening conditions; disease management for serious conditions; solution shops for significant, undifferentiated problems; focused factories for high-risk, high-cost conditions; and facilitated networks for complex, chronic diseases that require peer-supported, interdisciplinary care (see chapter 11).

Thus, so-called patient-centered care will not merely take individual considerations, values, and preferences into account when providing healthcare. Instead, it will be the ultimate transfer of control from physicians and healthcare organizations back to consumers, beneficiaries, and patients. Patients will make rational healthcare decisions based on the best available information, enabled by physicians, healthcare organizations, payers, accreditors, and community agencies.

Stand-alone healthcare organizations will not be capable of providing the comprehensive and varied services discussed in this chapter. At a minimum, they will need to collaborate with, align with, or join larger networks that can support the full complement of HIM, population health, and actuarial management infrastructure.

Thus, healthcare will increasingly be provided through sophisticated and fully integrated networks or systems that can link patients with healthcare resources in a coordinated and seamless way to produce optimized, cost-effective outcomes. While the twentieth century featured the cottage industry model of independent physicians working around a stand-alone hospital, the twenty-first century will be about comprehensive, clinically integrated systems built to serve the greater good of patients and aligned with payers, creating innovative ways to deliver improved services at ever-lower costs. The remainder of this book addresses that vision.

REFERENCES

Centers for Medicare & Medicaid Services. 2018a. "Innovation Models." Accessed February 21. https://innovation.cms.gov/initiatives/index.html#views=models.

———. 2018b. "NHE Fact Sheet." Modified February 14. www.cms.gov/research-statistics-data-and-systems/statistics-trends-and-reports/nationalhealthexpenddata/nhe-fact-sheet.html.

Chernew, M. E., K. Baicker, and J. Hsu. 2010. "The Specter of Financial Armageddon: Health Care and Federal Debt in the United States." New England Journal of Medicine 362: 1166–68.

Christensen, C. M. 2011. *The Innovator's Dilemma: The Revolutionary Book That Will Change the Way You Do Business.* New York: Harper Business.

Christensen, C. M, J. H. Grossman, and J. Hwang. 2009. *The Innovator's Prescription: A Disruptive Solution for Health Care.* New York: McGraw-Hill.

Christensen, C. M., and M. E. Raynor. 2013. *The Innovator's Solution: Creating and Sustaining Successful Growth.* Boston: Harvard Business Review Press.

Ehrenreich, B., and J. Ehrenreich. 1969. "The Medical Industrial Complex." *Health/PAC Bulletin.* Health Policy Advisory Center. Published November. www.healthpacbulletin.org/healthpac-bulletin-november-1969.

Emerick, T. 2016. "Walmart Expands Its Center of Excellence Program." The Doctor Weighs In. Published October 12. https://thedoctorweighsin.com/walmart-expands-its-center-of-excellence-program/.

Fernandez, K. 2013. Personal correspondence. Memorial Hermann Physician Integrated Group.

Francis, D. R. 2018. "Why Do Death Rates Decline?" National Bureau of Economic Research. Accessed January 22. www.nber.org/digest/mar02/w8556.html.

Gawande, A. 2009. *The Checklist Manifesto: How to Get Things Right.* New York: Henry Holt and Company.

———. 2004. "The Bell Curve." *New Yorker.* Published December 6. www.newyorker.com/magazine/2004/12/06/the-bell-curve.

Himmelstein, D., D. Thorne, E. Warren, and S. Woodhandler. 2018. "Medical Bankruptcy: Fact Sheet." Physicians for a National Health Program. Accessed January 22. www.pnhp.org/sites/default/files/docs/Bankruptcy_Fact_Sheet.pdf.

Kaiser Family Foundation. 2017. "Key Facts About the Uninsured Population." Published September 19. www.kff.org/uninsured /fact-sheet/key-facts-about-the-uninsured-population/.

Kirsch, D. G., and K. Petelle. 2017. "Addressing the Physician Shortage: The Peril of Ignoring Demography." *Journal of the American Medical Association* 317 (19): 1947–48.

Knobler, S., A. Mack, and A. Mahmoud. 2005. *The Threat of Pandemic Influenza: Are We Ready?* Washington, DC: National Academies Press.

McGlynn, E. A., S. M. Asch, J. Adams, J. Keesey, J. Hicks, A. DeCristofaro, and E. A. Kerr. 2003. "The Quality of Healthcare Delivered to Adults in the United States." *New England Journal of Medicine* 348: 2635–45.

National Center for Health Statistics. 2018. "Mortality Data." Centers for Disease Control and Prevention. Updated January 4. www.cdc.gov/nchs/nvss/deaths.htm.

Organisation for Economic Co-operation and Development (OECD). 2018. "Health Status." Accessed March 9. www.oecd-ilibrary .org/social-issues-migration-health/data/oecd-health-statistics /oecd-health-data-health-status_data-00540-en.

Urbach, D. R. 2015. "Pledging to Eliminate Low Volume Surgery." *New England Journal of Medicine* 373: 1388–90.

US Government Accountability Office (GAO). 2018. "Fiscal Outlook: Understanding the Federal Debt." Accessed February 20. www.gao.gov/fiscal_outlook/understanding_federal_debt /overview.

Woodman, J. 2015. *Patients Beyond Borders: Everybody's Guide to Affordable, World-Class Medical Travel.* Chapel Hill, NC: Healthy Travel Media.

CHAPTER 2

Sustainable Change in Healthcare: Leadership for the Twenty-First Century

Tom Atchison

Leadership equals relationships.
Leaders have followers.
Leaders unleash human potential for the greater good of the individual
  and society.
Leaders are born and made.
We all have the capacity to lead—to inspire others—at some level.
Leadership is earned from followers. Titles are given.
There is no automatic connection between titles and leadership.
Leaders motivate through aligned values.
Leaders inspire though their vision.
Leaders sustain positive change through trust and respect.
Leadership is very different from management.
Leadership is the single most important factor in the successful creation
  of a high-performing organization.

These facts are some of the impermeable realities of leadership. These realities have not changed since the first follower committed to the vision of the first leader. So what's new in today's healthcare environment? Context.

The context for today's healthcare is characterized by rapid and unpredictable changes, disruptive technologies, social networks, political unrest, generational differences, and speed-of-light communications. Given these unprecedented dynamics, this chapter focuses on leadership in today's world. How do successful healthcare professionals lead sustainable change processes in this complex, unpredictable, ever-changing environment?

Today's context has changed the requirements for successful leadership. Clinically integrated networks, accountable care organizations, large multispecialty groups, employed physicians, and the ever-multiplying mergers and acquisitions are a few of the major realities confronting healthcare leaders today. Seldom has a single field experienced so many external pressures. In healthcare, we deal with governmental regulations, insurance companies, pharmaceutical corporations, consumer expectations, manpower shortages, an aging population, an obesity epidemic, and much more—all coming together to place extraordinary demands on the US healthcare field to transform itself. Leadership axioms such as "leadership equals relationships" must be carried in a world that demands constant innovation.

Several superb leaders have allowed their stories to be told in this chapter. From these high-performing executives, readers can learn the best applications of effective change processes in today's transformational environment. I have also included stories of failed attempts at sustainable change. In these cases, the facts have been altered to prevent exposure of organizational names and personal identities.

A MODEL FOR SUCCESSFUL CHANGE LEADERSHIP

Organizational and personal change has many moving parts. Some parts are independent; however, most are interdependent. To quote

H. L. Mencken (1920), "There is always a well-known solution to every human problem—neat, plausible, and wrong." In other words, simple change in not an option. This section presents a model that seems most effective in today's healthcare sector and has emerged from experience in the field. The variables that make up the model are highly influenced by the context of the change process. My own definition of *context* is the following: The environmental factors controlling a healthcare organization's ability to change and affecting the individual's ability and motivation to make changes a reality.

BEFORE THE FIVE FACTORS: CONTEXT AND VALUES

Few in the field argue with Peter Drucker's purported observation that "culture eats strategy for lunch." The power of culture trumps strategy. Context—the set of ever-transforming noncultural realities—can be even more damaging to change processes, however. In the healthcare field today, context mainly comprises economic and disruptive forces.

The change leadership model presented in this chapter can help leaders deal with the contextual pressures on culture that ultimately affect strategic success. Exhibit 2.1 shows a set of management factors (in the top half of the exhibit) and a set of leadership factors (in the bottom half) that contribute to successful change. The bridge between the two sets is values. When an organization has aligned values, the managers and leaders interconnect for optimal performance as they improve.

The following sections discuss the factors that leaders, either consciously or intuitively, work on to create a sustainable change process, along with practical applications and case data. This model places a strong emphasis on values and focuses on five main organizational variables: soul, history, capacity, self-image, and motivation. In the course of this discussion, I demonstrate the interdependent,

Exhibit 2.1: The Bridge Between Leadership Factors and Management Factors

Management
Rewards
Metrics
Tactics
Strategies
Vision

Values underpin the successful management of change

Leadership and culture define values-based behavior for sustainable change

Soul
History
Capacity
Self-image
Motivation
Leadership

sequential, and developmental aspects of ongoing, successful change. My ideas may be challenged on whether they are complete, in the right order, or universally applicable. However, one factor is not debatable: The critical success factor for today's healthcare leader is sustainable change.

A FOUNDATION OF VALUES

Sustainable change must be built on a foundation of values. Without aligned values, all attempts to change an organization will fail. Aligned values are the bedrock on which leaders move organizations forward. When values are aligned, employees can accept and handle the daily vagaries of any change process with a minimum of

Sturm und Drang (storm and stress). They understand the values as the context for the change process. When values are not aligned, physicians and staff have no organizing context, and they see daily vagaries as evidence that the change process is failing. Many times, the absence of aligned values results in self-fulfilling prophecies.

Values rule! Values are motivation. Values drive behavior and underpin decisions. Values guide us through life. Values are learned (there are no genetically programmed values). Values cause behaviors. Values are the reasons we engage in some behaviors and not others.

The importance of values has been obvious throughout history. How many wars have started because of a negative variance in a quarterly earnings report? On the other hand, how many wars have started (and continue) because of conflicting values? The US Civil War had economic antecedents, but the main reason for conflict was a difference in beliefs. Today, Shiite and Sunni Muslims in the Middle East are in constant conflict. Although war analogies might seem extreme, conflicts over values pit individuals and groups of people against each other.

In a healthcare organization, if any of the parties involved in a change effort have conflicting values, leading and managing change will fail over time. Without values alignment, all the parties need good legal and financial advice and strong contracts to reinforce a tenuous and probably uncertain connection. Change processes that did not consider values alignment early on have often led to collapsed mergers and acquisitions, executive terminations, and substandard performance from highly skilled professionals. Today, changemakers in the healthcare management field seem obsessed with the economics of changing structures, radical cost reductions in operations, reevaluating service lines to find cost savings, responding to governmental laws, rules, and regulations, and physician employment. Of course, decisions to change must comply with prudent business models. However, the best predictor of success and sustainability is a positive answer to the question, Does this change process match our beliefs of what is good and how best to proceed? If the answer to this question is no, then do not proceed.

Every year, hundreds of healthcare executives and trustees analyze a good business deal only to have it fail after many months of meetings that focus only on the costs and benefits. Beaumont Health and Henry Ford Health Systems are two of the more public healthcare failures stemming from a clash in values. In reality, leaders should complete a values alignment analysis before they even begin with the accountants and lawyers. This chapter's model shows where values lie in the change process and why this central location determines success or failure.

Consider exhibit 2.2 and note the line with an arrow pointing from core values (in the center circle) to manifest behaviors (in the outer circle). The closer a desired behavioral change is to the core values supporting that behavior, the easier the change process will be. Likewise, the greater the difference between the desired behavioral change and the core values, the harder the change process. Moreover, when the desired behavior change is in conflict with core beliefs, there will be no sustainable change. Remember that sustainable change starts (or stops) with values alignment.

To clarify, for the rest of this chapter, the words *executive* and *manager* refer to those individuals who get predictable results. A *leader*, however, is an individual who inspires followers. Managers focus on objectives, processes, and procedures; leaders focus on relationships, trust, and communication. Leadership scholar Warren G. Bennis (2009) stated, "Managers do things right and leaders do the right things." These are not mutually exclusive concepts—healthcare change needs them both. However, leading change and managing change are different, albeit interdependent, dynamics.

Change Process Variable 1: Soul

Leaders know that corporate soul has everything to do with organizational change. Soul, as it operates in a person's work, is the deepest sense of purpose. Mihaly Csikszentmihalyi (2003, 154) gives a great

Exhibit 2.2: Relationship Between Change and Values

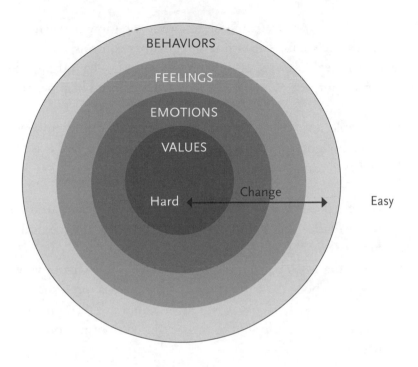

description in his book, *Good Business: Leadership, Flow, and the Making of Meaning*. He states that

> in many ways, the search for a life that "has relevance or meaning" beyond one's material existence is the primary concern of the soul. This is precisely the need that a person who is aware of his or her finitude feels, the need that motivates us to become part of something greater and more permanent. If a leader can make a convincing case that working for an organization will provide relevance, that it will take the workers out of the shell of their mortal frame and connect them with something more meaningful, then

his vision will generate power, and people will be naturally attracted to become part of such a company.

The contemporary overemphasis on profit and growth may have killed healthcare's soul. The business, regulatory controls, and economics of the healthcare sector—that is, the context—have trumped its existential purpose, which is to care for the sick and help people stay well.

For example, an excellent 2016 study by Merritt Hawkins explores the current thoughts of physicians concerning the perceived loss of soul. The key findings were the following:

- At 62.8 percent, a substantial majority of physicians are somewhat or very negative about the future of the medical profession.
- More than 53.9 percent of physicians feel somewhat or very negative about the current state of the medical profession.
- Half of physicians—49.2 percent—would not recommend medicine as a profession to their children or other young people.

What happens when work is soulless? An internist with decades of experience recently told me, "I used to be a doctor. Now I'm a pieceworker." An ear, nose, and throat specialist reported that he "believed that being a physician was a calling," but he had recently been told by the vice president of his system that he was an "economic unit." He commented, "I used to live for my patients, but now that I am an economic unit, I want to be paid for everything I do."

A sustainable change process starts with the soul because when a worker enjoys a fundamental connection between whom he believes himself to be and his work environment, he develops a sense of purpose that transcends self-interest. This connection "motivates us to become part of something greater and more permanent" (Csikszentmihalyi 2003). Can you imagine initiating an organizational change process with physicians and staff who see the change as creating something greater than themselves and more permanently beneficial for their patients? When they do so, leaders can make significant changes in a complex organization and enrich its soul in the process.

Can you think of a more complex organization than one consisting of a university hospital, medical school, and care network? How could any leader chart a new course for this veritable battleship in a bathtub? Larry Goodman, MD, president and CEO of Rush University Health System, has done just that. His knowledge of medicine and the workings of a medical school, as well as the complexity of delivering consistent, high-quality care in a busy urban setting, is second to none. But that skill set, while important to keeping the doors of the organization open, is not sufficient to move it forward. His leadership skills are the most important tool he has to create a sustainable change process that is truly exceptional.

His change process began with the trustees and executive team when they recognized that the organization's current vision had essentially been achieved. For Rush to continue to be successful in the next decade as it faced an unknowable future, a new vision was needed.

Dr. Goodman and his colleague Peter Butler, FACHE, the highly skilled and experienced chief operating officer of the system, are a great example of the required synergy for sustainable change—that is, change must be physician led and professionally managed. Together, Goodman and Butler, under the guidance of the board of trustees, began an effective change process focused on creating a new vision to guide the Rush enterprise for the next decade. The trustees and the executive leadership team laid out a several-month plan to engage the best thinking from all of the significant stakeholders. Exhibits 2.3 and 2.4 show the timelines, objectives, and milestones for this change process. Rush's perennial mission, as well as its new vision and values, are shown in exhibit 2.5.

Exhibit 2.3: Rush Governance Framework for Overall Vision and Strategy

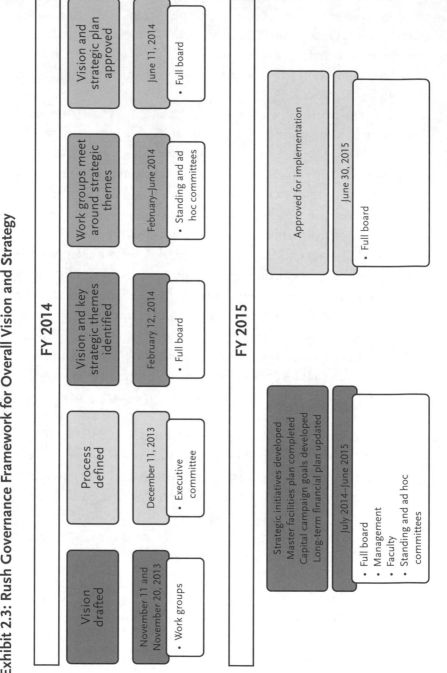

FY 2014

Vision drafted — November 11 and November 20, 2013 — • Work groups

Process defined — December 11, 2013 — • Executive committee

Vision and key strategic themes identified — February 12, 2014 — • Full board

Work groups meet around strategic themes — February–June 2014 — • Standing and ad hoc committees

Vision and strategic plan approved — June 11, 2014 — • Full board

FY 2015

Strategic initiatives developed
Master facilities plan completed
Capital campaign goals developed
Long-term financial plan updated — July 2014–June 2015 — • Full board • Management • Faculty • Standing and ad hoc committees

Approved for implementation — June 30, 2015 — • Full board

Source: Adapted from Rush University Health System materials.

46   *Essential Operational Components for High-Performing Healthcare Enterprises*

Exhibit 2.4: Rush Vision and Strategic Planning Framework

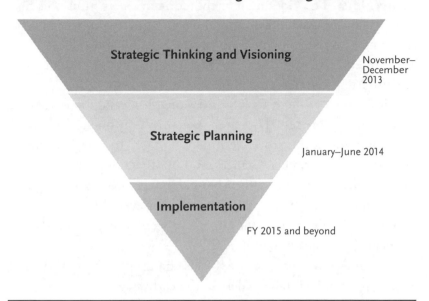

Strategic Thinking and Visioning — November–December 2013

Strategic Planning — January–June 2014

Implementation — FY 2015 and beyond

Source: Adapted from Rush University Health System materials.

Exhibit 2.5: Rush Mission, Vision, and Values

Mission: The mission of Rush University Medical Center is to provide **the very best care for our patients,** Our education and research endeavors, community service programs and relationships with other hospitals are dedicated to enhancing excellence in patient care for the diverse communities of Chicago area now and in the future.

Vision: Rush University Medical Center will be recognized as the medical center of choice in the Chicago area and among the very best in the United States.

Values:
- Innovation
- Collaboration
- Accountability
- Respect
- Excellence

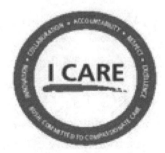

Source: Adapted from Rush University Health System materials.

Several important lessons are embedded in Rush's process of change. First, Dr. Goodman anchored it in the institution's history (or, as discussed previously, the soul) and confirmed that the visioning process would be built on the mission and values. Thus, the partners in the process were reassured that the important parts of Rush itself were not changing.

Moves such as these are a foundational leadership requirement for any change process. Too often, executives say only, "The world is changing and therefore we must change!" In this statement, there is no context, no assurances, and no direction. If you want to frighten physicians and staff early in a change process—and guarantee failure—declare a passionate need for everything to change. Remember to always give the change process context, boundaries, a timeline, and accountability.

A second powerful lesson of Rush's change process is maximum involvement of key stakeholders in the early stages.

In summary, the physician CEO at Rush developed trustee support, gained commitment from the executive team, and designed a sequential and developmental process that engaged departmental and service line leaders—all to craft the best possible ten-year vision. The final document was approved by the trustees and used as the basis for a strategic plan and an ongoing communication process, thereby turning a battleship in the bathtub and protecting the corporate soul throughout the process.

Change Process Variable 2: History

We are prisoners of our past. An individual's history with changes greatly influences her willingness to change today. Sadly, over the past several years, there have been many silver bullets that promised improved performance, higher quality, and the proverbial milk and honey. Quality circles, total quality management, Lean, Six Sigma, shared governance, Baldrige criteria, the seven steps of high performance, and many others promised the best way to change. In fact, a physician recently noted to me that every time the CEO went to a conference, the change "plan du jour" would be implemented—until the CEO went to a different conference! The desire to discover and implement the "one and only" or "best" program for change is a fool's journey.

The importance of history when discussing the problem of constant, failed change initiatives has been explained by a metaphor from child psychologist Dr. Rick Delaney. He says that multiple, unsuccessful changes create a powerful skepticism and even, in some cases, cynicism about another change. He calls it *foster child syndrome*. As a ten-year-old arrives at his fifth foster home in ten years, his new parents welcome him with open arms and all the right words—"We want you in our home," "We love you unconditionally," and so on. But after four previous times hearing the same promises, only to be given up to the system again each time, the child is reluctant to commit. After a while, the foster parents feel no reciprocation from the child and send him back, saying, "We did everything right and the child rejected us." Meanwhile, the child is thinking, "Yes, this is the way all these new placements end!"

A history of failed attempts at change predisposes individuals not to commit, to reserve judgment "until we see some success." By withholding their commitment, they ensure yet another failure. It's axiomatic that what people expect to happen, happens, and the implications of that human tendency for leaders wanting to change their organization are profound.

Change Processes and Guiding Coalitions

In John P. Kotter's (1995) classic article "Leading Change: Why Transformation Efforts Fail," the scholar recommends forming a guiding coalition to serve as the organizers and drivers of change throughout the organization. The selection of this group is one of the most important steps a leader will take to ensure a successful change process.

continued

continued from previous page

The following grid shows one way to think about the selection of members of the guiding coalition. It was designed several years ago in response to the often-used executive phrase "people are our most important asset." In reality, many leaders who use that phrase fail to give the selection process the attention it deserves. For instance, if a CEO is quizzed on her five human assets according to best performance, she might say, "All of the physicians and staff are good, or they wouldn't be here." If the same CEO is asked to name her top five service lines according to profitability, she could reel them off without hesitation. How can executives think that all physicians and employees are relatively equal but have detailed statistics on all major service lines? Organizations that rate physicians and staff by high, middle, and low cultural behavior metrics are much more likely to improve continuously in all areas of performance. Physicians and employees are not the most important asset; the right physicians and employees are the most important asset.

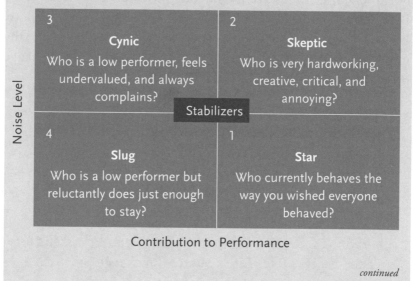

	3 **Cynic** Who is a low performer, feels undervalued, and always complains?	2 **Skeptic** Who is very hardworking, creative, critical, and annoying?
Noise Level	**Stabilizers**	
	4 **Slug** Who is a low performer but reluctantly does just enough to stay?	1 **Star** Who currently behaves the way you wished everyone behaved?

Contribution to Performance

continued

continued from previous page

Organizations can use the grid to classify high, medium, and low physicians and staff members by their behaviors. The horizontal axis represents contribution to performance, and the vertical axis represents noise level. In each of the four cells, there is a question that determines who is a star, a skeptic, a cynic, or a slug. People who do not fall clearly into one of those categories may be considered stabilizers.

All high-performing organizations have a set of core values and a list of behaviors that are driven by these values. Typically, these values-based behaviors are the cornerstones of a strong corporate culture. Leaders evaluate and rank individuals on the basis of the degree to which they routinely manifest the behaviors most reflective of the corporate culture. Therefore, the ranking of physicians and staff is not about the person; it is about the behavior. Effective leaders follow the mantra, "love the person, hate the behavior."

Behavioral rankings are contextual. A behavior that is considered undesirable in one healthcare system may be highly desired in another. For example, an executive who has a dominant behavior pattern of control and command might be ranked high in an organization that focuses mainly on profit; the same behaviors might cause the executive to have low rankings in an organization that emphasizes teamwork and consensus building. Remember that a behavior is defined as a physical expression that is observable, repeatable, and measurable.

To test the notion that "people are our most important asset," I asked two CEOs and two human resources (HR) professionals to count how many minutes per day they

continued

continued from previous page

spent engaging and re-recruiting their stars. For the sake of this small beta test, we used 600 minutes (i.e., a ten-hour day) as the numerator. I asked them to measure their minutes with stars for ten days (i.e., two workweeks). After two weeks, the CEO average was six minutes a day, and the average for HR professionals was zero minutes per day. One of the HR professionals commented that when she was with an employee or physician, it was mostly dealing with problems or complaints (i.e., cynics and slugs). Though this sample is extremely small, it suggests that the pronouncement "people are our most important asset" may not always be true.

The relevant point in using this grid to select your guiding coalition is that the initial coalition group must contain physicians and staff from cell 1 only—the stars. I suggest a four-step process for the creation of a guiding coalition for change. First, bring your executive team together. Second, ask them to write down the names of the physicians and staff members who come to mind when answering the question, Who is currently behaving the way we wished everyone behaved? Third, identify the persons whose names are written on most lists. Last, personally invite these individuals to become part of the guiding coalition.

All successful change programs are driven by the stars of the organizations. Frequently, the question arises of whether putting one or more skeptics or cynics in the group is a good idea. The answer is always an emphatic no. Don't introduce negative thoughts into the initial part of a change process. A counterpoint is that these folks will feel alienated and therefore will not commit—but that's

continued

continued from previous page

okay, because they were not going to commit anyway. Great teams, great orchestras, and great companies are great because they focus on the stars and drive all change through them.

The history of star performers is much more likely to be minimally negative and, in fact, most likely positive. The selection and early training of this group are a major determinant of whether the change process will succeed.

Let's put the first two variables together. As a leader interested in a change process, you must first determine whether those leading and managing the change process have aligned values and the appropriate set of desirable behaviors. Once the values-based behaviors are aligned, then it is important to anchor the desired change to the soul or purpose of the organization. Then, the senior leadership team identifies the stars to form a guiding coalition, which is trained on change management processes and communication strategies. (See Kotter [1995]. Also see Atchison [2004], which contains a case study in which the guiding coalition was instrumental in leading and sustaining a three-year postmerger change process in a hospital.)

Change Process Variable 3: Capacity

Capacity is one factor that is often ignored—even more than history. Capacity is, quite simply, the ability to change. A capacity analysis helps determine how fast and how far the change process can proceed with the current composition of physicians and staff. All humans cannot move in one direction at the same pace, so how can a leader of change expect equal performance from, quite possibly, thousands of diverse physicians and staff?

Humans vary widely in intelligence, energy, motivation, talent, creativity, and many other genetic and experiential factors. Therefore, an ongoing assessment of where, and with whom, change will happen most easily and where it will be difficult must be part of the implementation strategy. The following case, in which the capacity to change was not analyzed prior to implementation, shows the significant consequences of such an omission.

This story is about a talented medical/surgical nurse manager. Let's call him Peter Principle, MSN, MBA. He had a pleasant personality, though some might have described him as timid or shy. As a nurse manager for a large medical/surgical unit, he was exceptionally skilled. Staff, physicians, and patients all responded favorably to Peter, but he had one problem. He had reached the maximum compensation and benefit package for his academic credentials and years of experience.

Along came a merger of three highly specialized service units. These one-time competitors were combined into one corporation for the purposes of delivering trauma care to a large geographic area. The senior executives of the system thought this would be an excellent opportunity to promote Peter to vice president of the new service line, giving him a much larger compensation package. However, no one ever posed the basic question of whether he was capable of leading this group of subspecialists with a history of competition. The system executives did not assess his capacity to change from a linear, inpatient medical/surgical unit to a nonlinear, decentralized trauma provider group. If they had done even a rudimentary capacity assessment, they would have saved a great deal of heartache, money, and organizational trauma.

It soon became obvious that Peter lacked the capacity for dealing with verbal, aggressive, competitive personalities. Following the classic human response of fight or flight, he stayed in his office with the door closed and wrote emails—which produced counter-emails, all in caps! The whole unit had run amok.

The several-day corrective intervention began with a temporary suspension of the use of emails when dealing with interpersonal issues. Several cathartic sessions convened in an effort to eliminate the conflict and begin the healing, but it was clear that Peter could not continue as the vice president of the service line. The healing phase included his face-saving return to the medical/surgical unit as well as a process to identify the optimal characteristics and capacity for a leader of this complex and volatile trauma service line.

The financial and human costs of this lack of a capacity assessment process were huge. The repair phase took months. It required many difficult interventions to align the diverse, aggressive, and highly skilled specialists. Regrettably, two of these physicians were so conflict oriented that they had to be permanently separated from the organization.

The alignment of these professionals would have been difficult under the best of circumstances, with the right leader in place at the inception of the merger. The system executives exercised poor judgment in assuming that Peter's capacity to deal with change was equally applicable to trauma as it was to medical/surgical matters. Lesson learned: The capacity to lead change is strongly influenced by human and professional factors. Always assess the leader's capacity to lead change and the organization's capacity to change.

Change Process Variable 4: Self-Image

Over the years, people have begun to think of *self-image* as a "soft" concept best left to the world of psychobabble and self-help texts. However, in the ever-changing context of today's healthcare system, self-image can advance or restrict a leader's ability to implement sustainable change.

Self-image is our own estimate of personal capability combined with expectations from personal, interpersonal, and professional situations. It's where we see ourselves as most effective in life. Let's return to a couple of earlier comments: "I used to be a doctor. Now I'm a pieceworker" and "Being a physician was a calling . . . now I am an economic unit." Now imagine that you are an executive trying to manage change with these two physicians—not a good prognosis. Their estimation of their personal effectiveness (i.e., their self-image) has been destroyed by environmental circumstances (i.e., context). Whom they believe themselves to be and the organizational messages about how they are expected to behave are in conflict.

Personal estimates of competence are extremely important in leading and managing a change process. Significant research, as well as common sense, says that when self-image and organizational expectations are aligned, success is very likely. The converse is also true—when self-image and organizational expectations are in conflict, then success is very unlikely and certainly unsustainable.

The general malaise among physicians detailed in the Merritt Hawkins data mentioned earlier in the chapter is troubling because the need for significant change in healthcare delivery is undeniable. So how does a leader incorporate the building and maintenance of strong self-image during a comprehensive change process? Britt Berrett, FACHE, is an excellent example of a leader who understands the power of personal expectations. Britt is the coauthor of a book with the provocative title *Patients Come Second* (Spiegelman and Berrett 2013). His philosophy and approach have served him well in both for-profit and not-for-profit delivery systems. When Britt says patients should come second, he is encouraging healthcare leaders to put the physicians and staff first, the patients second, and finance and business operations third—and, if you follow this sequence, finances will be healthy. This notion runs counter to the dominant, more popular notion that money comes first, patients come second, and staff and physicians are the economic units that make the first two possible. Think about your 600-minute, 10-hour day—do you invest most of those minutes building a strong culture with the physicians and staff? Or do you spend your time with finance and business operations?

Take a look at your past several executive team agendas and past several board agendas—what is the ratio of topics dealing with financial capital to the amount of time spent on your corporate culture and on staff and physician engagement? Trying to lead and manage change without a strong corporate culture and significant commitment from staff and physicians is impossible, and full engagement is enhanced during the process of change. If the change process erodes or contaminates an individual's sense of self, the process will fail.

Change Process Variable 5: Motivation

Ask any executive group to list the leadership problems they are dealing with currently. Typically, more than 50 percent of the issues center around motivating staff during these complex and ever-changing times.

The term *motivation* is often used incorrectly. Motivation is what causes our behavior. Motivation is complicated, and understandings of it are saddled with two powerful myths:

- *Myth 1: People can be motivated or unmotivated.* The fact is that all humans are 100 percent motivated 100 percent of the time. Motivation cannot be increased or decreased; it can only be unleashed or directed. Staff members are motivated when they come in late, leave early, and take long lunches—the manager and the organization have not created an environment in which corporate goals trump personal motives.
- *Myth 2: All people are motivated by money.* In reality, money only motivates in one set of circumstances; it depresses motivation under two circumstances. First, if the money offered is perceived to be too low, then the amount demotivates; second, if it is perceived to be too high, it demotivates. (The latter is sometimes called *golden handcuffs*—perks offered to highly skilled employees that can only be redeemed while the employee stays with the company.)

It seems intuitive that if you pay people more, they will produce better results. However, compelling research suggests an insignificant relationship between money, performance, and job satisfaction. A meta-analysis by Timothy A. Judge and colleagues (2010) reviewed 120 years of research, synthesizing 92 quantitative studies. The final study included more than 15,000 people and 115 correlation coefficients. The reported correlation (.14) indicates that the overlap between pay and job satisfaction levels is less than 15 percent. In fact, research strongly suggests that money can depress motivation. Another meta-analysis by Edward Deci, Richard M. Ryan, and Richard Koestner (1999) revealed that incentives had consistent negative effects on intrinsic motivation.

The most important idea among these is *intrinsic motivation*. The vast majority of healthcare workers go into the field with a powerful intrinsic motivation to help others. The current obsession with money corrodes this internal motivational pattern and thereby depresses intrinsic motivation.

The main leadership lesson here is that people in healthcare *want* to do good work. Of course, we all need to make a living and provide for ourselves and others. But leaders understand the power of intrinsic motivation and create environments that unleash and direct it in order to promote and sustain positive change. In fact, the degree to which a system needs to use threats and or money to motivate effort is proportional to the degree to which intrinsic motivation has been corrupted.

Chris Dadlez, FACHE, is the former president and CEO of St. Francis Health in Hartford, Connecticut. I have watched and admired Chris's ability to tap into the intrinsic motivations of a wide variety of people over many years. The first thing that comes to mind when describing his leadership style is the phrase "genuine humanity." He cares about the people who are responsible for living the corporate values and achieving the mission of St. Francis. It would be impossible for Chris to call a physician an "economic unit" or to put profit before a caring, professional staff.

When his leadership team comes together to lead a sustainable change process, the energy in the room is palpable. During a strategic-thinking session with dozens of leaders from throughout the system, several motivational dynamics were obvious—some by their absence. Chris set the tone and the broad objectives. Then he became just another participant. There was no hierarchy in the room, no egos—just a bunch of smart, caring, highly engaged professionals trying to discover optimal avenues for change. Throughout the two-day session, there was never a mention of compensation for this extra service. Many of the physicians had to forgo office practice, surgeries, and patient visits to participate, but their motives for doing so were completely intrinsic.

Would money have increased the energy, commitment, and achievement of this leadership team? The answer is an emphatic no. In fact, my suspicion is that, had money been presented to members of this group, they would have wondered why they were being paid to do what they wanted to do anyhow. Intrinsic motives are deep and powerful. Money as a motivator is a slippery slope.

ASSEMBLING THE INDIVIDUAL FACTORS INTO A CORPORATE CULTURE

The five factors of soul, history, capacity, self-image, and motivation are the building blocks of sustainable change. Like any building, the structure is only as strong as its foundation. In organizational change, the organizational values must align with those of the physicians and staff to create a strong foundation. This foundation-building is a developmental, sequential, hierarchical process. For example, motivation is only as strong as the four other factors beneath it.

Leaders who understand the importance of the five factors meld them into a unified dynamic called *corporate culture*. This dynamic should be strong yet nimble enough to accommodate strategic changes—as long as the strategic changes are consistent with the cultural imperatives. When the organizational strategy is firmly built on the foundation, sustainable success is inevitable. Likewise, when strategy is disconnected from the individual factors, sustainable success is impossible. You may observe initial success, but it will result from the temporary presence of the leadership; it will not be inherent and will last only six to eight weeks.

Culture is another term that is used often without a clear definition. As I attended a recent two-hour lecture, I noted that the presenter used the word 12 times and never defined what she meant. The word was used differently in almost each sentence. When asked for a definition, she said, "It is what corporations do with people to get them to do what they want them to do." An understanding this vague will not help an organization build change. Culture has a precise definition.

The concept of a culture has arisen from anthropology. My basic definition is as follows: culture is "anything we do that is not genetically determined." The ability to produce sounds at birth (phonemes) is not cultural, but the language we speak is defined by the dominant culture—in fact, language is a significant part of culture.

A simpler way to define culture is that it is anything we do when no one is watching. Culture is the reason we dress the way we do, eat the kinds of food we eat, and speak and write in our primary language—all because "that's the way we do it here." This phrase is the most common way culture is defined. Most behavioral differences are a function of varying cultures.

Corporate culture is a subset of the greater concept of culture. It has all of the elements of the anthropological concept of culture, but more specifically, it is the organization's personality. Every company has essentially the same business components: finance, information technology, human resources, marketing, planning, executive management, and so on. So why are companies so different? How have Starbucks, Zappos, Patagonia, Google, Ritz-Carlton, and Amazon been successful in a rapidly changing and highly competitive environment? Each of them is known for its strong corporate culture.

An individual's personality is the manifestation of behaviors driven by core beliefs (values). Organizational personality—the corporate culture—has the same dynamic, writ large. It is behavioral consistency in all of the employees, determining how they behave and why.

When no corporate culture defines the corporation's personality, it has as many subcultures as it does employees. And, as for human beings, it is a really good idea just to have one personality! The subcultures in an organization define its potential for dysfunction. No change can be successful until there is a strong, single corporate culture.

Corporate cultures, whether in healthcare organizations or non-healthcare organizations, have the same four components: mission, values, vision, and trust. A mission statement answers the question, Why do we exist? A list of values answers the question, What beliefs drive our decisions? The vision answers the question, What is our destination? And trust answers the question, Do we give each other the benefit of the doubt? These four questions are fundamental to sustainable change. Their answers give the change process a context—something concrete that provides meaning to the individual during change. Leaders always anchor any change process in one or more of these cultural elements, just as Dr. Goodman anchored Rush's change in its history, mission, and values.

Without this context, employees anticipate change that is episodic and reactive. No change process can survive if leaders cite external perils, saying, "We are changing because the government is forcing us to change!" or "If we don't change we won't survive!" Even if these are statements of fact, they will not ignite the intrinsic motivations necessary to move forward. In fact, these statements are more likely to create fear and anxiety that will interfere with the change process.

The American College of Healthcare Executives (ACHE) is an example of an organization with a strong corporate culture. Its CEO, Deborah J. Bowen, FACHE, CAE, works closely with the ACHE Board of Governors on mission, values, and vision statements. The comprehensive and consistent communication of these cultural elements engenders a great deal of trust among staff members, who consistently live the values in the context of the mission in order to achieve the vision (see exhibit 2.6).

Exhibit 2.7 shows the three cornerstones of mission, values, and vision. These three factors are held together by trust. As a small test of trust, time yourself as you write out the mission, core values, and

---

Exhibit 2.6: ACHE Cultural Elements

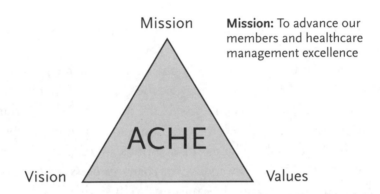

Mission

Mission: To advance our members and healthcare management excellence

ACHE

Vision

Values

Vision: To be the preeminent professional society for leaders dedicated to improving health

Core Values: We are committed to and live out our core values through our work

Integrity: We advocate and demonstrate high ethical conduct in all we do.

Lifelong Learning: We recognize lifelong learning is essential to our ability to innovate and continually improve ourselves, our organizations and our profession.

Leadership: We lead through example and mentoring, and recognize caring must be a cornerstone of our professional interactions.

Diversity and Inclusion: We advocate inclusion and embrace the differences of those with whom we work and the communities we serve.

Source: Adapted from ACHE (2018).

vision of your organization. Continue with the challenge as you write a 50-word statement about how you build and strengthen trust. If the entire process takes longer than five minutes, you may want to think about the strength of your corporate culture. Remember that change is only sustainable in a strong corporate culture; in a weak culture, intrinsic motivation is unlikely, and the organization is capable of episodic change at best.

Trust is the glue that binds leaders and followers. At the same time, trust is a lubricant that keeps the natural interpersonal friction of change from becoming full-blown conflict. Trust can be defined as the perception of honesty, openness, and reliability. Followers need to believe that the leader is telling them the full truth consistently.

When trust is present in an organization, physicians and staff give each other the benefit of the doubt. When an organization is mired in mistrust, staff and physicians are always looking for the hidden agenda. Imagine two staff meetings—one where levels of

Exhibit 2.7: Strength of Culture

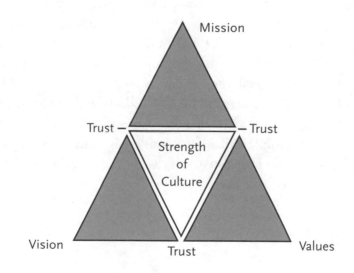

trust are high and another marked by great mistrust. These two meetings have the same agenda: How can we can change to better meet today's healthcare delivery needs? The trusting team will most likely brainstorm, challenge, and develop what-if scenarios. The mistrusting group will most likely sit quietly, waiting to discover the "real" reason for this move to change. After the meeting, the members will subdivide into cliques and gossip, and they will do whatever is necessary to protect their silos. In *The Five Dysfunctions of a Team*, Patrick Lencioni (2002) lists mistrust as the largest driver behind failure.

I recently heard of an egregious example of broken trust with the CEO as the culprit. He initiated a reduction in force of 60 clinicians and support staff members in mid-December—about two weeks before Christmas. The CEO said that the reduction in force was the result of the Affordable Care Act, state government payment reductions, the anticipation of a census decline during the holidays, and other negative reasons. He had a litany of justifications for his timing. What he didn't mention was that by cutting these workers in mid-December, the CEO came in underbudget, meaning that he could receive his own $100,000 performance bonus.

The physician members of the board were livid and, in an unusual move, publicly discussed the CEO's private salary information with colleagues and staff. His bonus didn't just break trust—it atomized trust! The organizational trauma that resulted required the CEO and most of the executive team to be replaced. As you might imagine, the new senior team started in a deep hole of mistrust.

Trust, in its simplest manifestation, is engendered by character, communication, and consistency. Trust takes a long time to develop but can be broken in a heartbeat.

CONCLUSION

This chapter shows that fundamental leadership dynamics have not changed over time but that the context for today's healthcare field means that leaders must apply these dynamics with a significant emphasis on innovation. A model for this new application is based on the notion that the deeper dimensions—soul, history, capacity, self-image, and motivation—are foundational to sustainable change.

The healthcare delivery system in the United States is experiencing a period of transformational change. Governmental regulations, new payment mechanisms, consumer activism, an aging population, a new emphasis on population health, disruptive technologies, and staffing issues will continue to fuel transformation. Leadership that is creative, nimble, and focused—that inspires followers with a powerful vision—will be successful regardless of the complexity of context in our changing times.

REFERENCES

American College of Healthcare Executives (ACHE). 2018. "ACHE Strategic Plan." Accessed March 12. www.ache.org/abt_ache /planning.cfm.

Atchison, T. 2004. *Followership: A Practical Guide to Aligning Leaders and Followers*. Chicago: Health Administration Press.

Bennis, W. 2009. *On Becoming a Leader*, rev. ed. Reading, MA: Addison Wesley.

Csikszentmihalyi, M. 2003. *Good Business: Leadership, Flow, and the Making of Meaning*. New York: Penguin.

Deci, E. L, R. M. Ryan, and R. Koestner. 1999. "A Meta-analytic Review of Experiments Examining the Effects of Extrinsic Rewards on Intrinsic Motivation." *Psychological Bulletin* 125 (6): 627–68.

Judge, T. A., R. F. Piccolo, N. P. Podsakoff, J. C. Shaw, and B. L. Rich. 2010. "The Relationship Between Pay and Job Satisfaction: A Meta-analysis of the Literature." *Journal of Vocational Behavior* 77: 157–67.

Kotter, J. P. 1995. "Leading Change: Why Transformations Fail." *Harvard Business Review* (March-April): 1–9.

Lencioni, P. 2002. *The Five Dysfunctions of a Team: A Leadership Fable*. San Francisco: Jossey-Bass.

Mencken, H. L. 1920. *Prejudices: Second Series*. New York: Alfred A. Knopf.

Merritt Hawkins. 2016. *2016 Survey of America's Physicians' Practice Patterns and Perspectives*. The Physicians Foundation. Accessed March 12, 2018. www.merritthawkins.com/uploadedFiles/Physicians%20Foundation%202016%20Survey%20of%20Americas%20Physicians.pdf.

Spiegelman, P., and B. Berrett. 2013. *Patients Come Second: Leading Change by Changing the Way You Lead*. New York: Inc.

CHAPTER 3

Governing the Future of Healthcare Systems

James E. Orlikoff

GOVERNING A SYSTEM of hospitals is different in form, function, and complexity from governing a single, stand-alone hospital. Similarly, governing a healthcare system that comprises disparate organizations and functions—a system driven by purposes that extend beyond hospital-based care—is very different from governing a multihospital system. Effectively governing large, complex healthcare systems of the future will require an intentional evolution of governance. We must address the new challenges in the healthcare market and master the new systems of care that are emerging in response.

Healthcare systems struggle with the immense and confusing challenges presented by changes in the sector and in society as a whole. Such challenges include, but are not limited to, the following:

- The shift from volume-based payment to more at-risk, value-based payment models
- The broadening definition of healthcare delivery, from case-by-case sickness care to population health, along with

a growing focus on social and economic determinants of health
- The evolution from silo-based organizational structures (and the reimbursement models that reward them) to structures that focus on the seamless integration of care provided in disparate organizations and settings
- A reversal of the economic model that maximizes profit by emphasizing intensive, expensive care to a model that generates margin by caring for people in the least intensive and expensive environments
- The movement from a wholesale market for healthcare to a retail market for healthcare; the transfer of financial risk to patients, providers, and key stakeholders; and the resultant rise of consumerism
- The challenge of dealing with traditional competitors while recognizing and responding to the rapid growth of disruptive competition
- The change from competition among geographically proximate organizations to competition among regional and national supersystems
- Rapid and revolutionary changes in the regulatory system
- Changing demographics and the aging of the US population
- Economic pressures to achieve more with less

To address such daunting and unprecedented external challenges, while at the same time attempting to balance crucial internal interests, is to disrupt and remake the very organizations that have defined American healthcare. Doing so requires a very different approach to governance. For these new twenty-first-century systems of care to succeed, effective governance is both more important and more challenging than ever.

THE EVOLUTION OF SYSTEM GOVERNANCE

The evolution of the majority of healthcare organizations has generally progressed from relatively simple to highly complex. Stand-alone hospitals and other care delivery organizations have yielded to multihospital systems, which in turn have added provider organizations such as skilled nursing facilities, inpatient or outpatient rehabilitation facilities, and so on. These organizations pioneered clinically integrated networks, employed physician groups, and accountable care organizations, growing from systems with insurance functions requiring the assumption of contractual risk to systems that assumed responsibility for the health of defined populations and covered actuarial lives. As healthcare delivery organizations evolved, so did the models and mentalities of governance.

Most multihospital systems over the twentieth century began with a *holding company*—a decentralized governance model in which corporate governance structure reflected the organization's strategic attempt to capture systemwide efficiencies while preserving the integrity of subsidiary organizations at all times. In essence, the goal of this approach was the best of both worlds. In such a model, optimization of the system as a whole, along with a focus on creating system synergies, was a foreign (or, at best, nascent) concept among system boards and leaders. The vast majority of multihospital systems had multiple boards that were decentralized in structure and function.

As the economic and environment changed, recognition grew that to capture the deeper and more challenging benefits and efficiencies of a true system, it was necessary to become truly integrated. The strategy and structure of systems began to change from a holding company model to an *operating company* model. In the latter, the system attempts to function as a single integrated organization rather than a collection of independently functioning pieces. When leaders began to push their systems to the progressive end of the continuum, older governance mentalities came under stress and scrutiny.

There are two broad categories of system governance structure: *centralized* and *decentralized*. A pure centralized model of governance means that the entire system is governed by a single board; multiple boards constitute a decentralized model. In the late twentieth century, the most common healthcare system governance model was decentralized, and this governance persists today.

A decentralized structure has several components. First, it has multiple boards. Second, it has a hierarchical structure and levels of governance, meaning that it has boards that are subordinate and that report to other boards. Third, it subdivides governance authorities and functions among the different boards in the system. Fourth, it has a "parent," or system, board, which is the ultimate authority in the system, and therefore has the unique role of overseeing and directing the other boards.

The decentralized system model has four subtypes: organizational, regional, functional, and combined. In an organizational model, each separate organization in a system has a board, and all share a parent board. In a regional model, a large system operating in diffuse geographic regions has several regional boards and a similar parent board. In a functional model, the system organizes its governance along functional or business lines; that is, it may have a single board that governs all the hospitals, a board that oversees all the insurance companies and functions, a board that oversees all the nursing homes, and so on. In the combined model, a system is a mishmash of all of the previous models. For example, it may have separate boards for all of its hospitals (organizational model) and have these boards report to a regional board (regional model), while it has several functional boards, such as an insurance company that provides services across the whole system, along with a parent board.

Though the dominant governance model of systems has historically been decentralized and organizational, as the holding company model lost currency in the market, system leaders began to realize that this approach to governance structure and function was both limited and limiting and was a major barrier to any significant movement toward an operating company model and true functional "systemness." One impracticality, for example, was that as the number of organizations in a system grew through acquisition and merger, the number of boards in the system multiplied. In fact, in many of these systems, executives and parent board leaders were (and are) unable to accurately identify exactly how many boards existed in the system without concerted effort and a detailed review of multiple documents. Many board members found that an inordinate amount of their time was consumed by preparing for, attending, and following up on board and committee meetings. Further time was wasted dealing with redundant governance structures, resulting in repetitive, board-by-board communication and turf battles between boards.

The largest drawback was the often interminably long time it took to make and implement significant system strategic decisions and to establish major directional changes. The delay resulted from the need to involve all or many of the boards and from the vague nature of the boards' roles and authorities. (Was the subsidiary boards' approval necessary to make a system strategic decision that affected them? Or were they just to be informed? Or were they to be consulted and their input on the proposed decision sought? Did their input have to be followed?) As the markets became less forgiving of this slow decision-making and less-than-nimble implementation, the frailties of the decentralized, organizational model of governance were exposed.

Another weakness, from a legal and regulatory standpoint, was the inevitable variation in policies, standards, and criteria applied by each board regarding its unique medical staff credentialing, privileging, and peer review structures. This discrepancy became problematic when courts scrutinized systems following adverse events and chose to use the highest or strictest standards to apply to any given case. The lack of a uniform approach unnecessarily placed each organization and the system itself at risk.

Perhaps the greatest weakness of this model, and the one that most inhibited the movement toward true, functional systemness, was the mechanism of choosing members for a board. In the past, stand-alone hospitals served defined communities, with the underlying assumption that governance on behalf of a specific community necessitated governance exclusively by members of that community—and board members should be drawn solely from the community served by the hospital. Further, board composition models were typically based on representational governance, where some or all members of the hospital board were selected, either explicitly or implicitly, to represent specific constituent groups (e.g., medical staff, auxiliary groups financially supporting the mission, hospital foundation) or regions in the service area. As systems developed, this model of representational governance persisted and usually included parent boards that were largely or exclusively composed of individuals drawn from subordinate or partner boards. The common downfall of such representational governance occurred when the board members tended to represent the interests of their component organization or constituent group rather than focusing on the interests of the system as a whole.

Representational governance is the antithesis of integrated, strategic governance based on systemwide thinking, and it almost always impedes the performance and advancement of the system as a whole. The source of the dysfunction is a core principle of systems thinking: If the system as a whole is to be optimized, then some of the pieces of the system must be cut back. According to this line of thought, the reverse is also true: If the pieces of the system are optimized, then the system as a whole will be less than optimal. Representational governance models and mind-sets always result in a focus on protecting the organizations within a system, on optimization of the pieces. As a result, representational composition models inhibit system optimization and present unnecessary roadblocks to effective governance and leadership. Such models, although still common today, are inappropriate for governance of twenty-first-century systems of care.

EFFECTIVE SYSTEM GOVERNANCE FOR THE FUTURE

As stated, the vast majority of multihospital systems began with a holding company approach, resulting in a decentralized organizational model of governance that relied on representational composition of the parent and other boards. This pattern was rarely, if ever, based on explicit principles developed by leaders. Rather, the model simply evolved, based on history and happenstance, from unspoken expectations and implicit assumptions.

To govern twenty-first-century systems effectively, the parent board of each system must ensure that its model of both governance structure and function is based on explicit, transparent, shared principles. I recommend the following principles as a foundation for best practices in twenty-first-century healthcare governance systems:

- *Consistency.* Governance structures are consistent throughout the system. Further, leadership models and structures (governance, management, clinical) are consistent throughout the system.
- *Leadership.* The purpose of governance is to lead the system, not to represent the interests of constituencies, stakeholders, regions, or pieces of the system. Therefore, governance composition models are competency based, not representational.
- *Authority.* System governance operates on the principles of centralizing authority and decentralizing decision-making. This rule is clarified and operationalized through the development and use of an authority matrix, a map that lays out the structure of power and responsibility.
- *Balanced power structure.* No individual, committee, or group of individuals is allowed to hold too much power.
- *Minimalism.* Fewer governance entities are better. Every effort is made to have as few boards and board committees

as possible to help maximize governance efficiency and reduce decision-making cycle time.

- *Intentionality.* Whatever model of governance structure and function is chosen, it is based on conscious choices and explicit principles, not on chance or precedent.

The concepts behind consistency, leadership, authority, and balanced power structure, as well as approaches to realizing them, are explored in greater detail in the following sections.

Consistency

The principle of consistency is fairly straightforward, and recognition of its value emerged through the frustration and governance gear grinding that was evident in systems that did not practice it. The result of a decentralized, organizational model of governance ranges from inefficient governance to organizational chaos.

Why? Imagine a system with ten subsidiary organizations and ten governance structures and processes. Each subsidiary board has a different size, a different mechanism for composing itself, different meeting frequencies and lengths, different approaches to board orientation and continuing education, different numbers and types of board committees, different terms and term limits for members and officers, different processes for making decisions, and different ways of framing the distinction between governance and management. From a governance perspective, this variation is inherently antisystem—by maintaining the idiosyncratic nature of each organizational board, the leadership focus on the pieces of the system is perpetuated, which weakens the system as a whole. Further, making this inconsistent governance model work requires inordinate amounts of system executive time for lubricating the different governance gears of each organization, adjudicating tension between boards as resources and services are allocated and consolidated, and achieving any coordinated movement toward systemness. Excessive drag on the time of the system executives, as well as the system board, diverts their attention from critical external issues and from striving to ensure that the system is strategically positioned to best achieve efficiency and deal with a transforming market.

Usually, this model results from systems that allow each organizational acquisition to maintain its own governance model as an inducement to join the system. The paradox is classic: What is necessary to consummate a deal from a governance perspective becomes an immediate impediment to making the deal work after it is done. If allowed to maintain its own governance model, the newcomer may be persuaded to join a system, but after it has done so, its governance model will pull the system toward antisystem behavior. As a result, potential benefits are rarely fully realized or, if they are, realized slowly.

For systems with a decentralized model of governance that wish to maximize effective system governance, mandating consistency in governance structure, process, and function is a critical initial step. Examples of such consistency in governance structure and function among all the boards in a system include standardization of the following:

- Board sizes and term limits
- Committee structures and functions
- Job descriptions (e.g., for the positions of board chair, vice chair, board member)
- Self-evaluation models and schedules
- Policies and practices for individual board member performance evaluation, pursuant to term renewal
- Board policies (e.g., conflict of interest, confidentiality, member removal, chair selection, new member orientation)
- Annual calendars and work plans

Further, in effective twenty-first-century systems, the consistency principle is also applied to all leadership models, meaning that the structures of management, governance, and clinical groups are also the same throughout the system. For example, all of the medical staffs in a system will have the same number, type, and size of committees; the same leadership positions, job descriptions, and terms of office; and similar bylaws, policies, and procedures. Management of each organization in the system is affected similarly—they have the same number and type of management positions, job descriptions, and human resources policies as well as similar performance expectations. The rationale for this consistent structure is the same as that outlined earlier, but there is an important evolutionary trend behind it and a common hurdle to overcome.

Many systems attempt to get the benefits of systemness without making all of the difficult leadership changes necessary to do so. That is, they try to gain the functional benefits of centralization and systemness while maintaining decentralized leadership structures. They do this by centralizing management but allowing governance and clinical structures and functions to remain varied.

In this model, the system is structured so that the executives of all of the subsidiary organizations report to, and can be hired and fired by, the CEO of the system. But, each separate organization in the system is allowed to maintain its own board and its own medical staff, clinically integrated network, or other clinical organization. The implicit strategy is to burden executive management with realizing the benefits of centralization while allowing the perception of independence to persist via decentralized governance and clinical structures.

While very challenging for executive management, this inconsistent model works for a while—until the market begins to require increasingly effective and efficient system performance and ever greater degrees of operational nimbleness. At that point, the painful drawbacks of this approach inevitably manifest and efforts are made to align the leadership models in the system. As a result, many systems have gone, or are going through, a staged model of leadership evolution:

- *Stage 1.* All leadership structures, including management, are decentralized. Typically, this is only seen at the very beginning of system formation.
- *Stage 2.* Management is completely or partially centralized, while governance and clinical structures and functions are decentralized. This stage tends to persist until the inefficiencies and tension created by this model make it difficult for the system to respond appropriately to external market pressures.
- *Stage 3.* Governance is centralized and made more consistent with management structures, but clinical structures are allowed to remain decentralized. Again, this stage tends to persist until market demands for clinical centralization are undeniable.
- *Stage 4.* Clinical structures are centralized to be consistent with management and governance structures. The structure of all leadership in the system is consistent.

Thus, effective twenty-first-century systems adopt a principle of governance and leadership consistency. All governance models are consistent throughout; further, all leadership models are consistent throughout. Systems that are in the early stages of evolution tend to devote energy to moving forward as quickly as they can.

Leadership

If the governance principle of leadership is adopted—the philosophy that the purpose of governance is to govern and lead the system, not to represent the interests of constituencies, stakeholders, or pieces of the system—then the member selection for system and subsidiary boards must emphatically reflect this. No other characteristic so directly and immediately affects the function of a board than who the members of the board are. Why and how the individual members are chosen, and how their skills, qualifications, experience, expertise, and backgrounds are balanced and blended, has a monumental impact on all governance functions and effectiveness and must therefore be a major component of effective governance. This is especially true in times of significant environmental change and challenge to the system. Many systems that developed with representational models of governance either have moved or are moving toward what is commonly called a *competency-based model* of board selection.

Competency-based board composition is a method of developing criteria for members, who must have specific skills, experience, characteristics, and attributes needed to facilitate the board's basic tasks and functions, and its development and accomplishment of strategic goals. These criteria are then used as the basis for the identification, evaluation, nomination, and selection of the members of the board. *Competency-based* composition is often regarded as an unfortunate term: "If we don't use that model, does that mean that I and my fellow board members are incompetent?" The unfortunate nature of the phrase notwithstanding, it is the shorthand term to describe a critical best practice, and no other term has yet replaced it in the governance lexicon.

Competencies are typically divided into three broad categories. The first is general competencies and characteristics; these are skills and traits that every board member must have. They might include the ability to disagree without being disagreeable, past board or leadership team experience, a defined level of professional accomplishment, big-picture thinking, comfort with ambiguity, the ability to support board decisions with which one disagrees, discretion, effective membership on a decision-making team, and the ability to fulfill the time commitment required of board service.

The second category is specific competencies at the individual level. Here, the board develops criteria for the selection of board members that reflect the formal priorities for characteristics, skill sets, professional positions, and specific expertise relevant to the current and projected strategic needs of the system. These are the characteristics necessary to build the ideal board at some point in the future. For example, a board might determine that it needs one financial expert, one expert in strategic planning, one expert in safety and quality improvement, and one expert in population health. When most people think of competency-based selection, they think of individual skills and characteristics that combine to create an effective board that is competent relative to the current and future goals and strategies of the organization.

The third category is desired diversity on the board, including such criteria as ethnicity, gender, geography, and age. Typically, a board will balance diversity criteria with specific skill-based competencies to develop prioritized criteria for the selection of board members. For example, one board might be seeking a new member who is (1) an information technology expert, (2) female, and (3) African American; another board may seek a new member who is (1) African American, (2) female, and (3) an information technology expert. If each board is not able to find a candidate with all three desired competencies, it will select the candidate with its first and second prioritized competencies, and so on. Thus, each board will likely recruit members with different characteristics, but each characteristic will be relevant to that specific board's needs.

A critical component of the competency-based model of board composition is not just to focus solely on the individual competencies of board members but also to think foundationally about the competency of the board as a whole. In fact, this is a good starting point for developing specific criteria for each of the three categories. Foundational questions regarding the competency of the board as a whole include, What are the primary areas of focus of the system board? How are the areas balanced? How might these competencies change? How can appropriate governance work be "pushed down" to subordinate boards? Two perennial governance questions also arise: What is the difference between the work of the system board and that of the CEO? How might that relationship change in the future?

It is important to consider competency-based board composition in the broader perspective of board development by identifying two categories of skill sets: expertise and literacy. Briefly, expertise relates to skills and characteristics that can only be found through recruitment of individuals with clearly defined skills gained through formal education and professional development. On the other hand, literacy refers to skills and knowledge acquired through a continuing governance education process. For example, a board cannot educate an individual to a standard of financial expertise, but it can educate a board member to a standard of financial literacy that undergirds good governance decisions. So, while individual criteria typically relate to expertise, it is critical to board composition and development that system boards and their governance committees constantly balance the needs of a board. What expertise should *some* individual members have? What must *every* member be literate in?

This approach should also be applied to board committees. For example, a system board's audit committee might be required to have one or two financial experts as members (one of whom is the chair) while the other members of the committee are required to be both literate in finances and in the audit function (with its attendant regulatory and legal requirements). The expertise is acquired through a competency-based process, while the literacy is acquired through a mandated continuing education plan. The latter element is also a characteristic of effective twenty-first-century system boards. They do not simply offer discretionary governance education to their board members. Rather, they establish it as a formal performance objective to be used in performance evaluation, pursuant to renewal of terms.

To govern twenty-first-century healthcare systems effectively, not only must board composition be based on a rigorous competency-based model, but new types of expertise must also be sought and new types of literacy developed in board members. Just as governance function should drive governance structure, so should system strategy and changing market conditions drive the development of competency-based criteria for board composition. For example, parent boards are currently seeking new competencies (expertise), such as the following:

- Systems thinking
- Population health
- Quality improvement and safety systems (often not from healthcare but from other fields, e.g., nuclear power, commercial aviation, or industries using Lean and Six Sigma models)
- Executive management oversight, evaluation, and compensation
- Change management
- Changing values and culture
- Information technology, telehealth, e-commerce
- Retail
- Group decision-making and decision theory
- Market disruption
- Innovation
- Enterprise risk management
- Mergers and acquisitions

Effective boards in the best-practice healthcare world believe that their purpose is to govern and lead the system, not to represent constituent or component interests. They translate this principle into action via a rigorous, competency-based model of board composition by developing and prioritizing their own list of desired competencies. These competencies are tailored to strategy, market driven, and focused on future needs. Boards then strive to balance individual expertise through the recruitment and selection process, engendering shared literacy through mandatory continuing education. Thus, the board helps ensure that governance is effective, efficient, and ahead of the curve. Leadership teams such as these are best able to effectively guide their systems into the future, rather than be dragged behind.

Authority

Having a system with multiple boards and board committees requires that governance authority and decision-making be clearly divided and assigned to the different bodies. The principle of centralizing authority while decentralizing decision-making addresses this need, concentrating strategic, policy, and executive oversight in the system board and then diffusing tactical and programmatic decision-making to board committees, subordinate boards, and others. The system board provides strategic and policy direction as the basis for the decisions and recommendations made by the entities under the board. Further, the system board makes sure that such decisions and recommendations are consistent with the strategic directions, goals, and parameters established by the board and takes appropriate action when it determines that they are not.

While this principle of effective system governance may seem obvious, it was often not recognized or employed in system governance in the past—and even in the present. In fact, systems built on a holding company model often have the opposite implicit principle. They tend to decentralize authority and centralize decision-making, a pattern that means that the authority to make major system decisions and approve significant strategic initiatives rests with subordinate boards in the system. Executives and system board leaders must get buy-in or consensus from the subordinate boards, if not their explicit approval, for decisions and strategies. If they are implemented without consensus, internal resistance builds and turmoil often results.

Meanwhile, the parent board, unable to set or approve strategy or make big system decisions, often finds itself occupied with making tactical decisions. As this governance dysfunction plays out, the system is stuck in neutral. Markets, of course, require high gear. Often, the system bylaws and governing documents do not explicitly assign this authority to the subordinate boards; rather, it is a cultural expectation that no decisions affecting them can be made without their approval or input. This dichotomy between the governance culture and the governing documents creates confusion and mystery. Where there is mystery there is no mastery, and there is no effective system governance.

It is important to remember that governance structure, including the number of boards in a system, does not in itself determine governance function. Structure can only facilitate or inhibit effective governance. Within limits, the governance structure for each system should be influenced by the unique and individually defined needs, culture, strategy, and mission of that system. However, even with appropriate variation in models from system to system, there are approaches to help ensure that different governance structures function at optimal levels. Thus, systems that opt to have decentralized, multiple-board models should adopt the principle of centralized authority and decentralized decision-making to make this model operate as well as it can.

One of the ways to operationalize this governance principle and to ensure that governance decision-making culture is consistent with the bylaws and other governing documents is through the development and use of a governance authority matrix.

The concept of an authority matrix arose to describe complex management structures with shared decision-making and accountability and a matrix model of management with multidirectional accountabilities. It is now being applied to healthcare systems with decentralized governance models. A governance authority matrix defines how decision-making is divided among different boards in a system (as well as between the system board and the CEO, and even between boards and their committees).

This clear map of leadership authority specifies diverse issues, including which board or group has the ultimate accountability for making a specific decision; what other board, committee, or group might have the ability to *recommend* a decision or course of action to a superior board; and which subordinate board, if any, must be *consulted* before a specific decision is made by a superior board. The governance authority matrix also makes clear whether the subordinate board's *approval* is required for the superior board to make a particular decision, or whether the subordinate board's input must be sought but not necessarily followed. In addition, it defines what boards or groups must be informed of a decision before it is publicly announced.

For maximum clarity, effective system boards will identify and define key roles used in their governance authority matrix (e.g., approve, recommend, consult, inform). Then, they will list each different governance decision, issue, or function and assign a role to each board, board committee, and relevant executive. (See chapter appendix for a sample authority matrix that addresses the relative authorities of a system board, system CEO, subsidiary board, and subsidiary CEO. It also provides definitions of *approve, recommend, consult,* and *inform.*)

For example, a classic area of tension between system and subsidiary is the hiring and firing of a subsidiary organization's executive. In many systems, this authority is vague, and when the situation arises, it can create open conflict and turmoil. Can the system CEO fire the subsidiary CEO? Must the subsidiary board be consulted about the decision? Must the subsidiary board concur with the decision? What happens if the system CEO wants to fire the subsidiary executive, and the subsidiary board strongly disagrees? These are just a few of the many vexing questions that can arise.

To avoid conflict, and to facilitate the mastery of effective governance, the governance authority matrix should clearly address this issue. For example, the ability to hire and fire the executive of a subsidiary organization might be assigned to the system CEO, but the CEO might be required to consult with the subsidiary organization's board and get its agreement before making the final decision. Alternately, the authority to hire the subsidiary executive might be separated from the authority to fire the subsidiary executive so that hiring a subsidiary executive might require consultation with the subsidiary board, but the same system CEO has exclusive authority to fire. The key is to prospectively identify these issues and assign clear, unambiguous authority and roles for each area of governance and system CEO authority.

The matrix is a cheat sheet that summarizes the multiple bylaws, policies, and procedures in the system. It is a self-contained, pragmatic document that lends clarity to the responsibilities of governing bodies in a complex system. However, simply having a governance authority matrix is not enough; it must be used routinely throughout the system. In effective systems, the matrix is always on hand and frequently consulted at all meetings of the various boards. It puts the principle of centralizing authority and decentralizing decision-making into action. It prevents mystery in system governance and facilitates governance mastery.

Balanced Power Structure

A core principle of effective governance is that the authority of the board derives from the group as a whole. If a single committee or individual is vested with too many powers of the system board, effective governance is usually severely compromised. Effective system boards, therefore, consciously and explicitly balance their governance power structure. That is, they do not allow the various critical powers, functions, and authorities of the board to reside in a single committee or an individual. As the growing scope of responsibility assigned to today's system boards increasingly requires that they delegate governance work and perhaps even some governance authority to committees, it is crucial that the board effectively oversees and controls its subordinate structures.

Typically, if such governance power or authority is inappropriately concentrated in a board committee, it is in an executive committee or equivalent group. When consolidated in an individual, it tends to be the board chair. To achieve better balance of power and effort, effective boards identify key areas of authority and responsibility and assign them to various committees. Likewise, effective system boards define and codify the duties and functions of the board chair, making it abundantly clear that she is accountable to the board and does not have the authority to direct or control the board or to individually exercise any powers of the board.

In twenty-first-century healthcare system governance, some of the disparate power functions that the system board has responsibility for and thus must strive to balance include the following:

- Hiring and firing CEOs
- Setting CEO performance objectives, evaluating CEO performance, and establishing CEO compensation
- Governance, including board composition, board evaluation, individual board member performance evaluation pursuant to term renewal, conflict-of-interest and director independence monitoring, corporate bylaw revisions and approval, board job descriptions and governance policies and procedures, and oversight of subsidiary boards
- Audit oversight and approval; compliance
- Quality and safety
- Financial oversight, including monitoring of debt covenants, stock purchases, and divestments
- Strategic planning and monitoring
- Integration and oversight of businesses, including strategic allocation of resources, adjustment of capacity, and consolidation of services to optimize the system
- Enterprise risk management

To optimize the system as a whole, effective system boards define their own power functions and authority and explicitly choose how to balance them. They hold discussions every year or two (frequently as part of board self-evaluation processes) to decide whether and how to rebalance or how to add new functions and responsibilities to the governance mix, as mandated by the market or by new regulations. The board decides which functions should be performed by the board as a whole or by a committee. It makes certain that these functions are distributed evenly among the committees and that key areas of authority are retained by the board as a whole. The latter is crucial to bearing out the principle that the authority of the board derives from the board as a whole. The decision-making authority that should be held and exercised by the board as a whole includes the following:

- System CEO hiring and firing (this clearly sends the message that the CEO is supervised by the board as a whole and not the board chair or the executive or compensation committees)
- Appointing, reappointing, and removing board members and officers, including the board chair
- Corporate bylaw revisions and approvals
- Mission revisions and approvals, mission loyalty (duty of obedience to a charitable purpose in a not-for-profit health system)
- Strategic plan approval
- Sale of assets, merger or affiliation, and consolidation of system components

Balancing the governance power structure takes time and labor, and it could unfold in many ways. In one method, the board begins by explicitly retaining the powers listed earlier and then documents these functions in the corporate bylaws. The board then subdivides the remaining functions among board committees as follows:

- A committee with responsibility for recommending CEO performance objectives, conducting CEO performance evaluation, and recommending CEO compensation adjustments to the board
- A committee with responsibility for board composition; continuing governance education; and evaluation of the board, board members, and board officers

- A committee with responsibility for strategic planning (the members are required to engage the full board in key steps of the process, and board approval is required for the final draft)
- A committee with responsibility for oversight of finance (though final approval authority for budgets and financial plans rests with the board)
- A committee with responsibility for audit and compliance (often with specific and ultimate authority for decisions regarding the acceptance of the audit opinion letter and the hiring and firing of the audit firm)

This hypothetical board has chosen not to have an executive committee. It strives to ensure that the composition of its committees is largely distinct—that is, the same board members do not serve on multiple powerful committees.

Great twenty-first-century system boards are effective teams that share the workload and balance decision-making responsibility. Such boards carefully avoid consolidating power among a few members to preclude the development of an inner circle. They identify and reserve the most critical decision-making authority for the board as a whole, and they make certain that other critical functions and delegated decision-making are distributed evenly among several board committees. Executive committees, if they exist at all, have clearly defined—and limited—authority and scope of responsibilities and are held accountable to the board as a whole. The important tasks of board member recruitment, board development, and board and board member evaluation are assigned to a separate committee, such as a governance committee, and are not performed by the executive committee or the committee overseeing CEO performance evaluation and compensation. Importantly, it is made abundantly clear that the boss of the system CEO is the full board and not any individual, committee, or informal group of board members.

EMERGING CHALLENGES TO EFFECTIVE SYSTEM GOVERNANCE

Several worrisome trends are on the healthcare horizon that may pose severe challenges to the effective governance of systems in the future. Even thoughtful, principle-based system governance may be inadequate in the face of continuously accelerating change and increasing complexity in the healthcare market. Similarly, as the size, scale, and scope of healthcare systems grow, so does the complexity of effective system governance. These changes and challenges inexorably present increasing demands on system boards and their members, and they are discussed in the following sections.

Time Pressures

Take, for example, the lament heard from members of system boards around the country: "Governance is taking too much of my time— we can't really address key strategic issues." This seeming paradox can partially be explained by the growing list of regulatory requirements for healthcare boards, as well as the considerable complexity of overseeing the governance structure and function of increasingly large and complicated systems. These challenges take much board time, which can easily inhibit market awareness, analysis, and strategic planning and decision-making.

The board can address time shortages by adopting and implementing the principles discussed earlier: board competencies, delegation, and consistency.

Volunteer Boards

Though excessive time demands are disquieting, they give rise to even more worrisome questions that challenge the deeply embedded not-for-profit tradition of the volunteer board member. Can society expect professionals and businesspeople to devote—on a voluntary basis—excessive amounts of their time to governing health systems? Will compensation of system board members be necessary in the future? This issue seems even more acute when the increasing pressures of work life and family responsibilities in today's hectic and disruptive environment are considered. In the face of these challenges, a question arises: Whither the soul of voluntary governance of not-for-profit health systems?

In addition, the pool of qualified board members may significantly diminish in the near future. We may be looking at a future in which the only individuals who can afford the time to serve as volunteer members of healthcare system boards are retired, are independently wealthy, have the luxury of working for generous employers or owning businesses that essentially run themselves, or are employed by the healthcare system itself. Add to this the emerging concern that generations following the baby boom may not have the same cultural commitment to volunteerism or the same tolerance for the group process involved in challenging and effective decision-making. Meanwhile, baby boomers are aging and cannot be the primary source of system board members for much longer.

Further, many board members are becoming concerned that the complexity, regulation, quality, and safety challenges of governing a health system expose them to inordinate amounts of liability and reputational risk. Many of them say, "I can volunteer to serve on the boards of other organizations that require less of my time and have much less liability exposure. Why should I serve on the board of a healthcare system?" In short, a crisis may be brewing in healthcare system governance.

If this scenario is accurate, is the solution to simply compensate the members of the boards of not-for-profit systems at a level commensurate with their for-profit cousins? Perhaps, but compensation of board members of not-for-profit, charitable organizations—no matter their size and scope—comes with several challenges. First, no empirical evidence exists that board member compensation improves the quality of governance. While it is possible that compensation in exchange for aggressive board member performance objectives, required individual performance evaluation, and a willingness to remove nonperforming board members would increase system governance effectiveness, the subject requires more research. It is equally plausible that compensation may denigrate the quality of system governance, as it risks diverting the board from pursuing a charitable mission toward an overemphasis on growth and financial success. One of the key fiduciary duties of the board of a charitable organization is obedience to its charitable purpose. Such a board is legally required to be primarily loyal to and focused on the mission of the system rather than on the success or growth of the system solely. Could board compensation subvert this fundamental requirement of not-for-profit governance?

By the same token, compensating board members risks aligning the interests of the board too closely with those of executive management, blurring the distinction between governance and management. Finally, remuneration—especially at levels commensurate with that of Fortune 500 boards—risks attracting people who primarily seek the benefits of the compensation and not candidates committed to governing a charitable healthcare system.

Another challenge to board compensation is that, while it is currently legal to provide compensation to the boards of not-for-profit charitable organizations, doing so carries questionable optics and has raised opprobrium from the media and members of Congress. Also, it is worth noting that compensation results in loss of the statutory immunity from liability, from both the federal government and state government, granted to uncompensated trustees of not-for-profit charitable organizations.

As we consider governance issues, we soon encounter another question: Should large, diverse, multibillion-dollar healthcare systems really be not-for-profit, charitable entities? At what point do they transcend the boundaries of community-based organizations? At what point should they convert to for-profit entities? While such a shift might address some of these governance challenges, and while such a shift is inexorably intertwined with the issue of effective system governance, the question is well beyond the scope of this chapter.

The problem of effective governance of healthcare systems can only become more difficult and complex as the century progresses. Thus, to be a truly effective board of a twenty-first-century system requires an impatience with the inefficiencies of the governance models and an unwillingness to be bound by the mind-sets of the past. Equally important, it requires that system boards cast a critical eye on the emerging challenges of governance and adopt intentional strategies to master them.

Appendix

Appendix
Sample Authority Matrix for System Board with Subsidiary Organizations

Decisions/Authority	System Board	System CEO	Subsidiary Organization Board	Subsidiary Organization CEO
System Mission, Vision, and Values				
1. Mission, vision, and core values of system	Approve*		Inform**	Inform
2. Missions of the subsidiary organizations	Approve		Recommend***	
New Organizations and Major Transactions				
3. Formation or acquisition of a new subsidiary organization	Approve	Recommend		
4. Sale, transfer, or substantial change in use of all or substantially all of the assets of system and merger, dissolution, consolidation, or disposition of assets on dissolution of system	Approve	Recommend	Inform	Inform
5. Sale, transfer, or substantial change in use of all or substantially all of the assets of subsidiary organizations and divestiture, dissolution, closure, merger, consolidation, change in corporate membership or ownership, or corporate reorganization of subsidiary organizations	Approve	Consult and/or recommend	Consult****	Consu t
6. Formation of all other legal entities	Approve	Recommend	Recommend and/ or inform	Recommend and/or inform

Governing Documents				
7. Articles and bylaws of parent organization	Approve	Recommend	Inform	Inform
8. Governing documents of subsidiary organizations	Approve	Recommend	Consult	Consult
Appointments/Removals				
9. Members of board of directors of system	Approve	Inform		
10. Core competencies for board members of both system and subsidiary organizations	Approve	Recommend	Recommend and consult	Recommend and consult
11. Selection and removal of system board chair	Approve	Inform		
12. Selection and removal of system president and CEO	Approve	Inform	Inform	Inform
13. Selection and removal of system board members	Approve	Inform	Inform	Inform
14. Selection and removal of members of a subsidiary board	Approve	Recommend	Recommend and consult	Recommend and consult
15. Selection and removal of subsidiary board chair	Approve	Recommend	Recommend and consult	Recommend and consult
16. Hiring and firing of subsidiary organization CEO	Consult	Approve	Inform	
Evaluation				
17. System board, board chair, and president/CEO	Approve	Inform		
18. Subsidiary board and board chair	Approve	Inform	Recommend	Inform
19. Annual performance objectives, performance, and compensation of subsidiary CEO	Inform	Approve	Inform	Inform
Debt				

20. System debt limits	Approve	Recommend	Inform	Inform
21. Subsidiary organization debt	Approve	Recommend within guidelines	Recommend within guidelines	Consult
Strategic and Financial Plans				
22. Vision statements of subsidiary organizations	Approve	Consult	Recommend	Consult
23. Subsidiary integrated strategic and financial plans, annual scorecard targets, and initiatives (budget)	Approve	Recommend	Recommend	Recommend
24. System integrated strategic and financial plan, including annual system integrated scorecard and system initiatives (budget)	Approve	Recommend	Inform	Inform
25. System auditor selection; receipt and acceptance of audit report	Approve	Inform		
Assets				
26. Transfer of assets and reallocation of debt among subsidiaries	Approve	Recommend	Inform	Inform
27. Projects or transactions involving expenditure of funds or divestiture of assets not otherwise addressed in this system authority matrix	Inform up to $XX million; approve more than $XX million	Approve up to $XX million; recommend more than $XX million	Inform	Inform
System Policies and Procedures				
28. System policies and procedures	Approve	Recommend		

Authority of Subsidiary Hospital Board		
29. Establish system goals and targets; set policies for credentialing, quality, and patient safety	Approve	Recommend
30. Granting of privileges and credentialing		Approve
31. Oversight of quality and patient safety		Approve
32. Regulatory compliance and accreditation		Approve
33. Community needs assessment		Approve

Definitions

*Approve: Review and either adopt, amend, disapprove, or send back for further consideration; includes authority to appoint individuals to offices or positions.

**Inform: Must be formally informed of action after a decision is made by superior board or executive.

***Recommend: May initiate action for consideration or a decision, but action may be taken by superior board or executive without recommendation from this group or executive.

****Consult: Must be sought for advice or information before a decision is made by superior board or executive.

CHAPTER 4

The Evolving Role of the Physician, Nurse, Medical Staff Services Professional, and Organized Medical Staff

Jon Burroughs
Kathleen Bartholomew
Mary A. Baker

TRADITIONAL HEALTHCARE BUSINESS models are evolving from the physician's office and the stand-alone hospital to an integrated delivery system with aligned physicians. Therefore, readers will not be surprised to learn that the traditional role of physicians, nurses, medical staff services professionals, and other practitioners must evolve as well. The images of the autonomous physician, subordinate nurse, clerical medical staff services professionals, and self-interested organized medical staff are all twentieth-century oversimplifications—negative stereotypes that must be discarded in favor of new models of leadership, management, business, and clinical savvy. Alongside other organizational executives, aligned medical professionals will manage increasingly complex healthcare organizations, successfully improving the care of the individuals and populations they serve.

This chapter explores the specific changes that are taking place in support of new roles and organizational structures. How will the current transition influence the success (or failure) of healthcare organizations? We will answer this question by examining the past and future of physicians, nurses, medical services professionals, and the organized medical staff.

THE EVOLVING ROLE OF THE PHYSICIAN IN THE TWENTY-FIRST CENTURY

Jon Burroughs

The role of the physician is coming full circle in a new context. Traditionally, physicians served as executive professionals, both caring directly for patients and managing a clinical practice as business owners. As reimbursement stagnated and overhead costs climbed, the business model of private practices began to fail, and physicians either struggled to support their enterprises through a focus on high-volume, high-margin cases or sought employment. (Currently, more than two-thirds of US physicians are employed [see Accenture 2015]). Unfortunately, both choices had unintended consequences that undermined both the physician's professional standing and the way in which physicians viewed their profession (and how they were viewed in return).

For those remaining in private practice, the pressure to meet the rising overhead forced a focused-factory model that resulted in spending less and less time with more and more patients. The focused factory also resulted in an overemphasis on the well-reimbursed procedures and tests that became the economic engine driving a failing model. These physicians left or largely abandoned the organized medical staff to devote all of their energies to their shrinking operating margins. Any potential obstruction to their efficiency and productivity was seen as a professional threat, which became the source of potential conflict with healthcare management;

nurses; and even patients, who began to feel shortchanged by the shrinking time spent with their physicians during a period of increasing costs. On one hand, management liked the operating revenue (including ancillary and elective revenues) that physicians brought to their organizations; on the other hand, they also needed physicians who would be willing to work with them to achieve aligned organizational goals.

Thus, self-employed physicians found themselves increasingly marginalized in favor of employed physicians, thought to be more loyal and more easily controlled through contractual arrangements. This preference frustrated and angered independent self-employed physicians, who saw themselves as the bedrock of their profession and the most committed members of the medical staff. Conflict would sometimes stimulate physicians to compete with healthcare organizations, such as the establishment of competing economic entities such as ambulatory surgery centers, imaging centers, and larger physician practices designed to divert profitable cases and ancillaries. Physicians' defiance and solidarity would, in turn, lead to significant political, economic, and clinical schisms in many communities.

For those who sought employment—and its supposed alleviation of administrative and nonproductive pressures—there was often deep frustration at the amount of nonclinical, non-revenue-generating activities required by the ever-growing and complex requirements of meaningful use and clinical data entry through the electronic health record. In addition, employed physicians often deeply resented leaders with little or no clinical experience managing their practices and overseeing the implementation of contracts that were essentially clinical in nature. Employed physicians also balked when clinical and operational processes were more complex, difficult to manage, and inadvertently undermined by nonclinical management as a result of a lack of understanding of clinical delivery and of how these services could be optimally provided.

The frustrations of both employed and self-employed doctors lie at the heart of the widely publicized phenomenon of physician burnout. Unfortunately, many well-meaning healthcare leaders treat only the symptoms of this growing syndrome through psychological counseling without addressing the root of the problem—restoring physicians to clinical executive roles that satisfy their underlying ambitions, values, and desires to lead healthcare again and regain both self-esteem and public respect.

Fortunately, organizations throughout the country are committed to restoring the physicians' traditional role as a clinical executive through several strategies. The overarching idea is to think of physicians as potential clinical executives and leaders who can work directly with management to drive clinical, operational, and business outcomes through aligned arrangements. Such arrangements generate operating revenue, superior clinical outcomes, high productivity, and aligned goals and objectives by focusing physicians' efforts on only those decisions and tasks requiring physician-level expertise. Helping physicians be physicians again improves engagement, morale, and cooperation. The strategies discussed in the following sections can help bring about that vision.

Recruit Advanced-Practice Professionals

Hospitals and health systems can take a multipronged approach to narrowing physicians' duties. For example, using clinical pathways and algorithms, they can delegate healthcare encounters that are high volume and low complexity to advanced-practice professionals (APPs) with physician oversight and medical direction. This shift enables physicians both to spend more time in a consultative role and to care primarily for patients with complex, difficult-to-manage conditions. The use of APPs lowers cost and improves accessibility for patients who suffer from more common, easier-to-manage conditions. Physicians can earn a percentage of the reimbursement for the care they oversee through specific Centers for Medicare & Medicaid Services (CMS) billing policies while earning higher direct reimbursement for the more complex care they personally deliver.

Accomplishing such a large-scale change requires many significant changes. To delegate responsibilities in this way, physicians must acquire oversight management skills, commit to working collaboratively with management, and be willing to assume increasing management and leadership responsibilities. Healthcare organizations will need to develop clinical triggers that stimulate immediate physician consultation. The process also requires clinical algorithms and protocols for physicians as they examine patients who return with a similar complaint within a defined time frame or who require a more in-depth clinical evaluation. Physicians should also participate in the recruitment, orientation, training, and ongoing supervision of APPs.

Recruit Scribes

Free physicians from data entry by providing scribes who are appropriately trained and managed—nonphysicians with clinical expertise (typically nurses with specialized clinical knowledge in a specific area) who are certified coders. This work reassignment enables clinical documentation to be completed in a far more comprehensive and timely way in order to optimize reimbursement. Scribes enhance physician productivity; increase returns per error-free ("clean") claim; and improve the revenue cycle through decreases in net days in accounts receivables, higher case-mix index, and higher revenues per case. Imagine a highly compensated CEO using half of her time to enter operational or financial data into spreadsheets instead of providing leadership and executive direction. It seems unlikely, yet physicians do it every day, at the cost of both revenue and physician morale.

There are two key reasons to hire or train scribes. The first is revenue. Physicians engaged in documentation activities do not generate operating revenue and may be creating an opportunity cost of up to 50 percent. The second is reimbursement. Physicians generally are not trained to include comorbidities in clinical documentation because of their focus on the primary, specialty-specific problem; thus, their documentation may include lower acuity and severity scores. Lower acuity documentation has a negative impact on allowable length of stay, quality scores, expected cost per case, and pay-for-value contracts.

Many organizations develop ongoing contracts with regional vocational schools to provide training to interested clinical specialists in exchange for an equivalent number of years of service to the healthcare organization. Organizations that do this successfully not only optimize productivity but also improve potential reimbursement by 15 to 25 percent (depending on the study). According to a 2015 systematic review of studies on the use of scribes in the healthcare setting, scribes improved physician satisfaction, increased the number of patients seen, increased the number of work relative value units (wRVUs) generated, increased net revenue, and improved physician–patient interaction (Shultz and Holmstrom 2015).

Develop Physician Leaders

To let doctors be doctors, hospitals and health systems use leadership academies to provide physicians with executive management skills. In the twenty-first century, doctors will need to collaborate effectively in an effort to address operational, financial, and strategic challenges. This empowers physicians to collaborate with management on key initiatives. Well-prepared physician leaders will be able to better direct care delivery settings such as clinics, multispecialty practices, or service lines.

High-performing organizations such as Baylor Scott & White (Dallas), Allina Health (Minneapolis), Memorial Hermann (Houston), and Intermountain Health (Salt Lake City) establish physician leadership academies as a regular part of their operations. Baylor Scott & White goes even further by underwriting master of business administration degrees for physicians who demonstrate leadership aptitude in exchange for equivalent years of service back to the sponsoring organization. Physicians who wish to test their interest in leadership without a multiyear commitment to school may be best served by the 150-hour certified physician executive program offered by the American Association for Physician Leadership.

Determining the return on investment (ROI) for such programs is an easy calculation, given that physician leaders drive improvements in case-mix index, length of stay, labor, and supply chain ratio. Baylor Scott & White management uses a group of qualified physician leaders as its organizational pipeline for prospective medical directors, chief medical officers, chief operating officers, and CEOs throughout the system. Physicians who can oversee both clinical and business performance are invaluable to pay-for-value agreements, in which significant dollars may be at risk based on clinical and business outcomes.

Reorganize Units

Optimizing the performance of physicians and organizations may also require reorganizing clinical departments into integrated clinical delivery units. Such units contain dyad or triad teams of physicians, nurses, and executive managers who manage quality, safety, service, and cost-effectiveness through the creation of integrated business units. With pay-for-value reimbursement, the ability of physicians to work with nursing and executive leaders to reach key clinical and business goals is key.

Develop Outstanding Comanagement Agreements

Savvy healthcare leaders of the twenty-first century collaborate with physicians to develop innovative engagement and alignment contracts. The new model for physician engagement and alignment includes comanagement agreements with physicians, who participate in activities such as direct care of difficult cases, oversight of or consultation with nonphysician staff, and management.

Obviously, each of these components has a fair market value (FMV) that can be assigned as appropriate incentives in the quest to achieve strategic organizational goals. Many legal advisers fall into the trap of assuming that all components of a *comanagement agreement* (agreement that includes both clinical and managerial goals and objectives) constitute a clinical contract that must be compared with benchmarked FMV surveys, rather than a combination of responsibilities, each of which has an FMV calculation of its own.

For instance, one large for-profit healthcare entity recently created a comanagement agreement with an obstetrician gynecologist that included the following sections, each with its own calculated FMV:

- Clinical productivity based on wRVUs for patients directly seen by the physician
- Oversight responsibility for four APPs (maximum allowable under that state's law)
- Medical directorship of a free clinic designed to care for uninsured patients and undocumented workers
- Medical directorship of a service line in women's health, with responsibility for key clinical and business indicators (e.g., lengths of stay, quality scores) that had a monetized value

The final compensation represented a summation of all FMVs, each prorated according to mutually agreed-on benchmarks. This lucrative arrangement was created at the request of the physician, who desired a seven-figure-plus income. This arrangement had an ROI for the healthcare organization of 3:1 ($3.9 million incremental revenue to the organization and $1.3 million potential revenue to the physician).

Parenthetically, every contractual agreement with physicians should be conceived of as a business unit that creates a positive ROI for the organization and above-average compensation for physicians willing to learn new skills and actively support enterprise-wide initiatives.

Self-employed physicians can be similarly incentivized through comanagement relationships that enable the physician-led practice to access many of the healthcare organization's resources:

- Leveraged reimbursement contracts
- Group purchasing organizations
- Information technology (IT) and analytics
- Revenue-cycle support (per FMV arrangement)
- Access to capital at a lower cost (as a result of the healthcare organization's bond rating and lower cost of capital)
- Practice management support
- Preferred referrals through narrow or tiered networks, contracted large employers, and payers
- Potential physician leadership roles at the highest level for those committed to working with management on mutual goals

Collaborate for New Revenues

Physicians do more than provide medical expertise; they are also a potential source of new ideas for revenue streams. Disruptive innovation occurs when healthcare organizations and physicians focus only on high-margin services and inadvertently abandon the low end of their industry, enabling new entrants to work their way upstream toward higher-margin services. Doctors can help offset these threats. Current examples include retail medicine and e-health, both of which require significant physician leadership and participation. Healthcare kiosks, smartphones, and other devices have been the platform for more than 100 million e-health visits in the United States alone over the past four years, and there are currently more than 3,000 retail facilities in the United States (it is predicted that there will be 50,000 worldwide by 2021) (Ahmed and Fincham 2011). Many exciting opportunities are available to entrepreneurial physicians and management teams willing to explore ventures in serving value-starved healthcare consumers.

Collaborate for Population Health

Perhaps the most important work today is the potential collaboration between physicians and healthcare executives as the architects of a new care delivery system capable of achieving high quality under pay for value. Organizations such as Intermountain Healthcare and St. Luke's Health System (Boise, Idaho) are taking on this challenge and have become national models for how a new healthcare delivery system can work. However, this radical change cannot be accomplished by physicians or management alone and requires creative individuals who are willing to transform both the clinical and business models of care. Chapter 11 describes the form that many of these new population health models will assume in the years to come.

The physician of the twenty-first century will regain his role as a clinical and executive leader adept in both clinical management and delivery. The contemporary challenge is to recruit early-adopter physicians who understand the necessity of gaining operational, business, management, and leadership skills and can convince other physicians of the value added for themselves, their profession, their organization, and their community.

THE EVOLVING ROLE OF THE NURSE IN THE TWENTY-FIRST CENTURY

Kathleen Bartholomew

By 2008, it was clear to prominent nursing leaders that a major "disconnect" existed between nurses' perceived role and their real ability to affect quality, cost, and access. Hospital leaders—as well as the general public—did not see the link between excellent nursing care and quality and safety outcomes (Kover and Spetz 2011). Other problems overshadowed the field as well. There was still no consensus on the number of years of college for entry into the profession; the pipeline of nurses was at a bottleneck as older nurses delayed retiring; and there was a critical shortage of nursing faculty, who tended to be poorly paid. In addition, experts noted a critical shortage of nurses in leadership positions. For example, nurses accounted for only 5 percent of hospital board membership.

The launching point for nursing in the twenty-first century began in 2010 with the Institute of Medicine's (2010) report *The Future of Nursing: Leading Change, Advancing Health.* This report contained four key messages:

1. Nurses should practice to the full extent of their education and training.
2. Nurses should achieve higher levels of education and training through an improved education system that promotes seamless academic progression.
3. Nurses should be full partners with physicians and other healthcare professionals in redesigning healthcare in the United States.
4. Effective workforce planning and policy making require better data collection and information infrastructure.

Implementation of these four recommendations is currently driven by the Campaign for Action, which is a network of coalitions in every state working with local leaders in health, education, and business to build healthier communities. For example, the campaign works with policy leaders on state and federal laws that decrease barriers to pursuing a bachelor's degree in nursing, advocating for funding, and approving five specific models of education to move nurses efficiently through the curriculum. It also formed an action coalition that obtained grants to implement interprofessional practice teams at community health centers. In addition, 19 nursing organizations came together with AARP and the Robert Wood Johnson Foundation to form the Nurses on Boards Coalition with a goal of placing 10,000 nurses on healthcare and hospital boards as well as other influential bodies by 2020.

Despite these important initiatives and actions, there are still multiple challenges facing the 3.2 million nurses in the United States today. While nurse practitioners relish their autonomy and advocate to practice at their full capacity, hospital nurses struggle with high acuity and heavy patient loads. Today, nurses are experiencing the best of times or the worst of times—depending on where they practice in the panorama of healthcare. It's important to learn from both extremes to build a promising vision for how nurses can potentially change the trajectory of illness and disease to promote health and wellness—by 2020 and beyond.

Nursing Today

Presenting to various nursing and healthcare organizations across the country has afforded me access to nurses in a variety of settings. Nursing professionals in every area of practice cite inadequate staffing as a primary concern. Having adapted to an increased workload as a result of decreasing length of stay and increasing acuity, hospital nurses are often task saturated. At any given time, hospital nurses have 7–8 stacking (simultaneous) tasks to be done; they perform more than 160 tasks in an eight-hour shift, with the average task time less than three minutes (Tucker and Spear 2006). This cognitive shift exceeds any other profession.

Physicians' chief nurse-related complaint is that they cannot find a nurse or that nurses are focused more on tasks than on therapeutic interactions. This situation is no surprise, as a study of medical/surgical units found that nurses spend less than 7 percent of their time reading vitals and assessing the patient and 35 percent of their time documenting details on patient charts (Hendrich et al. 2008).

Over the past 15 years, the time nurses spend with their patients has insidiously eroded as the business model has been forced to become leaner with every political swing. Electronic health records now take up nearly a third of nurses' time and have failed to increase the amount or quality of time with their patients (except in high-functioning emergency departments [EDs] and operating rooms, where the addition of scribes has been met with great success). In addition, 12-hour shifts, originally designed to increase nurse retention, are proving mentally and physically exhausting and are linked to poorer outcomes. Nurses are sleep deprived (Geiger-Brown et al. 2012). The combination of high stress, insufficient downtime, lack of sleep, and lack of power and autonomy has resulted in a depression rate for nurses that is double the rate for the population—18 percent compared with 9.4 percent (Letvak, Ruhm, and McCoy 2012).

The current impact of the healthcare-industrial complex and dysfunctional political landscape on the practice of nursing is often minimized or misunderstood because of poor role clarity in the eyes of the public, who still see nurses in subordinate service roles rather than as clinical leaders. Because the general public views nurses as obedient and invisible workers rather than independent, autonomous professionals, nurses have no power or voice in the business of healthcare. For example, nurses must currently fight for adequate staffing resources. The organization views staffing as an increased cost, while the healthcare complex is content with the monetary status quo. Role confusion has been compounded by a lack of consensus on college-entry requirements and the rise of medical assistants, who often inaccurately tell the public that they are "nurses," when in fact they have attended a six-week course. The media's inchoate or invisible portrayal of the nursing profession in television shows such as *ER* and *Grey's Anatomy* does not help. While Nurse Jackie (in the show of the same name) showcased much of the autonomy, creativity, and critical thinking skills of a professional nurse, the very human but uncharacteristic traits the writers gave her (e.g., drug addiction) undermined this positivity. This role confusion has resulted in a lack of public and political support.

The increasing number of admissions, discharges, and transfers, promulgated by a system focus on maximizing revenue, has created extreme stress. One of the most rewarding parts of nursing is the relationships nurses have with their patients and each other. This social capital—determined to be far more important to nurses than financial capital as a primary motivator and source of commitment to their practice (Putnam 2000)—has decreased rapidly, a trend exacerbated by 12-hour shifts. This decrease is critical because the patient experience is, and will always be, directly related to nursing job satisfaction. The pace at which many nurses (and physicians) have adapted to the recent changes in the medical field is unsustainable and harmful to caregivers and patients alike. Moral distress is rampant in the ED, where mentally ill patients may be kept in the hospital for observation for days, and in the intensive care unit (ICU) and oncology unit, where nurses prolong the painful final days of patients when they would never do so for their own family members.

Yet nurses have also seen many improvements in the first part of the century. Over the 2010s, autonomy has increased as nurse-led councils identify opportunities and implement strategies for improving the experience of care for both patients and providers. Education that has linked disruptive behavior between nurses and physicians directly to sentinel events has improved the physician–nurse relationship, and hospital boards have taken a stronger stance against disruptive behavior and for optimizing communication among healthcare professionals. More nurses are pursuing advanced degrees, especially because of easy access to online courses, and a goal has been set in *The Future of Nursing* report to increase the number of bachelor of science in nursing degrees to 80 percent of the current workforce by 2020 (American Association of Colleges of Nursing 2015). Interdisciplinary teams frequently round now in ICUs and high-acuity settings, and nurses are active participants in rounds, hospital committees, and initiatives.

The number of advanced-practice registered nurse practitioners (NPs) has grown to 234,000 in the past decade, as advanced registered NPs move out to the community to fill the gap left by the critical shortage of primary care physicians. More than 89 percent of NPs are certified in primary care, with nearly three-quarters accepting Medicare patients and 78 percent accepting Medicaid patients. More NPs are needed now in geriatrics, mental health, and oncology.

More consumers are paying out of pocket for complementary and alternative medicine, and in response, nurses are opening up independent practices when certified in these specialties, which are typically not reimbursed by insurance plans. Certification programs have graduated hundreds of nurses as skilled healthcare coaches, and nurse entrepreneurs are inventing exciting and innovative partnerships with their communities. The number of DNPs (doctor of nursing practice) is increasing to address the impending faculty shortage, with numerous programs now offered nationwide. Because only 1.9 percent of NPs have been named as a primary defendant in a malpractice case, malpractice insurance rates remain low. NPs now have admitting privileges in all 50 states and Washington, DC.

Nursing in 2025

What will the nursing field of the future look like?

Imagine the year is 2025. Today, a complex-labor-and-delivery nurse has observed that a new mom rarely makes eye contact with her newborn daughter but instead spends hours on Facebook. So the nurse writes a referral to the new mother unit, where the mother volunteers to stay for further relationship coaching. Society now understands the vital importance of the primary nurturing bond for the future health of both mother and baby and has reallocated resources to add additional nursing support.

After her assessment, the social media nurse helps the new mother better understand the effect of digital media addiction on her parenting skills, specifically how a lack of eye contact creates a deficiency of mirror neurons and decreases the child's ability to be empathetic. Each night, the new baby's family comes to the hospital to eat dinner together and learns how they can all build strong, nourishing relationships with each other. Following the discharge of the mother and infant, a home health and safety nurse is available as needed to coach and provide emotional as well as educational support for the new family. The response to this program has been a rapid and sustained decrease in infant mortality.

Or, after a complicated organ transplant, a transplant nurse notices that his patient, a woman with diabetes, has asked the family to sneak in fast food—which explains her erratic blood sugar levels. So the nurse writes a referral to the diabetes unit for a three-week stay (research has validated the 21 days it takes to change habits) where his patient will learn healthy cooking and lifestyle tips and bond with other people with diabetes to hardwire habits, creating a community of support that will extend long after discharge. Not only are nurses excited about their pivotal new roles in patient care, but also role clarity for nursing has increased tremendously, as patients now have a very visceral and practical idea of exactly how nurses facilitate healing and health.

As incentives are shifted to wellness and quality outcomes, hospital nurses slowly transition to the prevention of disease, teaching healthy lifestyle choices to the general population. Per the American Pediatric Association recommendation of 2016, all schools now have a nurse who is actively engaged in teaching netiquette (internet etiquette), relationship, and resiliency skills as well as identifying the early onset of physical and mental disease. The rate of depression among girls younger than 17 is now slowly trending downward as their self-esteem and coping skills increase through nurse education.

Nurses who practice in the hospital care primarily for patients with complicated comorbidities, provide ongoing intense education, and pioneer research on helping people with chronic illnesses live longer lives. They will work four ten-hour shifts a week: eight hours of clinical duties and two hours of outreach, education, streamlining processes, and documenting outcomes. Instead of being glued to a computer, nurses are present to their patients. Scribes do all the data entry for nurses now, as healthcare executives had noted the vast amount of time devoted to charting. High-security cameras in the ED have decreased violent episodes, and in the operating room they are used by the team to improve communication and teamwork. Drones bring needed medications and supplies. Every day the NP, registered nurse, and patient meet for 30 minutes to discuss progress on the plan of care they created together.

The role of the nurse navigator, who helps patients through care transitions, has evolved into caring for patients with multiple illnesses. For example, a patient with Parkinson's disease, spinal stenosis, and a rare eye disease could not possibly navigate his own hospital stay without someone to coordinate tests, medications, and education for the orthopedics, cardiology, palliative care, and ophthalmology departments.

Life-or-death decisions no longer rest solely on the shoulders of patients and their families with the support and counsel of physicians and legal institutions. Through their work on the healthcare team, nurses help both patients and their families to reconcile and come to peace with the dying process and to understand that death is as much a part of life as birth. They are key resources in assisting patients and their families with documenting end-of-life wishes to support the values of patients and their families. Practitioner orders for life-sustaining treatment and advance directives have become accepted tools, and the cultural code that Americans must fight death with all their strength is being rewritten.

Nursing in 2030

By now, the public has realized that unless a nation spends as much on the social determinants of health as it does on actual medical costs, the economy suffers. After the opioid epidemic of 2017 claimed more than 60,000 lives, Americans were forced to widen their very narrow definition of health and began addressing the causes of death and disease. Recognizing that cancer was estimated to increase worldwide by 70 percent by 2034—from 14 million to 25 million cases (World Health Organization 2018)—changed America's national strategy to focus on the cause of cancer instead of the cure. A holistic nursing approach now addresses the multiple causes of disease, especially nutrition, the environment, and psychological well-being.

More than 50 percent of all nurses now work in public health. Uniformed nurses have taken an active role in the mainstream media, with public service health announcements every hour on the radio, television, and social media. This broad-based education has been made possible by the Pharma Tax of 2020, which instituted a 5 percent tax on all pharmaceutical advertising for use in educating the general public. The national nurse, who is the recognized nurse leader, works closely with the surgeon general to prevent disease and suffering. Healthcare is viewed as a public utility, delivered by a team that identifies the geographic threats and norms by zip code. The nurse and her team members then devise a plan with physicians, businesses, and governments to incite and sustain change.

Education for nurses has doubled as they realize that before they can become true experts in wellness to the public, they first need to act as role models in their own wellness. Physical and mental criteria and a master's degree are now prerequisites for the nursing profession. Physicians and nurses are educated in the same classes for the first two years of college. Since 2010, nurses have worked passionately in the Campaign for Action to change the laws that supported unhealthy American lifestyles. As a result, the Food and Drug Administration has doubled its resources, food regulation has tripled, and the nation has fallen from 30 percent obesity to 10 percent. The number of people with diabetes has been cut in half, and childhood obesity has gone from one in five to one in ten. It took 13 years, however, for the life expectancy of Americans to change course after the downward trend began in 2017.

Nursing in 2040 and Beyond

The United States suffers from a noticeable lack of imagination and inspiration when it comes to describing the future of nurses as the primary leaders in managing the patient experience. Nurses could one day work in partnership with patients, families, and the healthcare team to ensure cost, quality, and safety outcomes. Imagining this future is critical. As Carl Sandburg once said, "Nothing happens unless first a dream." Now is the time to dream of an era in which the profession of nursing takes its rightful place and significantly improves the health and well-being of all Americans.

THE EVOLVING ROLE OF THE MEDICAL STAFF PROFESSIONAL IN THE TWENTY-FIRST CENTURY

Mary A. Baker

Editor's note: The medical staff services professional is the right arm of the organized medical staff, often working with the chief medical officer on credentialing, privileging, peer review, meetings management, and overseeing practitioner performance management. The medical staff office has grown both in size and complexity, making up the nerve center of every organized medical staff. It now increasingly works with payers, regulators, and accreditors to optimize medical staff performance and compliance. The medical staff could never function optimally without these valued and dedicated professionals.

The Task and Functions of the MSP in the Presoftware Era

Before the 1960s, credentials verification consisted of collecting a copy of a state medical license, a task performed by the CEO's secretary when time allowed. A decade later, there were no primary sourced verification requirements (direct confirmation of professional education, licensure, and other materials) and no National Practitioner Data Bank (NPDB). Therefore, the early MSP was focused on collection and verification of medical licenses, education records, and professional references to create a formal file. In the mid-1980s, credentialing software emerged, which allowed for mass production of verification documents and formalization of a repository for information such as education and training, work history, licensure, malpractice insurance coverage, and peer references. Soon, MSPs were able to more easily detect falsification of credentialing documents, which led to identification of practitioners who hurt patients. Credentialing verification then focused on proving credentials, and the importance of MSPs' efforts was more readily recognized.

The Effect of Software on the MSP

As credentialing software became more common and more sophisticated, these systems were used not only to generate documents and hospital information but also to reach out to the primary source verification sites, such as the AMA Profiles, and pull the verified information back to the computer system. This retrieval is done by web crawlers and other automated systems—for example, the required query (at least every two years as required by federal law) from the NPDB. Information that took four to six weeks to retrieve in the early years can now be verified and obtained in 30 minutes or less.

MSPs can now send letters to educational and training organizations, acquire peer references (to establish clinical competency), and query licensing agencies (for license status) automatically from the system electronically. These same systems allow responses to be delivered and downloaded directly. The application process timeline can also be reduced significantly by allowing the practitioner to complete her materials online rather than submitting one (or more) applications on paper. These systems can be programed to require certain questions to be answered before allowing the practitioner to continue. This improvement reduces the submission of incomplete applications.

Credentialing systems also play a vital role in managing so-called *expirables* (items—such as licensure, Drug Enforcement Administration, malpractice insurance, board certification, and visa status—that expire any time within reappointment cycles). MSPs can use systems to generate reports summarizing not only when each expirable is due to be reverified but also when verification was retrieved, which employee is working the application, how long he has been working on verifying the application information, and the current status of the application verification process.

The Whys and Hows of Credentialing Verification Organizations

With hospital acquisitions and mergers on the increase since the early 2000s, healthcare organizations began to recognize the need to consolidate and standardize the credentialing process. Initially, for-profit credentialing verification organizations (CVOs) were used to help reduce duplication and redundancy in the verification process. Eventually, larger healthcare systems (typically organizations with three or more facilities) developed system CVOs that absorbed responsibility for the credentialing verification process for all facilities in the organization. This innovation allowed for standardization and consolidation of processes, not to mention a great reduction in duplication of effort. These CVOs also allowed more time for the in-house MSP to concentrate on hospital-specific responsibilities, such as privileging request assessments for new or different clinical activities and application processing, bylaws maintenance, meeting management, assisting with medical staff–related responsibilities, and serving as liaison between administration and the medical staff.

How Are Large Systems Organizing the MSP Function?

Over recent years, many organizations began to think differently about how the MSP should and could function. In healthcare systems where a system CVO exists, the CVO can perform both the credential verification process and the appointment or privileging process. However, some healthcare organizations want to keep the privileging process within the individual organizations; therefore, the system CVO may only perform credentials verifications, with the work product of member organizations being an administratively complete application ready for medical staff–specific privileging or appointment consideration. The healthcare organization remains responsible for analysis of the application content, with verifications, privileges and appointment requests, and the medical staff leader–approval process and governing board–approval process.

In smaller organizations without a CVO, the MSP performs many tasks, including, but not limited to, credential verification and privileging, the application approval process, meeting management, bylaws maintenance, ED call schedules, dues, and accreditation compliance.

MSPs Taking the Lead

Many larger healthcare organizations are involving their management services organization (MSO) in credentialing practitioners on behalf of health plans and other payers, with the goal of consolidating efforts in this era of shrinking resources. This initiative has resulted in the MSP becoming more knowledgeable in multiple accrediting agencies, such as the National Committee for Quality Assurance (NCQA), URAC, and others. The role of the MSP will continue to expand as healthcare organizations and providers develop customized strategies for clinical care redesign and healthcare reform—clinical integration, patient-centered medical homes, and accountable care organizations (ACOs). The role will continue to be focused on baseline patient safety by streamlining the verification process and validating clinical competence using a standardized and efficient approach.

The MSP's Role in Monitoring Contractual Terms and Metrics for Quality, Safety, and Service

In most organizations, the MSO had little involvement in monitoring contractual terms between practitioners, payers, and the healthcare organization. In recent years, the MSO has started to work more closely with the organization's clinical contracting, as well as human resources and legal departments, to develop contracts that ensure compliance with eligibility requirements for various health plans, accreditors, and payers.

The MSO has become much more involved in managing practitioner quality, especially with the implementation of The Joint Commission's focused professional practice evaluation (FPPE) and ongoing professional practice evaluation (OPPE) in order to assess the performance of all licensed practitioners granted clinical privileges on the organized medical staff. For many years, MSO leaders have been monitoring accreditation compliance for the medical staff, leadership, performance improvement, and human resources accreditation standards. Years ago, the MSO received quality data only at the time of reappointment. However, in the twenty-first century, many surveying bodies require continuous quality improvement and validation of ongoing clinical competence with standards that cross departmental lines. The MSO, the quality improvement department, and the human resources department have become more collaborative in the exchange of competence and behavior information, within the legal specifications of information-sharing agreements.

The Evolving and Future Role of the MSP

Over the years, the MSP's role has evolved from primarily a clerical job to a position that requires special management skill sets, critical thinking, and specific knowledge and professional leadership competencies. Although the role of the MSP has changed substantially, patient safety was, is, and will remain the primary focus of all efforts.

For continued professional growth in today's rapidly changing healthcare environment, the MSP must continue to develop efficient, economical, standardized processes; collaborate with multiple departments and organizations; and continue to educate herself on the evolution of traditional and nontraditional medical staff services. Working on task-oriented, diverse teams is now usual and expected.

The MSP role has evolved to include not only credentialing, privileging, and appointment to the hospital's medical staff but also oversight of compliance with accreditation and regulatory requirements—for medical staff as well as for leadership, human resources, medical records, and more. The MSP's role and ever-changing responsibilities will expand to include myriad projects: practitioner onboarding (orientation); provider enrollment in health plans; recruitment; federal provider–based designated location management to meet payer eligibility requirements; standardized credentialing initiatives for systems and health plans; investigation of legal, peer review, and malpractice issues; risk management; performance and quality improvement; patient safety; and project management.

As a greater number of healthcare organizations employ and contract physicians, MSPs become more knowledgeable about recruitment, hiring, and termination processes, typically managed through the human resources department. Healthcare mergers and acquisitions require today's MSPs to shift their processes from a single-facility thinking to systems thinking. This increase in responsibility and knowledge has elevated the MSP from a clerk to a leader with a key role in ensuring patient safety.

THE EVOLVING ROLE OF THE ORGANIZED MEDICAL STAFF IN THE TWENTY-FIRST CENTURY

Jon Burroughs

Since the organized medical staff was pioneered in 1919 as a part of the American College of Surgeon's Minimum Standards for Hospitals, the organized medical staff has been the bedrock of the profession for hospital-based physicians. Originally created as a means to improve the quality of care, the organized medical staff quickly evolved into a source of professional identity and protection for physicians who were sometimes at odds with professional management. An organized medical staff is now required by all organizations that are deemed status accreditors as well as by the CMS Conditions of Participation.

Prior to physician employment, the organized medical staff was an entity separate from management, reporting directly to the healthcare governing body. The president of the medical staff had a role parallel to that of the CEO. With the emergence of employed physicians nearly 40 years ago, these parallel structures blurred. Most physicians found themselves accountable to both the organized medical staff (through the medical staff bylaws) and management (through their employment or other contracts). This ambiguity was often the source of misunderstanding and conflict— self-employed physicians increasingly saw themselves as isolated defenders of the traditional model and values, while employed physicians felt torn between their loyalty to management and loyalty to their peers.

With the evolution of the healthcare business model, from the physician's office and stand-alone hospital to an integrated delivery system, the organized medical staff must adapt once again to a rapidly changing environment. The following sections represent the many changes facing the medical staff in the early twenty-first century.

A System Focus, Not a Hospital Focus

The organized medical staff was founded as a hospital-based organization, eventually becoming the wellspring of physician-based inpatient activity. Physicians would meet between rounds, discuss hospital-based cases, and work with management on operational and clinical issues. As hospitals expanded into integrated delivery systems, the medical staff expanded as well. Currently, physicians may be a part of operational subunits of healthcare organizations as varied as health plans and outpatient rehabilitation facilities. In the future, most physicians will be practicing in ambulatory or outpatient environments, so excluding them from most of the traditional hospital models would be self-defeating. The organized medical staff is becoming system based and must incorporate all components of a healthcare system to remain relevant, inclusive, and reflective of medicine as it is today—not how it was structured in the past.

Many medical staffs redesign their committee structures to reflect this rapidly evolving organizational structure. For instance, the medical executive committee (MEC) was traditionally made up of medical staff officers and department chairs, along with ex officio members of the management team. Today, many organizations rework this model to more accurately represent their organizational structures and demographics. For instance, many organizations have a physician or practitioner employment group or an ACO, and it may make sense to have a representative leader from each of these operational subunits as a voting member of the MEC. Other organizations are replacing a complete roster of department chairs with at-large members from representative specialties who are committed to representing the interests of the medical staff and organization as a whole.

Each healthcare organization must customize its medical staff; a one-size-fits-all approach does not work. Whatever the structure, the medical staff should represent all physicians, dentists, psychologists, podiatrists, advanced-practice nurses, and physician assistants throughout the system in a way that makes sense to its members and enables seamless communication between the organized medical staff, management, and the governing board.

Pursuing Ambulatory Quality *and* Hospital Quality

The traditional medical staff functions of credentialing, privileging, and peer review must now go beyond the old-model inpatient focus. These functions once only pertained to what practitioners did in the hospital itself and did not include or incorporate the majority of care delivered in clinics, offices, or ambulatory settings. However, physicians must now oversee all clinical quality throughout the system.

To expand this focus, it is necessary to build an IT infrastructure with clinical and business analytics that can capture outcomes across the continuum of care, not merely within the hospital. This way, OPPE (the ongoing assessment of practitioner performance) and FPPE (a more focused and short-term assessment of practitioner performance) can be conducted throughout the system. NCQA will increasingly use—and modify—ambulatory indicators such as the Healthcare Effectiveness Data and Information Set to capture quality data, primarily focusing on patient care in the ambulatory environment. Many organizations today are accredited by The Joint Commission, the Healthcare Facilities Accreditation Program, or Det Norske Veritas (for inpatient programs), NCQA (for ambulatory or managed care programs), or URAC to ensure comprehensive oversight throughout the system.

Many systems create a CVO in order to coordinate the credentialing, privileging, OPPE, and FPPE processes among multiple organizations. This ensures the uniformity of criteria across the system. Consistency is particularly important in multifacility systems with multiple medical staffs, as courts do not appreciate multiple standards in the same system (particularly with a single corporate governing structure). As discussed by Dr. Baker earlier, many experienced MSPs now oversee and manage large CVOs that serve multiple facilities, health plans, payers, accreditors, and other key stakeholders.

Operational challenges for these more complex organizations are multiple. For example, they must grapple with new administrative burdens from stakeholders. Increasingly, health plans and payers are delegating the rating of practitioners and organizations to the organizations themselves. A typical payer rating may include average adjusted cost per case, morbidity and mortality indexes, and rate of upcoding. This important process often determines which practitioners and organizations will be in or out of network and at what level practitioners and organizations will be reimbursed. Delegated credentialing, in which stakeholders may use the clinical and economic credentialing functions of the organization as a proxy to meet their own network requirements, adds to the burden.

Another challenge is the question of clinical credentialing versus economic credentialing. Today's environment requires physicians and other healthcare practitioners to participate in highly evolved and competitive operational units, each with its own credentialing requirements and standards. For instance, an organization may have an ACO that participates in at-risk contracting with large payers or employers and may expect a higher standard of qualifications in exchange for premium reimbursement. Thus, healthcare organizations increasingly impose requirements on physicians and other practitioners—that they be parties to exclusive arrangements or service lines, that they meet higher eligibility criteria, or that they use evidence-based approaches. Requisites such as these go far beyond the traditional standard of "clinical competence" and are referred to as *economic* or *non-competency-related credentialing*.

As healthcare systems and payers continue to evolve, increasingly complex sets of data and analytics need to be monitored, tracked, trended, and reported for each payer, accreditor, and operating unit. This requires a sophisticated IT system coupled with a health information exchange to link information transmission among all operating units and analytics with an enterprise data warehouse to capture clinical and business information in real time.

Aligning quality improvement objectives with the goals of the organization's strategic plan is increasingly important. For example, many organizations incentivize physicians largely on the basis of wRVU productivity measures, as determined by benchmarking organizations such as the Medical Group Management Association. Unfortunately, focusing exclusively on productivity measures may inadvertently undermine quality, safety, service, and cost-effectiveness, thus inadvertently impairing pay-for-value contract metrics that may carry significant, monetized, at-risk values. For closer alignment, high-performing staffs create a medical staff strategic plan based on the organization's strategic road map and then generate an operating plan to determine which committees, expertise, structures, and resources are necessary to support the enterprise from a medical staff perspective.

Aligning the credentialing, privileging, and peer review functions and processes with the strategic goals and objectives of a healthcare system is increasingly important. It is also necessary to be able to compete in an increasingly pay-for-value world.

Shifting to Use of Nonphysicians, Fully Interdisciplinary Teams, and Physician Oversight

As physicians become increasingly able to perform more sophisticated clinical and managerial duties that require physician-level expertise, healthcare organizations will become dominated by advanced-practice nurses, physician assistants, and other healthcare professionals who perform functions that significantly free up physicians for more executive functions.

Nonphysicians provide care that can be standardized, such as screenings, routine follow-ups, treatment of minor acute conditions, care for chronic conditions, and minor routine procedures. They will also take over primary call functions to provide screening examinations with routine admissions of stable, acute emergencies and minor acute conditions. APPs assigned to hospitalist services enable larger physician-to-patient ratios than the traditional 1:15, with physicians serving in consultative and supervisory roles. APPs also play a key role in population health.

Health systems can engage APPs through the creation of a medical staff–APP interdisciplinary advisory committee that reports to the MEC. APPs bring a great deal of specialty-specific expertise that can be invaluable throughout the medical staff credentialing, privileging, and peer review processes. Physicians increasingly rely on APPs for their expertise, particularly on scope of care (which APP services should be provided) and scope of practice (which privileges should APPs be delineated and granted).

As described previously, scribes free physicians from data entry. They also optimize revenue cycle management by enabling accounts receivables to be generated the day of discharge. Organizations commonly employ scribes who lack either clinical or coding background; this is an error, as it largely negates their potential benefit. Scribes should always add expertise to their team and not merely serve as adjuncts. They do not simply constitute an added cost.

The care coordinator, often an advanced-practice nurse with a public or population health background, is a key leader in population health. The coordinator has significant expertise in the care delivery system as a whole and a working knowledge of stakeholders, facilities, payer contracts, health plans, regulatory requirements, and more. These workers often, with physicians, head up population health teams and represent the primary interface for consumers. Care coordinators maximize the cost-effectiveness of care given in the context of population health agreements.

Rural hospitals, which have difficulty recruiting physicians, already have medical staffs made up primarily of nonphysicians. These institutions are reaping the advantages that skilled professionals bring. Most other healthcare organizations will soon follow suit.

The Rise of Unified and Integrated Medical Staff Models

Healthcare systems are often the result of mergers, acquisitions, or affiliations with multiple facilities. Each component of the system may have its own unique provider number, organized medical staff, and medical staff bylaws. This discrepancy may be problematic when physicians and other practitioners migrate from facility to facility. For example, when adjudicating a medical negligence case that occurs in multiple facilities within a system, courts will often use the highest standards and eligibility criteria in the system to determine a standard of care. Many systems now seek to create a unified and integrated medical staff to eliminate this non-value-added complexity and to standardize and streamline traditional medical staff functions. How does a unified and integrated medical staff work?

First, each facility with a unique Medicare provider number must have its own organized medical staff controlled by bylaws and overseen by a governing body. That being said, the creation of a unified and integrated medical staff enables all medical staffs in a system to have the following:

- Standardized medical staff bylaws, regulations, and procedures
- Standardized credentialing and privileging criteria (possibly customized for different facilities based on the availability of clinical specialties and the existence of exclusive agreements)
- Standardized criteria for peer review through the creation of review, rule, and rate indicators
- Standardized OPPE or FPPE processes across clinical specialties
- Systemwide credentialing and peer review committees to generate and oversee facility-based functions

When creating such a medical staff structure, the key is to enable physician leaders from each facility to work with management to design standardized structures and processes that respect the cultural differences of each facility. However, these structures and processes must at the same time standardize whenever possible, aiming to minimize ambiguity and cost while optimizing quality and consistency throughout the system.

Since 2014, CMS has had a condition of participation that requires medical staff bylaws to include the opportunity for medical staffs within a system to both become unified and integrated but to dissolve the unified and integrated model if so desired. The relevant CMS Conditions of Participation outlining these requirements are summarized in the following sections.

Interpretive Guidelines §482.22
The hospital must have one medical staff for the entire organization (including all campuses, provider-based locations, satellites, and remote locations). For example, a multicampus hospital may not have a separately organized medical staff for each campus. On the other hand, in the case of a hospital system, it is permissible for the system to have a unified and integrated medical staff (hereafter referred to as a *unified medical staff*) for multiple, separately certified hospitals.

Interpretive Guidelines §482.22(b)(1)–(3)
If the hospital uses a unified medical staff it shares with other hospitals that are part of a multihospital system, its situation does not change the requirement for the medical staff to be well organized and accountable to the system's governing body for the quality of care in each separately certified hospital.

If the hospital uses a unified medical staff, only one individual may be responsible for the organization and conduct of the unified medical staff; that individual may or may not hold privileges and practices at the hospital being surveyed. When the individual does not practice at the hospital being surveyed, and it is necessary to interview him as part of a survey, a telephone interview must be arranged.

If the hospital uses a unified medical staff, the medical staff continues to be accountable for the quality of care in each separately certified hospital that uses the unified medical staff.

Interpretive Guidelines §482.22(b)(4)

A hospital that is part of a system consisting of multiple, separately certified hospitals may use a unified medical staff that is shared with one or more of the other hospitals in the system. In other words, as long as the requirements of §482.22(b)(4) are met, it is not necessary for each separately certified hospital in the system to have its own distinct medical staff organization and structure, including hospital-specific medical staff bylaws, rules, and requirements; hospital-specific medical staff leadership; and hospital-specific credentialing and peer review. Instead, it may use one medical staff organization and structure for multiple hospitals, so long as all of the requirements of this section are met. However, separately certified hospitals that share a unified medical staff must also share a system governing body, in accordance with the provisions of §482.12, given that only one governing body may carry out the governing body's medical staff responsibilities for a unified medical staff.

Note that a multicampus hospital that has several inpatient campuses that are provider-based, remote locations is not a multihospital system. A multicampus hospital is one certified hospital, not several separately certified hospitals. It may not have separate medical staffs at each campus, given that each hospital must have no more than one medical staff. A multicampus hospital with one medical staff separate from that of other certified hospitals is not employing a unified medical staff, as that term is used in this regulation. However, one that is part of a hospital system consisting of multiple, separately certified hospitals may share a unified medical staff with other separately certified hospitals in the system.

The governing body in a multihospital system must elect to exercise this option. Because a number of hospital systems interpreted the medical staff condition of participation to permit a unified medical staff prior to publication of the final rule at §482.22(b)(4) on May 12, 2014, or its effective date of July 11, 2014, the existence of a unified medical staff prior to July 11, 2014, is considered evidence of the governing body's election of this option.

This fact does not relieve the governing body of the responsibility to conduct a review of all applicable state and local laws, including regulations, and make a determination that use of a unified medical staff that is shared by multiple hospitals does not conflict with those laws. The hospital must maintain documentation of this determination by its governing body.

This fact also does not relieve the governing body of the obligation to inform the medical staff of the right to vote to opt out of a unified medical staff arrangement. (See discussion of §482.22[b][4][ii], which requires notification of all members of this right. Failure to comply would be cited under the tag for §482.22[b][4][ii].) If a hospital is part of a multihospital system that wishes to establish a unified medical staff for some or all of its separately certified hospitals after the July 11, 2014, effective date of the final rule at §482.22(b)(4), then the hospital's system governing body must document in writing its decision to elect to use the unified medical staff option, conditioned on acceptance of a unified medical staff by the hospital's medical staff in accordance with §482.22(b)(4)(i). The governing body must also document its determination that such election does not conflict with state or local laws, including regulations.

Following is a summary of these regulatory requirements:

- The organized medical staff and governing body of each facility must decide to opt in or opt out of a unified medical staff model.
- If there is a single corporate governing body, then the organized medical staff of each facility must decide with the corporate governing body to opt in or out.
- CMS does not define specifically what a unified medical staff model must look like. Its structure should be

customized at the discretion of each organization with significant physician input.

- A unified and integrated medical staff may only have one president of the medical staff (physician, dentist, or podiatrist); the chosen individual is not required to have clinical privileges or membership at each facility represented.
- A healthcare organization that has a unified and integrated medical staff must have a single governing body for the entire system (in addition to optional advisory boards for each facility) to whom the medical staff is accountable. In other words, a unified and integrated medical staff cannot be accountable to advisory or local governing bodies at each represented facility.

A unified and integrated medical staff is an important model because it enables complex healthcare systems to standardize medical staff bylaws, rules and regulations, and policies or procedures so that medical staff functions will better align for pay-for-value contracts. Distinct medical staffs, on their own, are unlikely to be able to link quality performance to rapidly evolving incentives in the face of the bewildering array of quality metrics in payer and employer contracts.

Holding Physicians Accountable for Clinical Outcomes over Which They Have No Direct Control

Population health poses a challenge to physicians of the twenty-first century. One of the major features of population health discussed in chapter 11 is the heightened use of matrix management, through which population health contracts can be established. In matrix management, hospitals—and even integrated healthcare organizations—contract with entities ranging from schools to skilled nursing facilities to provide comprehensive population health services.

As clinical leaders and executives, physicians will be expected to work alongside the executive team to create mutually agreed-on quality, safety, service, and cost-effectiveness metrics that enable organizations to succeed with pay-for-value, at-risk contracts. Thus, physicians need to work with and significantly influence facilities that employ providers that may have no formal legal ownership or shared-asset arrangement with their healthcare organization.

The ability to influence and generate reliable clinical outcomes requires management skills and typically comanagement relationships, whereby physicians assume responsibility for both clinical and business outcomes. This shift requires an organization to create at-risk arrangements with every physician on its medical staff who is willing and able to be aligned. Parenthetically, a growing number of healthcare organizations are making the willingness to go at-risk a nonnegotiable part of membership on an organized medical staff.

For instance, Intermountain Healthcare has the following nonnegotiable requirements for physicians and healthcare practitioners participating in its organized medical staffs and population health agreements:

- Be willing to participate in at-risk contracts based on strategic goals and objectives developed and approved by physicians and management.
- Comply with clinical and business best practices, as determined by peer group and management (and be willing to be peer audited for exceptions).
- Agree to unblinded transparency of all clinical and financial data and analytics.
- Be willing to comply with a value-analysis process (multidisciplinary committee designed to make decisions regarding vendors, supply chains, and new technology or clinical paradigms).
- Disclose all potential conflicts of interest, and accept the determination of deliberative physician bodies.

Physicians who are unwilling or unable to comply with these non-negotiables are not eligible to participate on the organized medical staff. Thus, organizations are rethinking the old-model practice of generating operating revenue by recruiting as many physicians as possible on the medical staff. The more contemporary goal is to have the "right" physicians and practitioners on the medical staff—those who are able and willing to generate value for patients, payers, and the organization. This new approach represents a significant cultural shift that is necessary in order to pursue at-risk, value-based arrangements.

Taking an Assertive Role in Management

In the twenty-first century, physicians and executives will need to manage clinical care, operations, finance, marketing, and branding together. Clinical decisions have a profound impact on length of stay and morbidity or mortality rates, and conversely, operational and business decisions have a strong impact on clinical outcomes—all factors that are monetized in pay-for-value contracts.

A classic example of the necessity of focusing on the optimization of quality and the minimization of costs is the impact of the regionalization of healthcare for complex, high-risk, volume-sensitive procedures as articulated by John D. Birkmeyer and colleagues (2003) and many others over the past 40 years. The literature supports the adoption of narrower scopes of practice for healthcare facilities based on their institutional and practitioner volumes, expertise, infrastructure, and quality metrics. In his landmark *New Yorker* piece "The Bell Curve," Atul Gawande (2004) emphasized the significant difference in life expectancies for people with cystic fibrosis based on where, and by whom, the care is delivered.

The decision to offer certain services does not solely rest with physicians, management, or the board. It must be made collaboratively based on best available evidence, current metrics, and the implications for both the health of patients and the business.

Thus, the pattern of physicians making clinical decisions and leaving management to take care of operations is no longer a helpful model for the organization as a whole.

To better merge the decision-making by traditionally disparate and separate professions, many organizations are integrating the organized medical staff and the management team. Health systems have experimented with various initiatives, including a few discussed in the following paragraphs.

Some institutions have professionalized medical staff leadership positions into compensated management positions based on the leader's ability to generate clinical and business outcomes. This organizational shift requires converting a medical staff nominating committee into a medical staff leadership and succession planning committee, made up of physician leaders and management, to create job descriptions with eligibility requirements, selection criteria, ongoing 360-degree assessments with coaching and further leadership development, and appropriate incentives for mutually agreed-on goals and objectives.

Many health systems have transitioned physicians into clinical executive roles with both clinical and operational unit oversight responsibilities. As mentioned earlier, turning physicians into clinical executives involves creating FMV comanagement agreements based on the physician's level of motivation, professional interests, and abilities. But the nature of departmental structure has also changed. Clinical departments have evolved into service lines, which often have dyad or triad leadership, as well as compensated medical directors who work to standardize care and integrate clinical and business outcomes.

Organizations may be helped along in the process of physician–management integration if they promote transparent, dynamic payer contracts. Shared information is developed and managed collaboratively by physicians, managers, and payers. This constitutes a complete merger of interests between key stakeholders and effectively minimizes the traditional separation of clinical and business functions.

Conclusion

In the twenty-first century, the organized medical staff will undergo profound changes to remain relevant in a transformed clinical and business model. Institutions unwilling to change will increasingly find themselves at a significant disadvantage in pay-for-value contracts, and those willing to innovate and change will enjoy potential premium payments as well as the knowledge that they are supporting improved clinical and business outcomes.

REFERENCES

Accenture. 2015. "Many US Doctors Will Leave Private Practice for Hospital Employment, Accenture Reports." Published July 2. https://newsroom.accenture.com/news/many-us-doctors -will-leave-private-practice-for-hospital-employment-accenture -reports.htm.

Ahmed, A., and J. E. Fincham. 2011. "Patients' View of Retail Clinics as a Source of Primary Care: Boon for Nurse Practitioners?" *Journal of the American Academy of Nurse Practitioners* 23 (4): 193–99.

American Academy of Pediatrics. 2016. "AAP Policy Statement Recommends Full-Time Nurse in Every School." Published May 23. www.aap.org/en-us/about-the-aap/aap-press-room /pages/AAP-Policy-Statement-Recommends-Full-Time-Nurse -in-Every-School.aspx.

American Association of Colleges of Nursing. 2015. "Fact Sheet: Creating a More Highly Qualified Nursing Workforce." Updated May 19. www.aacnnursing.org/Portals/42/News/Factsheets /Nursing-Workforce-Fact-Sheet.pdf.

Birkmeyer, J. D., A. E. Siewers, P. P. Goodney, D. E. Wennberg, and F. L. Lucas. 2003. "Surgeon Volume and Operative Mortality in the United States." *New England Journal of Medicine* 349: 2117–27.

Gawande, A. 2004. "The Bell Curve." *New Yorker*. Published December 6. www.newyorker.com/magazine/2004/12/06/the-bell-curve.

Geiger-Brown, J., V. Rogers, A. M. Trinkoff, R. L. Kane, R. B. Bausell, and S. M. Scharf. 2012. "Sleep, Sleepiness, Fatigue, and Performance of 12-Hour-Shift Nurses." *Chronobiology International* 29 (7): 961.

Hendrich, A., M. P. Chow, B. A. Skierczynshi, and Z. Liu. 2008. "A 36-Hospital Time and Motion Study: How Do Medical-Surgical Nurses Spend Their Time?" *Permanente Journal* 12 (3): 25–34.

Institute of Medicine. 2010. *The Future of Nursing: Leading Change, Advancing Health*. Accessed February 5, 2018. http://floridasnursing.gov/forms/iom-future-nursing-info.pdf.

Kover, C., and J. Spetz. 2011. "The Future of Nursing: An Interview with Susan B. Hassmiller." *Nursing Economics* 29 (1): 32–41.

Letvak, S., C. Ruhm, and T. McCoy. 2012. "Depression in Hospital-Employed Nurses." *Clinical Nurse Specialist* 26 (3): 177–82.

Putnam, R. 2000. *Bowling Alone: The Collapse and Revival of American Community*. New York: Simon and Schuster.

Shultz, C. G., and H. L. Holmstrom. 2015. "The Use of Medical Scribes in Health Care Settings: A Systematic Review and Future Directions." *Journal of the American Board of Family Medicine* 28 (3): 371–81.

Tucker, A., and S. Spear. 2006. "Operational Failures and Interruptions in Hospital Nursing." *Health Services Research* 41 (3): 643–62.

World Health Organization. 2018. "Cancer." Published February. www.who.int/en/news-room/fact-sheets/detail/cancer.

CHAPTER 5

Strategic Planning for the Future Healthcare Enterprise

John M. Harris
Dan Grauman

THE TWENTY-FIRST-CENTURY HEALTHCARE enterprise embraces the transformation from volume to value, which necessitates greater financial risk for those who deliver care. It also likely involves physicians who are employed by the enterprise, as well as independent groups of physicians, who care for patients within the expanding boundaries of evolving and consolidating health systems.

Strong clinically integrated networks (CINs) are likely the closest current analog to the future healthcare enterprise described throughout this book. As in a CIN, each healthcare enterprise will likely focus on delivering improved value across the full continuum of health needs through more thoughtful use of resources and better coordination among providers. The healthcare enterprises will enter episode-based and population-based payment contracts to be rewarded for enhanced value, or they will incorporate the functions of payers into the enterprise, further extending their role. As is often the case in healthcare, models will vary based on local market characteristics. Healthcare enterprises will take a variety of forms, including the following:

- Health systems with employed physicians
- Health systems with employed physicians working closely with independent physicians (typical of many CINs in the second decade of the twenty-first century)
- Networks of multiple CINs sharing infrastructure and covering a broad geographic region
- Health systems that own and operate health plans

These organizational structure options do not represent a natural progression toward an inevitable end point of health systems that employ all of their physicians and also include a health plan. Rather, different models make sense in different markets, each reflecting different levels of integration (physician, hospital, other providers, health plan) and different degrees of risk. Furthermore, the same health system may serve different populations and employ a clinically integrated and coordinated model of care through multiple contractual arrangements, each with its own degree of risk. Exhibit 5.1 illustrates this point.

While these organizations take many forms, for the balance of this chapter, we use the term *healthcare enterprise* to refer to any of the organizational structures described earlier. In all cases, we are focused on providers transitioning from a focus on the volume to a focus on the value of services and competing on that basis.

CHANGES TO STRATEGIC PLANNING

The healthcare enterprise of the future will be different from current health systems in profound ways. Setting strategy for these future enterprises is complicated because these organizations incorporate many of the following factors:

- They offer physicians (both self-employed and employed) an expanded role in leadership and governance.
- They bear greater financial risk.

Exhibit 5.1: Example of Value-based Payment Arrangements by Population

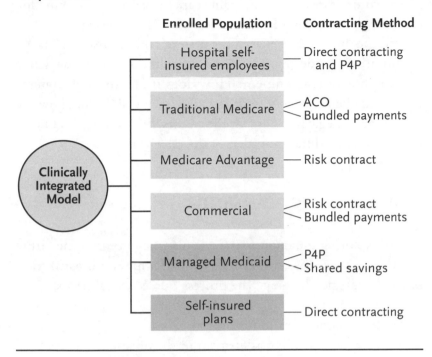

© 2017 Veralon Partners Inc.

- They engage in a broader span of activity than do traditional providers that includes operational, financial, strategic, and marketing oversight.
- They compete in an ever-more-demanding and -competitive market environment.
- They use a greater number of complex partnerships.

As a result, certain strategic issues will arise for the healthcare enterprise of the future that were not present, or at least were not as critical, for traditional hospitals and health systems. For example, delivering value to purchasers and engaging physicians become even more important in the future healthcare enterprise than in a traditional hospital or health system. At minimum, a healthcare enterprise must consider its size, scale, and market relevance, as well as new core competencies, including care management, information technology, predictive data analytics, and risk management.

But the differences between the present and future of healthcare organizations go deeper. How does a healthcare enterprise define its competitive environment? How does it identify key strategic issues and challenges and set its strategy? We will explore how the process of strategic planning for the twenty-first-century healthcare enterprise must differ from that of the past.

WHY STRATEGIC PLANNING?

Before exploring the unique strategic planning needs of the future healthcare enterprise, we must establish why any organization pursues strategic planning. The process fulfills several needs:

- Identifies opportunities and threats
- Provides a realistic assessment of the organization's strengths and weaknesses as well as its ability to address threats and pursue opportunities
- Sets a clear strategic direction
- Clarifies organizational goals and objectives
- Identifies specific initiatives to pursue
- Prioritizes resource allocation
- Inspires stakeholders
- Establishes clear measures of success (key performance indicators, or KPIs)
- Provides a road map and accountability for implementation

Effective strategic planning should achieve these results.

The strategic planning process is iterative, rather than linear. While each individual activity generally leads to the activity that logically follows, some back and forth occurs and, in particular, the process requires review and reconsideration even when the next activity is underway. So, rather than follow a linear, non-overlapping path from one activity to the next—where a given activity generally informs and leads to the next one—the activities actually overlap and interrelate as well as provide a foundation for what comes next.

Exhibit 5.2 illustrates a planning process that works well for healthcare organizations. Its four constituent activities are environmental assessment, organizational direction setting, strategy formulation, and implementation planning.

ACTIVITY 1: ENVIRONMENTAL ASSESSMENT

An organization's failure to respond to market changes can lead to organizational crisis or failure. Overcoming the inertia of incumbency is a key reason to complete an effective strategic plan. An environmental assessment, the initial activity of the strategic planning process, is the foundation on which strategy is developed.

A strong environmental assessment can make the case for the need for action. In particular, developing scenarios that predict the potentially negative results of inaction can break through the assumption that "things will be pretty much like last year." By identifying compelling critical planning issues, the environmental assessment can counteract the complacency of incumbents and stimulate consideration of the bolder strategies necessary for a changing and more competitive environment.

The core components of an environmental assessment are internal analysis and external analysis. Though these basic components are the same for a healthcare enterprise as for a more traditional health system, the new healthcare enterprise must analyze certain factors more deeply. Exhibit 5.3 describes the purpose and content highlights of the environmental assessment.

Exhibit 5.2: Strategic Planning Approach

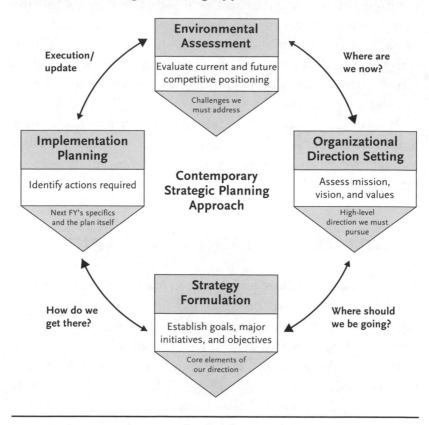

© 2017 Veralon Partners Inc.

External Analysis

Many strategic plans spend too much time focused on internal considerations and too little time considering the effect of external factors on strategy. A traditional health system external analysis would focus on competitors, payment rates, technological innovation, population demographics, and policy changes. A healthcare enterprise external analysis goes beyond these factors to dive more deeply into payer market dynamics; market share; primary care;

Exhibit 5.3: Environmental Assessment: Purpose and Desired Characteristics of End Product

Purpose	Desired Characteristics of End Product
• Identifies how external forces might affect the organization in the future • Allows the board and others less knowledgeable about the organization to obtain a solid grounding for constructive involvement in the process • Helps determine what factors are subject to the organization's control or influence • Clarifies past successes and failures; what has worked, what has not, and why	• External orientation • Broad and insightful competitive analysis • Focused analysis at operating-unit level in large organizations • Key findings summarized with comprehensible graphics

© 2017 Veralon Partners Inc.

and specialty physician control of attributed lives, benefit design, contractual options, and consumer preferences.

In the past, healthcare may have felt like a very complex environment to hospital leaders. However, for decades, the amount of true competition has been limited. Exhibit 5.4 illustrates how many of the traditional barriers to competition in healthcare are peeling away, resulting in a more contested environment.

Health plans were a relatively small consideration in traditional strategic plans. Typically, payment rates were either favorable or unfavorable, and insurance products allowed patients to choose from most providers without any financial penalty for choosing expensive providers.

Exhibit 5.4: Changing Face of Healthcare Competition

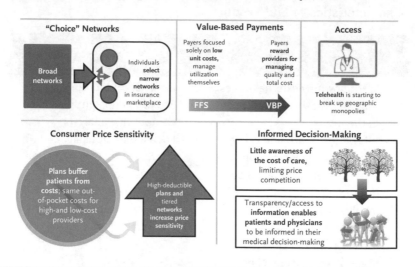

Source: © 2017 Veralon Partners Inc.

In a value-based payment environment with high-deductible health plans, payer relations become much more complex. Rather than simply trying to maximize payment rates and volume, providers must consider strategic dynamics that include consumers with increased price sensitivity from high-deductible health plans, health plan and large employer readiness to contract with value-based models and narrow networks, competing healthcare enterprises wooing physicians away through better value-based payments, and competition from nontraditional providers who may attract patients and steer them to specific aligned providers before they even have a primary care physician (PCP).

Traditional providers are not always ready for this unsheltered marketplace and the challenges from a more diverse range of competitors. Traditionally, hospitals were in competition with other hospitals. Now, a myriad of niche players compete with hospitals, taking advantage of newfound consumer price sensitivity and provider efforts to manage total population health costs in shared-savings or risk contracts. These niche players include the following:

- E-health platforms
- Retail clinics
- Freestanding outpatient imaging, surgery, endoscopy, and other diagnostic and treatment centers
- Specialty surgical hospitals
- Freestanding emergency departments
- Microhospitals

In addition to these competitors, new types of entities compete with healthcare enterprises to control referrals and market share, including independent physician entities seeking to manage care and reap rewards from payers, sometimes with an adversarial tone toward hospitals. Sometimes, these are innovative primary care practice models that focus on managing population health. In other instances, these may be health plans building their own primary care networks. Competition from nonprovider entities is also growing. Some large retail and technology companies (e.g., Amazon, Apple, Google, Facebook) may use their relationships and skills engaging consumers to disrupt healthcare and take the lead in care delivery and management. They may engage consumers before they even see a PCP and steer them to lower-cost providers. They may also use artificial intelligence to provide a first line of primary care that is cheaper and more convenient than current points of access. In addition to these less traditional competitors, healthcare enterprises still face competition from their traditional competitors. These dynamics force healthcare enterprises to continuously strive to deliver better results to their affiliated physicians.

To make anticipated changes in the external environment more tangible and compelling for planning participants, it is helpful to develop potential market scenarios. In a volume and fee-for-service world, scenarios were focused on payment rates and potential competitor actions that might drive volume. Scenarios in a value-based environment are more complex, incorporating payer market dynamics, physician population health strategies, market pricing, competitor healthcare enterprise strategies, and innovators that are redefining care delivery models. Planners should identify the most likely market scenario, as well as less likely scenarios that are also possible, to ensure that the organization's strategic direction considers the range of possible futures.

Internal Analysis

Complementing the external analysis is the internal analysis, which takes stock of the organization itself. A typical internal analysis for a health system has included an assessment of the following organizational characteristics:

- Financial performance and position
- Operational performance (e.g., labor, supply chain)
- Market position
- Service line strengths and weaknesses (e.g., quality, safety, service, cost-effectiveness)
- Medical staff characteristics
- Facility condition and needs
- Information technology resources

With the shift toward large systems that bear more financial risk and accountability, additional factors must be considered in the internal analysis. These new issues include population health capabilities, performance on value-based contracts, engagement of physicians to achieve success in value-based contracts, and pricing of services.

As part of internal analysis, the healthcare enterprise should take an honest look at its capabilities and staff expertise, particularly in those areas not traditionally a focus for providers (e.g., care management, risk management, predictive analytics).

Even areas such as information technology infrastructure that have long been covered in an internal analysis look different for the future healthcare enterprise. The question is no longer simply whether the electronic health record (EHR) and billing system are good enough. A healthcare enterprise needs to integrate payer claims data with EHR data and deploy information technology, establishing the analytics to track and improve performance in risk contracts and other value-based payment arrangements.

The ultimate goal is real-time integration of clinical information, claims data, mobile health data, and other patient information through an enterprise data warehouse. This merging will support effective and efficient treatment. With a strong information technology backbone, the data will help to predict patient needs and tailor care. However, the path to this goal can be long and winding. A wide range of approaches may be pursued, with successes and failures in both expensive and inexpensive efforts. Ongoing partnerships with sophisticated national vendors through purchase or lease arrangements are likely to be a hallmark of future information technology strategy.

For the purpose of the information technology component of the internal analysis, the focus should be on current status and needs as well as any potential shortcomings in the face of future needs.

The nature of physician alignment will transform. When contracts were based on fee-for-service, physicians got paid whether the hospital succeeded or not. Under risk contracts and other value-based contracts, a sizeable portion of physician revenue may come through success in healthcare enterprise contracts. These results will affect revenue for both hospital-employed and independent physicians.

Many healthcare enterprises are likely to involve some independent and self-employed physicians. Unlike the solo and small independent practices that have been typical in many markets, over time these physicians may be part of larger private groups. If these physicians do not see the results they are seeking with one healthcare enterprise and its value-based contracting, they are likely to shift their alignment to healthcare enterprises that are delivering positive clinical and business results that physicians can share. Therefore, a key aspect of the internal analysis is the organization's ability to succeed in risk and value-based contracts and to deliver rewards from that success to share with physicians.

Finally, pricing of services becomes increasingly important—and in a different way from what was previously the case. In the past, providers sought to get the highest payment rate and most possible unit revenue from each service. However, in a more competitive, value-based, risk-contracting world, high unit prices (in the form of high contracted rates) are likely to drive away volume. The assessment of pricing must consider its impact on the attractiveness of the healthcare enterprise, and specific services it offers, to price-sensitive consumers with high deductibles and to cost-sensitive physicians trying to succeed in value-based contracts. A clear and honest analysis of pricing based on actual costs is, therefore, an essential part of the environmental assessment. Transparency will help calibrate pricing with value-based contract goals.

The environmental assessment should be summarized in a few key analyses: strengths, weaknesses, opportunities, and threats (SWOT); scenarios; and critical planning issues.

The SWOT analysis is a familiar first step, identifying strengths and weaknesses (which are internal), opportunities (which can be both internal and external), and threats (which can be both internal and external).

Building on this assessment, it is helpful to identify a range of scenarios that may occur in the future and consider the most likely future environment. In the context of healthcare enterprises and risk contracting, these need to include a wider range of potential changes than for a traditional health system. Payer market dynamics must be considered in more depth. Will payers pursuing value-based payments outperform those that focus on traditional contracts? Will provider–payer partnerships block access to certain patients? In addition, it is important to consider the potential impact of poor performance on risk contracts. Because these contracts include more financial risk than do fee-for-service contracts, it is important to evaluate that risk and develop strategies that meet the organization's risk tolerance.

The last step in the environmental assessment must prepare for the remainder of the planning process by focusing on any critical issues. Being sidetracked by details and distractions is all too easy, particularly with the added dimensions of a healthcare enterprise described earlier. That complexity makes it all the more important to focus the planning, and the organization, on a small number of critical planning issues that must be addressed.

ACTIVITY 2: ORGANIZATIONAL DIRECTION SETTING

As health systems evolve into the healthcare enterprises of the future, they are building on a foundation that is sometimes decades or centuries old. These health systems are incumbents in a rapidly changing healthcare environment. There are some advantages to incumbency—a strong reputation, long-standing relationships, and resources to invest.

However, there are also perils to being an incumbent in a dynamic environment. It is hard for an incumbent to change the behavior of stakeholders or to change strategy rapidly if the market environment changes. Key stakeholders are likely to ask, "We've succeeded in the past—why do we need to change now?" Underestimating the threat from new competitors is easy, but they may be more nimble and able to focus on market opportunities without the burden of keeping current operations running smoothly or serving difficult populations. To survive in the future, healthcare systems must reset their organizational direction to aim toward becoming healthcare enterprises.

Exhibit 5.5 describes the purpose of setting your organizational direction and sets out the desired characteristics any statement of new plans. While the purpose of direction-setting is largely unchanged from that of traditional providers, the content can vary significantly.

Directional statements should be sharp and specific. In larger organizations (and even some smaller), all business units and entities must be aligned in pursuing a common direction. At a minimum, organizational direction for subsidiary entities cannot be inconsistent with organization-wide direction.

Revisiting mission, vision, and values is another vital step. Many health systems have taken a step toward becoming a healthcare enterprise by shifting from a focus on sick care to a focus on maintaining the health of a community, changing their mission statement as shown in exhibit 5.6.

However, these changes in mission or vision statements do not necessarily transform the organization from a focus on volume to a focus on value. Many organizations have changed the words but not the organizational commitment. Clearly stating why an organization exists (the mission statement) and what it seeks to achieve (the vision statement) only provides the foundation for achieving the vision and fulfilling the mission.

Exhibit 5.5: Setting Organizational Direction: Purpose and Desired Characteristics of End Product

Purpose	Desired Characteristics of End Product
• Establishes the overarching strategic path for the organization • Represents the policy dimension of strategy • Provides a framework for the more detailed goals and initiatives	• Sharp, tailored directional statements • One vision, one direction (operating unit direction must be consistent with corporate direction) • Clearly articulated mission, vision, and values

Source: © 2017 Veralon Partners Inc.

Exhibit 5.6: Example of Mission Statement Change

Original	Revised
Make a genuine difference by optimizing our patients' healthcare experience	Make a genuine difference in the health and well-being of the people and communities we serve

Source: © 2017 Veralon Partners Inc.

When establishing organizational direction, it is essential that organizational values be clearly articulated. Clearly stating the values and principles that will guide the behavior of all operating units, as well as physician members, can help support all future efforts. A clear statement of shared values and principles will prevent the need to reinvestigate whether each expectation or standard is appropriate.

In addition to the public articulation of the values of the organization, another type of values statement can be beneficial. A physician compact establishes a foundation for mutual understanding and trust between the enterprise and physicians and among physicians themselves (Kornacki 2015). It also helps the healthcare enterprise and physicians to agree on their shared commitment to improving the value of services provided.

In addition to reevaluating and revising the mission, vision, and values as necessary, the organizational direction phase of strategic planning should articulate the organization's overall strategy for achieving its vision. In the case of a healthcare enterprise, this overall strategy may focus on physician–hospital collaboration, a firm commitment to value-based contracting relationships, or similar broad approaches to achieving the vision. The overall strategy then becomes a foundation for setting goals and identifying initiatives that help achieve the vision.

ACTIVITY 3: STRATEGY FORMULATION

Once a distinct vision establishes the phase of organizational direction-setting, the organization is prepared to develop goals and objectives, identify strategies to achieve the goals and objectives, and establish milestones to track performance. This activity is known as strategy formulation.

Exhibit 5.7 displays the purpose and ideal outcomes of this step. Rather than try to set goals for all possible strategic issues, contemporary strategy development processes focus on setting priorities and making choices. As larger systems and networks develop, strategic planning increasingly occurs at multiple levels in the organization. In these settings, corporate or system leadership typically sets overall organizational goals, which then direct the development of the goals and objectives of operating units.

Gaining agreement on goals and objectives is key to maintaining accountability. Physicians and hospital leadership alike must be committed to the shared goals and objectives and understand

Exhibit 5.7: Strategy Formulation: Purpose and Desired Characteristics of End Product

Purpose	Desired Characteristics of End Product
• Develops the core content of the strategic plan • Addresses the most critical issues facing the organization directly • Forces prioritization and making choices to focus the organization and its resources on what matters most	• Broad involvement of internal constituents • Addresses a limited number (no more than ten and ideally as few as three to five) of the most critical issues • Directs operating unit goals and objectives via overall corporate goals

© 2017 Veralon Partners Inc.

the mutual effort and sacrifices being made to achieve them. For example, success in healthcare enterprises requires extra effort and increased accountability from physicians and willingness from hospitals to drive down utilization and provide competitive pricing, all to provide better value (quality and cost). When these goals are shared, the hospital and physicians are better positioned to succeed in a competitive market.

If physicians are actively engaged in formulating strategic initiatives, they are much more likely to want to see those initiatives succeed. While this is true of strategic planning for healthcare systems, it is crucial to the success of strategic planning for healthcare enterprises. Physicians must be committed or the enterprise will not succeed.

When evaluating risk contracts and other value-based arrangements, leaders have a tendency to focus on direct contract results (bonuses, surpluses, incentive payments) as the only measures of success. However, healthcare enterprises derive many wider benefits from success in value-based contracting. It helps reduce leakage of patients to competitors and improves cooperation on operational improvements that can reduce operating costs. It also furnishes a counterforce to competitor efforts to shift physician allegiances and builds an attractive financial model for physicians that may help to prevent physician shortages (Harris and Hemnani 2013). All of these benefits must be considered when evaluating strategies and setting goals for value-based contracting. Otherwise, it is easy for healthcare system leadership to shift its focus back to fee-for-service revenues and to undermine the enterprise's long-term market position.

ACTIVITY 4: IMPLEMENTATION PLANNING

In all strategic planning, one of the greatest challenges is to ensure that the good ideas developed are actually implemented. Failure to do so leads to frustration, apathy, and resentment among all stakeholders who spent time developing the plan. Implementation planning is worth every healthcare enterprise's effort.

Exhibit 5.8 displays the purpose and the implementation planning activity and the desired characteristics of its end product. As specific resource needs are identified and accountability is assigned, organizations often seek to launch too many initiatives at once. This is a good time to set priorities, trim some initiatives, and implement initiatives that match resources, rather than set the stage for failure and frustration. In larger systems, succeeding at activity 4 will require setting priorities among operating units.

The failure to effectively implement strategies can be more devastating for healthcare enterprises than for hospitals and systems. Physicians with a variety of bonds to the organization will be assessing whether the organization is delivering on its promises. Employed physicians may be frustrated and demoralized if a health system does not provide the tools for their success. Independent physicians have more options and may shift their allegiance to healthcare enterprises

Exhibit 5.8: Implementation Planning: Purpose and Desired Characteristics of End Product

Purpose	Desired Characteristics of End Product
• Bridges planning and implementation • Makes explicit the key steps, timelines, and incremental resources required for implementation • Identifies responsibilities and accountabilities for actions • Completes strategic plan and results in board approval	• Carefully thought-out plan to finish process and gain necessary approvals • Ongoing process-tracking system, defined and agreed on by leadership • Priorities set by top-level leadership, especially among competing needs of operating units

© 2017 Veralon Partners Inc.

that better support their risk-contracting success. Physician frustration leaves long-lasting scars in physician–hospital relations. It is, therefore, critical to actually implement strategy.

A clear implementation plan can help maintain focus and accountability for all involved—healthcare enterprise management, physicians, hospital leaders, and organizational partners. Given that healthcare enterprises will succeed based on mutual trust and mutual success, accountability and follow-through are extremely important.

CONCLUSION

Strategic planning can help drive an organization forward to address boldly a complex environment through a unified effort. As healthcare enterprises seek to deliver value and bear risk in an increasingly complex competitive environment, strategic planning is a critical tool for achieving success.

REFERENCES

Harris, J. M., and R. Hemnani. 2013. "The Transition to Emerging Revenue Models." *HFM* 67 (4): 54–63.

Kornacki, M. J. 2015. *A New Compact: Aligning Physician–Organization Expectations to Transform Patient Care*. Chicago: Health Administration Press.

CHAPTER 6

Models and Competencies for Clinical Integration

Jon Burroughs
Carl Couch

CLINICAL INTEGRATION BETWEEN healthcare organizations and physicians is a necessary condition in the twenty-first century—achieving any of the quadruple aim (cost, quality, patient experience, provider experience) will be impossible without it. This chapter discusses many of the elements of clinical integration, including legal definitions and current models. We also discuss the Baylor Scott & White Quality Alliance, an accountable care organization, to examine the finer details of its complex and challenging conversion to a more sustainable structure.

SEVEN LEGAL COMPONENTS OF CLINICAL INTEGRATION

In 1996, the Federal Trade Commission and Department of Justice created a legal definition of a clinically integrated network (CIN) that consists of seven fundamental components to support healthcare organizations' efforts to pursue this goal: legal structure, physician leadership, physician and practitioner participation, performance improvement, information technology, contracting options, and flow of funds.

Legal Structure

To qualify as a CIN, the health system and physicians must create an organized structure that supports its program objectives; these may include a physician–hospital organization (PHO), an independent practice association (IPA), or a subsidiary of the organization that requires participating physicians to sign separate legal agreements to participate. Typically, such an organization becomes a contracting entity to negotiate with third-party payers, large employers, health plans, or health maintenance organizations (HMOs) to achieve mutually beneficial clinical and business objectives. The entity typically focuses on the coordination of care through a partnership model, with both employed and self-employed physicians, to create and achieve performance improvement initiatives through the creation of risk-based contracts. These structures may be created de novo or built on the foundation of an existing structure, such as a legacy PHO, IPA, or HMO.

Physician Leadership

True physician–executive collaboration requires physician leadership and education in pursuit of enterprise business and management skills. Leadership training is an investment with a calculable return based on improved ability to lead other physicians to monetized quality outcomes. Both employed and self-employed physicians require alignment under the oversight of respected physician leaders.

To ensure accountability for organizational goals, clinical integration should be underpinned by a governance structure comprising physician and nonphysician executive leaders. Such governance may oversee diverse areas such as quality, safety, service, finance (compensation models), operations, marketing, contracting, and human resources. Such governing boards may have subcommittees that should ideally be integrated and aligned with existing structures on the organized medical staff and separate subsidiaries (e.g., employed physician groups) so that there is no duplication or redundancy. When an organizational layer is added, the existing structure should be simplified and consolidated to compensate so that the level of complexity does not become excessive. Common subcommittees include executive, quality, safety, compensation, and contracting.

Physician and Practitioner Participation

Organizations should require all physicians and practitioners who participate in a CIN to sign an agreement outlining expectations and requirements for participation. These agreements may involve any kind of legally binding document that sets forth the goals and objectives of the program and the obligation of all participants to adhere to mutually agreed-on guidelines and standards. Such requirements may include general guidelines and standards as determined by both physicians and management; full engagement with information technology; evidence-based guidelines as determined by physician leadership; use of transparent, unblinded clinical and business analytics; participation in all network contracts; and compliance with legal, regulatory, and accreditation issues.

Performance Improvement

Clinical quality and operational improvement projects are required in a CIN. Physicians are expected to both lead and to take an active role in the creation, development, and oversight of these important initiatives. The establishment of quality goals or objectives; performance metrics with benchmarks; and standardized reports to physicians, practitioners, and leadership are essential components. The ability to operationalize such aligned programs requires a robust health information management (HIM) infrastructure. Such programs are essential in pay-for-value contracts; metrics should be aligned with strategic organizational and payer requirements. Projects are varied and may include eliminating non-value-added clinical and managerial variation; optimizing quality, safety, or service; avoiding unnecessary services; reducing costs; transforming care or business approaches; developing population health services; and aligning organizational and community healthcare objectives.

Information Technology

HIM technology is a necessary foundation for the provision and tracking of quality healthcare services. Like every other industry, healthcare is becoming fully digitized. Its new frontier encompasses many innovations, including electronic health records (EHRs), practitioner and patient portals, and electronic decision supports to guide patient management and treatment. All practitioners, organizations, and facilities must use these tools to become seamlessly interconnected through health information exchanges (HIEs), permitting the treatment of individuals throughout the continuum of care.

The rapid growth of clinical and business analytics, supported by an enterprise data warehouse (EDW), is a mandatory component of clinical integration—they permit organizations to monitor the cost and quality of healthcare in real time; use predictive analytics to risk-stratify subpopulations; and contract with payers, large employers, and health plans. Many organizations adopt e-health strategies to permit routine healthcare services in real time at a cost far less than the cost of traditional services and to create greater convenience for patients. Accreditors increasingly require organizations to maintain databases of patients to support the early identification and treatment of potentially life-threatening diseases and complications. Disease management and palliative care programs use standardized evidence-based care pathways to promote a rule-based approach to the optimization of healthcare outcomes delivered through precision medical units.

Contracting Options

Pay-for-value contracts that place participating organizations at risk for clinical and business outcomes are a growing phenomenon. They are spurred by large employers and healthcare organizations, the Centers for Medicare & Medicaid Services (CMS), and commercial carriers interested in partnering with healthcare organizations committed to value. Value-based contracts may be for a population of covered lives (population health), a particular procedure across the continuum of care (bundles), or specific services to a defined population (e.g., advanced primary care, patient-centered medical homes [PCMHs], or accountable care organizations [ACOs]). Pay-for-value contracts often have a financial upside and a financial downside for contractual incentives or penalties (based on mutually agreed-on benchmarks) and increased rates (based on optimized quality and cost); they also have performance initiatives and sometimes shared savings or gainsharing as rewards for decreasing the total cost of care by a predefined amount. Some CINs act as for-profit or not-for-profit subsidiaries of a parent healthcare organization and contract with the parent entity.

Flow of Funds

A CIN must calculate and distribute funds based on quality and business outcomes prenegotiated with payers and other contractors. These distributions may be system based, network based, or organization based and are allocated according to predesigned contractual methodologies. Some distributions are based on specific quality, safety, and service metrics; a global budget for the total cost of care; or specialty, individual, or aggregate performance. Regardless of the methodology, it should be transparent to all parties, easy to understand, and monitored by all involved stakeholders. Ideally, all business and clinical analytics should be openly shared with relevant parties, and information-sharing agreements should be created to support the unencumbered flow of clinical and business information throughout the continuum of care on a need-to-know basis, according to professional roles and accountabilities.

CURRENT MODELS OF CLINICAL INTEGRATION

Several models of clinical integration are found throughout the country, including advanced primary care, PCMHs, the bundled-payment model, and ACOs. They are discussed in the following sections.

Advanced Primary Care

The advanced primary care model was developed by CMS to support a more comprehensive primary care delivery system, particularly for complex patients who require multiple community-based services. It is related to the PCMH. In advanced primary care, a patient is cared for by a primary provider and a care coordinator who manage the needs of patients who represent greater risk and cost and who can benefit from a more robust primary care model. This model works well with alternative payment models such as bundled care, population-based payments, global budgeting, or some form of capitation.

Care may be delivered through traditional practices or through alternative models such as an ACO, a PCMH, or a CIN. There may be multipayer participation with performance measures developed and monitored by clinicians, payers, and patients.

Patient-Centered Medical Homes

The PCMH is a care delivery model whereby treatment of a patient is coordinated through his primary care physician to ensure he receives the necessary care when and where he needs it, in a manner he can understand.

The objective is to have a centralized setting that facilitates partnerships between individual patients, their personal physicians, and, when appropriate, their family. Care is facilitated by registries, information technology, HIEs, and other means to ensure that patients get the indicated care in a culturally and linguistically appropriate manner.

The National Committee for Quality Assurance (NCQA) accredits organizations and practices that seek to become PCMHs through the following six standards:

1. *Patient-centered access.* Offer team-based care and provide convenient and readily accessible services to patients both during and beyond regular office hours. Patients should have prompt access to members of the healthcare team through direct, portal, and e-health access.
2. *Team-based care.* Meet the cultural and linguistic needs of patients through team-based approaches and customize the care to the patient's unique personal values.
3. *Population health management.* Collect and use data for population health management. This effort requires predictive clinical and business analytics supported by an EDW that can stratify populations of covered lives into subpopulations with unique clinical care plans.
4. *Care management and support.* Use evidence-based rules to optimize prevention and the management of individuals with acute and chronic conditions.
5. *Care coordination and care transitions.* Ensure seamless provision across the continuum of care through the

coordination and tracking of tests, treatments, handoffs, and care coordination.

6. *Performance measurement and quality improvement.* Use of performance improvement methodologies to upgrade the quality of care continuously.

Each of the NCQA's standards must be met to achieve accreditation. PCMHs can be organized in almost any setting, within almost any organizational structure, as long as the fundamental characteristics of patient centeredness, coordination of care, and team-based collaboration and a culture of continuous performance improvement are emphasized. Good examples include Martin's Point Health Care, ProvenHealth Navigator, Community Care of North Carolina, and the Integrated Behavioral Health Project.

Martin's Point Health Care, operating in New Hampshire and Maine, is a stand-alone primary care healthcare delivery system unaffiliated with any hospital. It boasts seven healthcare centers and two health plans. It is a physician-led not-for-profit whose modular office design ensures flexibility with onstage and offstage areas and collaborative work spaces for team-based care. Martin's Point has a low-cost structure with a Lean emphasis and provides data-driven care with informatics and analytics.

Geisinger Health System's ProvenHealth Navigator in Pennsylvania was initially focused on the elderly and then expanded to include all beneficiaries of commercial health plans. It now drives a significant drop in readmission rates, as well as reduced visits to emergency departments (ED) and physicians' offices, through a more comprehensive and proactive approach to individuals with chronic and high-risk diseases. It administers specialized programs that focus on cardiac care and elective surgery.

Community Care of North Carolina comprises 14 regional networks that serve the state's dual-eligible population (Medicare and Medicaid) with a specialized focus on children. Its care is targeted toward at-risk populations and specific diseases. Community Care features a well-developed palliative care program and works to identify high-yield transitional care opportunities, reduce ED utilization, and optimize screening rates. It also seeks to reduce Medicaid spending and preventable hospitalizations.

In California, the Integrated Behavioral Health Project focuses on accelerating the integration of behavioral health into primary care throughout the state. It features a data-driven strategic focus with clinical and business analytics, which it uses to focus on high-risk populations. The organization emphasizes care for patients with complex, difficult-to-manage conditions.

Key Trends

The challenge of the PCMH model is to drive the cost structure downward, which will, in turn, permit sustainable margins while improving outcomes. To drive costs down, organizations can employ every member of the healthcare team to the full range of his licensed duties. Successful PCMHs standardize, digitize, and commoditize the traditional primary care process so that it can be delivered effectively at a fraction of the cost.

The development of the PCMH has seen the emergence of a number of important trends. They include the following:

- Physician-guided, team-delivered care
- Data-driven policies with robust use of predictive and real-time clinical and business analytics; EDWs
- Integration of behavioral health with all clinical areas
- Team-based workflows to ensure comprehensive interdisciplinary input
- Alternatives to traditional, office-based visits, including e-visits, home visits, retail clinic access, and customized patient portals
- Price transparency, with at-risk arrangements for all parties (e.g., providers, payers, patients)
- Customized decision support tools for consumers

- Direct-to-employer and health plan contracting for population health services

Bundled-Payment Model

Bundled payments are another model of clinical integration. The Bundled Payments for Care Improvement initiative was developed by CMS in an effort to maintain or optimize healthcare outcomes while driving down costs. It was designed as a middle ground between fee-for-service and capitation to enable facilities and practitioners to work together to standardize care and business practices in a partial-risk situation and was originally organized into four evolving models.

Model 1 is a bundling of hospital-based care for inpatient visits using a discounted diagnosis-related group payment and traditional fee-for-service payments to physicians.

Models 2 and 3, on the other hand, are retrospective payment models. In model 2, actual expenditures are reconciled against a targeted cost for defined episodes of care. The episode is defined as acute care plus 90 days of post-acute care services. In model 3, the episode is triggered by an acute care visit but begins with the initiation of post-acute care, including skilled nursing facilities, outpatient rehabilitation facilities, home health care, and nursing homes.

Model 4 is a prospective payment system. It provides a single payment for defined episodes of care to hospitals, facilities, and physicians. The episode is defined as the inpatient visit. Models 2 through 4 cover 48 separate episodes of care, including problems such as joint replacement, stroke, renal failure, and gastrointestinal obstruction.

At the outset, CMS advocated the mandatory use of the bundled-payment model with the Comprehensive Care for Joint Replacement program. CMS then expanded the mandate to include the Advancing Care Coordination Through Episode Payment Model and the Cardiac Rehabilitation Incentive Payment Model. All three are designated as alternative payment models under the Medicare Access and CHIP Reauthorization Act, which entitles physicians to a potential 5 percent payment boost under Medicare Part B. Political pressures delayed the implementation of further mandatory bundled-payment programs through January 2018; however, at the time of writing, more than 500 healthcare organizations across the country had moved forward with these programs in an attempt to optimize both clinical and business outcomes. CMS is once again offering a care improvement initiative to further expand the number and varieties of bundled-payment programs available on a voluntary basis, optimizing quality and reducing costs.

What do bundled-payment programs require for success? The following are among the critical factors:

- An integrated and aligned physician staff with at-risk contracts
- Clinical and business analytics that provide real-time and predictive information to support at-risk contracts among key parties
- Robust clinical and business leadership
- Service line or institutional structures to support greater standardization and control over both clinical and business processes
- A culture of transparency, unblinded performance data, and accountability
- An interdisciplinary process of value analysis intended to optimize labor and supply chain spending through the use of relevant labor analytics and supply chain simplification

Regardless of the politics, the bundled-payment model represents an essential stepping stone in the transition from volume-based fee-for-service to the inevitable payment models that will evolve in the near future.

Accountable Care Organizations

The ACO is another model of clinical integration. Various definitions of the term all similarly describe bringing physicians, hospitals, and others into a clinically integrated organization willing to be held accountable for both the quality and cost of services for specific populations. Multiple organizational structures are possible for ACOs, including physician only, physician–hospital, and payer, to name a few.

The Affordable Care Act of 2010 encouraged the creation of ACOs for Medicare recipients and created shared-savings models that allowed some of the savings to be retained by the delivery organizations if quality parameters were exceeded. Clinically integrated organizations emerged and were required to meet substantial legal and regulatory requirements.

On closer examination, the disruptive nature of accountable care quickly becomes apparent: in a fee-for-service world, reducing unnecessary care, avoiding admissions, avoiding unnecessary procedures, and reducing ED visits all may result in lost revenue for either the hospital or the physicians, or both. Yet the movement to value is occurring rapidly and must continue.

Success as an ACO can be tricky, but many factors contribute to a positive outcome. For example, the healthcare system must take into consideration the disruptive impact of the ACO on other organizational components. Reasonable rewards and incentives will help along the way; however, participants must be committed to the journey toward value or incentives will be insufficient. Moreover, ACOs require accountable leaders at the physician, nursing, administrative, and payer levels—people who are willing to assume personal and organizational accountability for measureable clinical and cost outcomes.

As another example, the delivery of care must itself be transformed in successful ACOs. Care coordination, typically by a care coordinator who is a registered nurse with a deep knowledge and understanding of the healthcare system, will ensure cost-effective care and services. Relatedly, PCMHs, particularly for complex patients with multisystem or chronic diseases, can help drive an ACO toward success. To optimize clinical and business outcomes, it is helpful to integrate behavioral therapy into primary and specialty care. Wellness assistance and behavioral health should be a basic component of both insurance design and clinical care.

Clinical integration of all relevant participants, including self-employed and specialty physicians, is necessary to ensure comprehensive services and alignment of mutually agreed-on key performance indicators consistent with the organization's overarching goals and objectives.

Many of the elements of a successful ACO involve policies and administration beyond care provision. The organization must offer an insurance plan design that meets the needs of employers, payers, organizations, providers, and patients. It should also provide analytics on cost and quality at the payer, organizational, regional, and individual levels. Actionable information allows real-time modification of clinical and business practices to optimize quality and minimize costs.

AN IN-DEPTH LOOK AT THE BAYLOR SCOTT & WHITE QUALITY ALLIANCE

Texas is home to a particularly interesting example of clinical integration—the Baylor Scott & White Quality Alliance (BSWQA). The process began in 2012, when Baylor Health Care System in Dallas created an ACO—the Baylor Quality Alliance. Following the 2013 merger of Baylor Health Care System with Scott & White Healthcare, the organization was named Baylor Scott & White Quality Alliance, a wholly owned, not-for-profit subsidiary of Baylor Scott & White Health. Today, BSWQA is one of the largest ACOs in the country, with 5,200 physicians and 46 hospitals, providing post-acute care services to more than 460,000 patients. BSWQA has moderated the rise of healthcare costs by creating substantial savings while improving quality in many areas.

Fundamentally, Baylor believes that there are four key parts in the organizational design of the ACO: (1) point of entry for care, (2) clinical integration, (3) population health infrastructure, and (4) sustainable financing.

Point of Entry for Care

Today the healthcare industry boasts many options for patient entry, including mobile video or e-visits and retail pharmacy clinics, as well as traditional practices. Baylor created a new point of entry—the Member Solution Center at BSWQA, which helps people make optimal choices based on personal values and insurance coverage.

In general, contracts between an ACO and payers require a download of historic and ongoing claims data for any given population based on previous care. Today, most ACO contracts with payers are based on shared-savings financial models, where total actuary-predicted cost targets are measured annually against the actual spending. Any excess savings are shared between participants. Health insurance plan benefit designs offer the greatest financial benefit to patients for remaining in-network, with the remainder being an out-of-pocket obligation. In our experience, patients choose to remain in-network in significant numbers when they are responsible for at least 50 percent of the cost of out-of-network care. This limitation results in a significant number of patient choices to remain in network.

Beginning the patient–provider relationship with a solid PCMH is ideal. The benefits of coordinated care are significant, in terms of both cost to patients and better clinical outcomes.

Once enrolled in a benefit plan contracted with BSWQA, Baylor Scott & White found that an initial and annual proactive wellness and biometric assessment launches an identification of risks, allows closure of preventive care gaps, and initiates a therapeutic doctor–patient relationship once patients are enrolled in a benefit plan. Moving forward, patients have a comprehensive care plan for identifying clinical conditions. In addition, this assessment allows segmentation and predictive modeling of the population so that population health resources can be directed proportionally to those with the greatest need. In the broader healthcare field, patients with complex conditions may be referred to a nonintegrated specialist when more time and attention from a primary care physician (PCP) would be sufficient. Recognizing this, BSWQA has determined that additional reward allocation to primary care is necessary to support PCPs' function as "comprehensivists."

In BSWQA, shared-savings rewards disproportionately flow to PCPs. Those who have larger panels of complex patients are also disproportionately rewarded for the complexity of that care. The PCPs and specialists recognize the higher compensation to be necessary because of the additional work required to manage such patients, coordinate care between specialists and hospitals, and interact regularly with care coordinators.

PCMHs are a cornerstone of the entry point. Today, all BSWQA primary care practices—more than 600 of them—are level-3 NCQA certified (the highest level). The homes are structured around team-based care, evidence-based guidelines, data-driven performance improvement, continuous relationships with personal physicians, electronic and personal access to care, full adoption of EHRs, use of patient portals, freely available educational information, care coordination, and proactive outreach. BSWQA primary care practices complete all preventive services at a rate of nearly 90 percent. They exhibit an 86 percent control of hypertension to less than 140 over 90, exceptional diabetes scores, and high patient satisfaction. Allied services include advanced-practice providers, embedded care coordinators, behavioral therapists, scribes, electronic prescription-refill centers, and performance dashboards at the physicians' fingertips.

Transforming a primary care practice into a team-based, comprehensive care environment changes the role of the PCP, allowing all members of the team in a PCMH to perform the full range of duties they are licensed to do, freeing physicians to perform at the top of their license. The result is better access and team leadership by a PCP, with less need on her part to see every patient. In fact, delegation of work to lower-level providers has been shown to improve care. Most important of all, however, these transformed practices are restoring the joy doctors take in their craft.

Clinical Integration

Integration begins at the governance level. BSWQA's board of managers comprises 21 members, one of whom is a patient and 18 of whom are practicing physicians. A physician chair leads the organization, supported by the president and management team. Key committees include Membership and Standards, Finance, and Best Care. The Best Care Committee is essentially the quality heartbeat of the organization, defining, implementing, monitoring, and improving evidence-based care. Realizing that physicians want to define and approve the standards they hold themselves to, the Best Care Committee brings clinical expertise, national guidelines, specialty standards, and evidence to the table in creating every protocol. The ability to measure a protocol or guideline is important—nonmeasurable standards are frustrating to physicians, so the committee limits protocols and guidelines to objective, measurable criteria. Managing what can't be measured is an impossible task.

Integrated care must be built around patients, spanning the progression from wellness, through illness, and back to health and functional improvement. Wellness initiatives (historically an employer-offered benefit) have been shown to play a very large role in healthcare. Even CMS has begun to offer an annual wellness visit to enrollees. Most seasoned clinicians know that the wellness exam provides a comprehensive opportunity to assess risks, document existing problems, and establish care paths for those problems. This extended visit ideally engages patients around a shared decision-making process and an agreed-on care plan. Goals can be set for health improvement. Counseling regarding disease management and initiatives such as exercise, weight control, and drug misuse can occur during this important exam. Further, it offers an opportunity to coordinate input from multiple specialists, with the PCMH team serving as the coordinative resource for complex patients. BSWQA has made annual wellness exams a priority for all Medicare and Medicare Advantage patients.

BSWQA has made an effort to address handoff issues. In the current fragmented care world, handoffs between venues are treacherous. For example, BSWQA nurse care coordinators know that medication reconciliation problems are almost universal when patients transition from hospital to home. They now assume that there are disconnects, misunderstandings, or redundancies in complex medication algorithms, so they always begin a posthospital encounter with an attempt to reconcile those discrepancies. They report that, often, half of the care coordinator's first visit with any patient is devoted to solving medication issues. As a result, these professionals uncover major medication-related problems, prevent ED visits, and avert unnecessary admissions. One care coordinator discovered a single patient who had almost 40 medications on hand. A pharmacist was dispatched to the home, and an almost-certain bad outcome was prevented. These nurses represent the most important resource in delivering integrated care. Similarly, these nurses frequently find discordant advice from multiple specialists; lack of clarity about who is managing what; and even lack of clarity about diagnosis, treatment, and prognosis. Including these coordinators in the chronic disease management team dramatically improves integration.

At BSWQA, most care coordination is done remotely, but as primary care practices increase their proportion of ACO members, some are attempting to embed the nurse in the practice itself. However, he should not be used as an adjunct office staffer but rather as a specialized team member coordinating complex care. To leverage technology and extend the nurse's effectiveness, remote electronic and biometric monitoring should be deployed for the sickest patients, such as those with advanced heart failure and chronic obstructive pulmonary disease. Such technology is enabling closer, timelier, more objective monitoring of clinical indicators of deterioration. The costs are offset by a reduction in unnecessary services, resulting in global population cost savings. The possibility of extending the scope of disease management and gaining better clinical results with these technologies is promising.

At BSWQA, a team of advanced nurse practitioners, overseen by geriatricians, perform house calls for frail, elderly patients. Their patients are near the end of life, have mobility problems, and are cared for in the home setting. The results have been a notable reduction in ED use and hospital admissions, a near 100 percent completion of advance directives, and a large majority of patients electing to be at home as life ends. Patient and family satisfaction with this coordinated, hands-on care method is high.

Clinical integration between specialists and primary care is hard work. Protocols must be jointly developed by specialists and PCPs treating the same condition. BSWQA expects communication between providers, and it is facilitated when all practitioners are able to access the same EHR. The HIE described later in the chapter facilitates communication as well. As a result, BSWQA coordinates care paths more easily, averts redundant tests, and improves patients' understanding of their care. The organization created more than 125 care protocols in multispecialty and specialty subcommittees, all approved by the Best Care Committee and posted on its secure website.

Integration of behavioral health into care delivery is a critical success factor for true clinical integration. In the past, behavioral therapy benefits were carved out of insurance design and delivered in a fashion that did not blend with general care. BSWQA believed that this was unacceptable because primary mental health issues, as well as mental health comorbidity, require holistic clinical integration. For example, a patient with four or five chronic diseases is often depressed as she contends with daily illness. Complex patients are routinely screened for anxiety and depression in BSWQA, allowing early intervention. Healthcare economists rank behavioral or mental health costs among the three or four most expensive in the United States.

To integrate behavioral health and to escalate its implementation in the case of behavioral necessity and disease severity, BSWQA uses two strategies. It embeds a behavioral therapist into larger primary care clinics, and it employs a multilevel behavioral strategy using licensed professional counselors and family therapists at the lowest level of severity, psychologists at the next level, and psychiatrists at the highest level. Behavioral telehealth is being tried, with promising early results.

BSWQA's dedication to integration extends to contractual physician alignment. Merging primary care, specialty care, hospital care, ambulatory surgical center care, post-acute care, and home care into an accountable alliance is challenging. Before joining BSWQA, every physician must meet several demands:

- Agree to the values of transformational leadership and care
- Pay a one-time membership fee
- Be accountable for quality, safety, service, and cost-effectiveness
- Use an approved EHR

The cultural challenges inherent in bringing independent self-employed and system-employed physicians together were anticipated from the outset. Regardless of their employment status, from the outset, BSWQA insisted that all physicians needed to establish and use approved evidence-based guidelines. The organization needed to build electronic connectivity for the exchange of clinical data supported by an EDW and drawn from clinical and financial analytics.

Changing practice patterns, responding to data indicative of quality and cost variation, and creating a culture of accountability require time, vision, and committed leadership. For physicians who live in a fee-for-service world, the daily impact of an ACO is minimal until they accumulate a significant number of contracted lives. Currently in BSWQA, nearly one in four primary care patients is in the ACO, with most physicians increasingly mindful of alternative dispositions and value expectations when caring for these patients. BSWQA is delivering higher-quality care, and the market is recognizing that performance.

Population Health Infrastructure

To pursue the third key part in the organizational design of an ACO, population health infrastructure, BSWQA has used technological innovations, wellness initiatives, and staff-based solutions.

Technological Innovations

The first element of BSWQA's approach to population health is technology. For example, the alliance uses several risk-stratifying and predictive software systems but currently finds a home-grown system to be of best predictive capability for total expenditures, preventable hospital admission avoidance, and unnecessary ED use. Use of this predictive capability guides its care integration and deployment of coordination resources.

Good data and analytics are key to managing any population. BSWQA believes that data can be categorized in two general ways: data for care and data for performance. BSWQA collects these data via required EHRs and downloads of claims from payers for all ACO-contracted patients. However, one of the drawbacks of the Affordable Care Act of 2010 was that it generated a proliferation of different types of EHRs; as a consequence, BSWQA independent physicians were found to use 72 different brands. The problem of acquiring information in such a diverse electronic environment is immediately apparent. How can a patient's clinical information be tracked between sites of care or between physicians? How can their noncommunicating, stand-alone EHRs share performance data with the alliance?

One solution to the surfeit of record types has been the emergence of HIE tools. BSWQA purchased a good HIE that connects its diverse EHR sources well. A patient's information in any EHR is viewable in a drop-down menu that allows his problems, medications, allergies, recent X-ray and laboratory test reports, and visit summaries to be seen on the practitioner's own platform without launching an additional program. This feature has begun to cut down on redundant testing, save clinicians time retrieving essential information, and promote clinical integration. In an ideal world, every clinical site would use the same EHR, but a state-of-the-art HIE has proven to be the next best solution.

Collecting all of the clinical data into a common database and supplementing those data with a full download of claims for all patients from each contracted population allow construction of reports on both quality and cost data. These reports are produced in BSWQA for four types of data:

1. *Organizational data.* Performance dashboards measure the overall health of the enterprise and guide the leadership and management in understanding costs, cost-reduction opportunities, outlier performance, and progress on spending targets. Each population has a targeted annual expenditure determined by an actuary. Shared-savings rewards to BSWQA members depend on care delivery spending below that target.

2. *Regional and local data.* Because care is largely delivered on a local level, BSWQA is divided into nine geographic regions or "pods." PCPs, specialty physicians, and their nearby hospital facilities meet quarterly in pods to review comparative pod performance, as well as individual physician performance, in a transparent environment. These pod meetings generate both the interest and the engagement of physicians, capitalizing on their spirit of professional competitiveness and acknowledging high performers. Pod-to-pod comparison has sparked regional competitiveness and shared learning about processes of care and best practices.

3. *Specific physician performance data.* Statistics on performance are simultaneously viewable to all PCPs and

specialists in the system. These "Data at the Bedside" reports are available in password-protected physician dashboards on the BSWQA website. They are also individually reviewed with physicians by pod medical directors on a quarterly basis. Medical directors host lunch-and-learn sessions on improvement opportunities, which are well attended by both physicians and their practice administrators. Most physicians do not wish to be performance outliers and when shown credible data, most will engage in steps to improve their performance. However, BSWQA has the ability to review continually poor performance or noncompliance in a fair, peer-reviewed manner, resulting in exclusion from BSWQA if escalation progresses that far. Physicians come to trust the data, and they experience growing pride in knowing that their practices are delivering high-quality, cost-effective care in a manner pleasing to patients.

4. *Patient satisfaction data.* This information also is presented on a physician-by-physician basis, with comparison to peers.

Wellness Initiatives

BSWQA has put a variety of solutions in place to cultivate healthy behaviors. For example, it works with employers to create incentives for healthy eating, exercise, weight control, and smoking cessation for their workforces. When combined with wellness exams and biometric screening, these opportunities can be reinforced by the medical home team. Convenient access to information on healthy lifestyles from BSWQA and employers also helps patients be smart about well-being. Integration of wellness activities with community and public health resources—such as food banks, YMCAs, social services, transportation resources, medication financial assistance programs, and local public health clinics—can give at-risk strata of the population the tools they need to prevent disease. The BSWQA

Care Coordination Department employs several social workers who are integrally involved in care, particularly in complex cases.

Staff-Based Solutions

Many of the solutions that BSWQA has created have been staff based. As discussed earlier, the organization employs nurse care coordinators, who incorporate health and self-care tools into their encounters, often using motivational learning techniques. They are skilled in both primary and secondary disease prevention as well as the management of complex diseases. Primary care and specialty physicians regard the nurse care coordinators as valuable team members. In fact, all of its clinic physicians and nurses use techniques that effectively engage patients to perform self-care. All medical home team members can contribute, each working at the top of his license to reinforce healthy behavior at every opportunity. The care they give integrates behavioral therapy with primary care. BSWQA employees also furnish convenient access to educationally, culturally, and linguistically appropriate educational opportunities, including electronic patient education.

BSWQA's experience clearly shows that the three most effective elements of reducing cost and improving quality are (1) care coordination by nurses for highest-acuity patients, (2) PCMHs that deliver comprehensive care, and (3) actionable data and analytics that allow performance to be measured in real time. Although most care coordination initially centered on primary care practices, specialty-specific performance has begun to have a great effect. The BSWQA care coordination infrastructure is expanded to look at care across the hospital-to-ambulatory environment. At Baylor Scott & White Health, more than 200 inpatient care coordinators and more than 50 ambulatory care coordinators are under a common managerial structure. Today, the act of hospital discharge is regarded as a transitional event, not the end of care. Discharged patients are called promptly by ambulatory coordinators; care plans are reviewed by nurses and coordinated among primary care physicians, specialty physicians, and post-acute care facilities. All post-acute services (skilled nursing and home health) are provided by carefully selected BSWQA members who voluntarily join the organization, agreeing to be accountable for measurement and performance of goals (e.g., avoidance of unnecessary readmissions, falls, and pressure ulcers; completion of advance directives; adherence to care plans). They submit data to a post-acute care dashboard, viewable on the BSWQA website in a comparative performance format.

Sustainable Financing

BSWQA's fourth and final element of ACO success is sustainable financing. Across the United States, the most common method of ACO financing is to share the global population cost savings (shared savings plans, or SS) between payers (or employers) and the providers. The two original Medicare ACO plans are based on that model. Shared savings can be one-sided, with no financial risk to the provider organization, or two-sided, with greater opportunity for positive incentives but actual downside financial risk to providers if costs exceed targeted expenditures. BSWQA initially participated in only one-sided savings models, but it has recently begun to accept downside risk in select contracts (a two-sided model).

A second method of financing is to create bundled-payment methods. Participants are incentivized to produce high-quality outcomes at the lowest cost, avoiding unnecessary expenditures. Low quality and adverse outcomes are considered events that the providers must rectify without additional remuneration. Good outcomes, cost-effectiveness, and high patient satisfaction are necessary to sustain the bundling contract with the payer. If the provider is successful in delivering that bundled care, the ACO distributes any residual funds among participants. Bundled-payment methods can exist in a population-based ACO or as stand-alone payments to willing participants.

Risk-based payments for accountable care involve providers being at risk for both positive and negative financial outcomes in a population. Full risk (capitation) involves transfer of essentially the entire healthcare premium or budgeted amount to the provider organization, which in turn administers all expenses for the care of that population annually. It retains surpluses but absorbs excess expenditures. Stop-loss agreements can be purchased to deal with catastrophic cases. Risk agreements can involve full risk or partial risk (such as the Medicare Pioneer two-sided risk contracts) and may have defined risk-reward corridors that limit both the upside opportunity and downside risk to the organization. All of these models have further contractual requirements that quality thresholds must be maintained or exceeded, and many (such as measures required by the Medicare Shared Savings Program) include access and service expectations as well as patient satisfaction targets.

Each of these innovative payment models was created to align providers with incentives to deliver high-value care. The most successful methodologies involve clear assignment of patient care duties to providers as well as patient incentives and engagement strategies to induce them to remain in the network. Addition and removal of individual patients to and from the population cohort must be carefully monitored. For shared-savings programs, careful, actuarially determined targets must be established. The quality and service of the providers and the organization itself are important in order to keep patients in the network year after year, and the organization must both deliver quality and prove its value to the payer community.

Funding the services needed to provide quality healthcare, such as care coordination, initially requires willingness from the employer or payer to reimburse the ACO for those services. Most care coordination programs require ratios of 1 nurse for every 200 patients in the top 5 percent stratum of acuity. Funding care coordinators for those sickest patients costs between $2 and $3 per member per month. Yet it is critical that the coordination function be delivered within the ACO, and not by the payer. BSWQA found that engagement levels by patients with nurse care coordinators are 400 percent higher when the ACO assumes that function previously provided by insurance carriers. As a result, BSWQA patients regard their care coordinators as an extension of their physician's practice, and their level of engagement proves far superior to disease management systems under traditional health plans.

New data systems were required for BSWQA, including purchase of the HIE, predictive modeling tools, care coordination tools, and analytic software. ACO-specific physician leadership and management was created to both focus and perform the value-based work of transforming care. Initial capitalization was necessary to launch the ACO because in most shared-savings models, no rewards can be anticipated for at least 18 months (12 months of performance with an additional 3 months of claims washout and 3 months of reconciliation to break even). The infrastructure and organizational capability has to be of such quality to support the movement toward eventual risk assumption. Building the ACO infrastructure has to occur concurrently with the recruitment of a geographic and specialty access panel of providers for potential members. As a result of the geographic extent of the Dallas-Ft. Worth metroplex, currently almost 5,200 physicians are needed to provide sufficient access.

For financial sustainability through strong income streams, providers must observe proper coding procedures. For example, for Medicare Advantage patients, good coding is linked to accurate reporting for each patient, and it limits the number of patients for whom who must be recoded annually; otherwise, CMS assumes that the beneficiary's health diagnoses disappear on January 1. Educating physicians to properly capture these codes annually is vital because the severity codes generate a risk-adjustment factor score, which in turn determines the amount of money that the Medicare Advantage carrier receives for each patient that year. Failure to code properly results in a huge opportunity cost because the entire population looks healthier than it actually is (which also has an adverse impact on quality scores). In fact, BSWQA created coding seminars for physicians, and it uses professional coders to identify proper coding opportunities. However, the learning curve for adoption of proper coding often causes lower-than-expected financial performance during the first year of contracts, and that effect must be taken into account by organizations seeking to develop their own ACO.

Baylor Scott & White Quality Alliance and Employers

Commercial insurance in the Dallas-Fort Worth market is 75–80 percent employer funded rather than fully insured by the carriers. In such employer-funded plans, the insurance companies are merely third-party administrators, with the employers at full financial risk. The initial target population for BSWQA was Baylor Health Care System's 34,000 employees and employee dependents. In the first three years of care, the alliance generated more than 7 percent savings over target spending. The total savings amounted to more than $36 million over three years. Notably, BSWQA's annual cost increase is virtually flat in comparison with the 6 percent annual increase for the commercially insured population of Dallas-Fort Worth. The summary result of performance in the first three years is no increase in population cost versus an aggregated 18 percent cost increase for non-BSWQA patients in the community. As a result, BSWQA began holding employer forums, educating about insurance benefit design that can support these value achievements.

The seven key elements of benefit design that we asked employers to consider include wellness integration, the establishment of PCMH relationships, preferred or narrow-network plan design, claims receipt by the ACO, direct-to-employer contracts, state-of-the-art consumer-focused mobile apps, and other opportunities.

Wellness Integration

Wellness programs, health risk appraisals, and biometric testing are incorporated into the delivery model. Such offerings may be coupled with employer incentives to encourage patients to lose weight, exercise, or stop smoking. Historically, these benefits were not well connected to the healthcare system—information is given only to the patient, and with little or no clinical follow-up. However, ideally, the data should be incorporated into the patient's EHR and reviewed in her medical home.

Establishment of PCMH Relationships

PCMHs are proven to produce better outcomes at lower costs. Employer incentives through benefit design that encourage and facilitate participation (e.g., first appointment on enrollment in the plan is personally facilitated) are effective.

Preferred or Narrow-Network Plan Design

Another element of benefit design that BSWQA discussed with employers was narrow-network plans. Patients who drift geographically have the most disconnected care and often experience higher costs and poorer outcomes. In the 10-county metroplex of Dallas-Fort Worth, BSWQA made great effort to establish sufficient primary care and specialty physician coverage within these networks, easing access problems. To incentivize cost-saving, plans maximize coverage benefits when the patient remains in the network.

Employers worry that being too restrictive with a narrow network will result in higher employee dissatisfaction and turnover, but, at the same time, they want a healthier workforce and lower costs. In BSWQA's first years, a benefit payment differential of at least 50 percent between in-network and out-of-network coverage was sufficient to cause most patients to remain inside the network while still preserving a degree of choice. Having a high-quality, geographically accessible network of 5,200 providers has facilitated patient acceptance of the more limited choices.

Claims Receipt by the Accountable Care Organization

BSWQA cannot measure true cost performance without access to monthly claims downloads, and employers can require that of any reluctant carrier. The ACO has learned to aggregate claims from payers, in spite of varying forms of submission.

Direct-to-Employer Contracts

As an ACO grows, it discovers economies of scale and develops population management competence, resulting in opportunities for direct-to-employer relationships. The ACO must conform to state insurance regulations, of course, but the Scott & White Health Plan, which preexisted the merger of Baylor Health Care System and Scott & White, provides a vehicle for many new design opportunities. Integrating the financing of care with actual delivery of care via a captive insurer, such as the Scott & White Health Plan, offers an opportunity to remove non-value-added services as well as to reduce procedural and administrative hassles.

State-of-the-Art Consumer-Focused Mobile Apps

Baylor Scott & White created MyBSWHealth, a multifunctional mobile app available on iOS and Android platforms that allows consumers to make appointments, pay bills, seek care coordination, purchase insurance, view medical records, communicate with providers, and acquire health information. The program is constantly refreshed with new functionality via BSWQA's app store and has been received well by patients.

Other Opportunities

BSWQA has found that larger employers express interest in the development of on-site clinics. Provider-run wellness plans (using the Baylor Scott & White Health employee wellness plan for the employees of a commercial contract, help desks, member solution centers, and care navigators) facilitate appointments with providers and are well received by patients and providers. Opportunities for video visits, which significantly reduce the cost of care for minor ailments, are created for patients in specific contracts if payment for those visits is agreed on. E-visits are viable care options that are both more convenient and significantly less expensive. These structured e-mail visits boast lower cost and significant convenience. BSWQA created retail relationships with two national pharmacy chains, allowing frugal and convenient nurse practitioner–administered visits, yet integrating that care through HIE technology. All of these initiatives can be incorporated into thoughtful benefit design, and the employer can direct some or all of them to be administered through a relevant carrier.

CONCLUSION

Clinical integration represents a core competency of successfully managed healthcare delivery systems in the twenty-first century. The myriad structural and process considerations that must be made to achieve this competency apply to all clinical integration models and should be customized to organizational resources; regional market determination; payer, physician, or leader preferences; and the underlying values and culture of the organization's mission. Success factors include effective physician leadership and collaboration, committed physicians, a robust HIM system to support transparent clinical and business analytics, a culture of transparency and collaboration, and a willingness to be accountable to clinical and management processes that are standardized and evidence-based. However, most important is the alignment between the CIN and its parent organization on key performance indicators that support the organization's strategic vision.

CHAPTER 7

Taking the Service Line to the Next Level in the Twenty-First Century

William Vanaskie

THE SERVICE LINE model in healthcare, so vital to the field for the past three decades, was largely created to increase volumes in high-cost or high-margin areas. Organizations could succeed where they could make a distinctive impact on both the quality of the service provided and the cost of delivering the service. This tactic was particularly rewarding under a fee-for-service payment system. But how long will these tactics and their rewards last?

Healthcare is undergoing a revolutionary change away from fee-for-service, episodic delivery of care into a focus on enhancing the health of a distinct population, not just caring for hospital patients. In fact, the new consumer of healthcare is much more educated about, and involved in, his care than ever before. He is looking for ready access to efficient care in an appropriate setting that provides the highest value to him. Cost and quality alone are no longer sufficient.

It is not my intention to focus on the individual elements of the ongoing changes in healthcare in this chapter, but we do need to understand how those changes have affected, and will affect, our service lines and how we can adapt the service line to continue to be of strategic importance to the overall organization. Service lines will remain a key component of this changed delivery model only if they can evolve to meet the changing environment. Consequently, I will first discuss the current state of service lines and their underlying strategy before suggesting how they might change.

Next, we will look at why healthcare should use the service line model and the direction in which it needs to go to respond to the evolving environment. Form follows function, so once we get a clear look at where healthcare is with its service lines and where we want to go, I will discuss how best to organize the service line to meet objectives. This section will examine the various models employed and how to best fit the service line in the overall health system.

The essential element in the functioning of the service line is physician involvement. Success is dependent on their understanding of the strategy, the structure, and the need to alter their approach to care to meet the objectives. This part of the chapter will examine some of the key concepts and approaches to enhancing physician engagement and, as necessary, physician leadership within the service line.

The critical determinant in the success of the service line, however, is the leadership. The ability to facilitate change and succeed requires a unique skill set. It goes beyond pure management of day-to-day activities to providing a clear vision, directing collaboration, and facilitating coordination. In this section, I will examine the changes being felt in the healthcare environment and how leaders might alter their approach to leading the service line. In the final section, I will address some of the key impacts the service line approach will have on the organization.

THE STRATEGY BEHIND THE SERVICE LINE

The service line has long been a responsible model for growing profitable volumes in the fee-for-service payment environment. To put it simply, the service line bundles a set of organizational resources to focus care for a particular class of patients. Ideally, it also allows for decentralized decision-making, planning, and program development. It accomplishes all this by bringing elements of the diverse departments and services in the hospital together into patient-centered groups (service lines). This structure corresponds to the long-standing management philosophy of a strong form of product management, in which a single person has accountability and responsibility for cross-functional decision-making for a major portion of the business.

To develop strategy, every service line should have a vision and some defined, quantifiable objectives against which to gauge success. Let's begin with the vision. Is your vision that of being a local participant, a market leader, a regional leader, or a national leader? And, as of today, what are the objectives of your service line in regard to cost, quality, service, volume? Do the objectives include a focus on growth, improved financial performance, a reduction in unnecessary variations in performance, or some other market- or performance-based standard? Whatever the objectives are, it is just as important to know why you defined them and be able to measure your success at achieving them as it is to know what they are. We must clearly understand the original intent of the organization because as we refocus on meeting the demands of an altered payment system, those objectives, and even the vision, may need to change.

To fully understand how your strategy might need to change, you will also need to understand what constitutes a service line in your organization. Who is your patient or customer? Only then can you make appropriate decisions, define and quantify vision and objectives, and choose services. Once that question is answered, it needs to be followed by clearly defining what is "in" your service line. Are your service lines based on specialties, such as cardiovascular care, orthopedics, or neurosciences? Or do they treat specific diseases, such as cancer, diabetes, or behavioral health conditions? Or do you define your service line by the patient demographics, such as women's health, geriatrics, or pediatrics? There is no wrong answer, though the most common service lines are cancer, cardiovascular, orthopedic, and neuroscience, according to a survey conducted by HealthLeaders Media (2013).

It is important to understand that the service lines in your system are defined as either an organizational model or a clinical model. Organizational models focus on service delivery as well as on broader planning, management, and direction for a specific area of treatment throughout the institution. Clinical models focus strictly on service delivery, such as in a center of excellence, or on a defined program or department. It is best to clearly define your intent.

The terminology you use is important to helping employees understand the function and the goals of the service line. For example, a *center* is a place or facility where an expanded scope of comprehensive clinical services is provided, generally through an open staff model for the providers. A *program* is usually a coordinated, but limited, set of diagnostic and therapeutic services designed to provide care to a group of patients (also provided through an open staff model). By contrast, a *service line* is an operational unit designed to deliver care for a defined group of patients, the standard of which goes beyond that of a program. A service line involves a broad scope of services and is not limited to an open staff model.

These definitions are particularly important because understanding why certain services are to be included in the service line needs to be easy. An appreciation of why they are necessary to support the vision and the objectives will help everyone work together and overcome the normal barriers inherent in a departmental model. Formality eases this process.

There are many ways organizations have determined what "belongs" in a service line. Considerations include the percentage of volume or revenue and the cost attributed to service line patients. Healthcare enterprises must also consider the frequency with which the settings and services anywhere in the continuum are used to manage the care of the patient effectively. However, it is best to keep in mind that added responsibility for many hospital-based services that also treat other patients may hinder the success of the service line by directing administrative and management functions away from the service line patients and to a broader patient base. The rule of thumb should be, "If the service can be bought or coordinated effectively, then it should not be included in the service line." An example would be radiology services, which are typically considered a support service for multiple service lines. Despite the fact that every patient in a service line may need certain radiographic procedures, it is not necessary that the service line assume responsibility for the entire radiology department. Rather, it can cooperate with the department to acquire specific treatment and required reports.

For the purposes of this chapter, I will forgo the discussion of how to select service lines to start or to develop, as there are several other resources that can assist with that endeavor. Instead, we will look at what healthcare organizations' strategy should be for an existing service line in the transformed payment environment.

Service Lines in Systems

Service lines in large health systems require a thorough review of the appropriate strategy for integrating across the system or consolidating into a single site or a limited number of sites. Considerations might include the systemwide organizational philosophy with regard to control and direction, the existing market dynamics or geographic size of the market, the relationship among the various member organizations, and the balance between the need for organizational autonomy and the need for strategic interdependence.

In his book *The Service Line Solution*, E. Preston Gee (2014) discusses these alternatives in detail and offers advice. He suggests that if the organization has an approach similar to that of a clinical center of excellence, in which the majority of the resources are concentrated in one facility or campus, then it is probably best to centralize the responsibilities at the system level. However, if the system decides that, because of its culture and geography, it is best to maintain the service lines at each facility, then it is more likely that a decentralized reporting structure would be the most appropriate alternative. Regardless, the reporting structure should reinforce the strategy. In exhibit 7.1, I offer pros and cons for central, regional, and hybrid reporting structures.

In the hospital system, it is rare that service line reporting remains within the individual hospitals, mainly because of the need to migrate evidenced-based practices across the system to meet the demands of the new payment structures. I have observed that the central reporting structure is the most common today. It allows an opportunity to deploy integration strategies between the service lines at the individual locations. These strategies vary from one that allows the least system-level control and the highest level of organizational autonomy (coordination) to one that has the highest level of system-level control with the least organizational autonomy (consolidation). On the continuum between these two extremes is a point at which healthcare enterprises have a degree of organizational autonomy but

Exhibit 7.1: Pros and Cons for Central, Regional, and Hybrid Reporting Structures

	Central Reporting	Regional Reporting	Hybrid (Local and Corporate)
Description	Hospital and service line leaders both report to system leadership	Service line leaders report to regional leadership	Service line leader has dual reporting (hospital and system leadership)
Pros	Facilitates consistency and coordination	Facilitates coordination across geographic area	Strengthens service line leader visibility and accountability
Cons	Potential disconnect between hospitals and corporate	No incentive to cross regional boundaries	Potential for mixed signals (system vs. hospital)

are still synchronized in their functioning and outcomes through a single, system-level lead.

Coordination involves an agreement between the organizations in the system to work together, with no shared risk between the organizations. It is best used when the entities exist in diverse markets with a large geographic dispersion. For example, before 2015, Banner Health was a 17-hospital system spread over several western states, with hospital sizes ranging from 100 to 600 beds. It developed clinical consensus groups to coordinate its service lines. Each group comprised 15–20 members, both independent physicians and hospital representatives. Each group was chaired by a physician, and it reported directly to the system chief medical officer. The purpose of each group was to share best practices and adopt standard protocols to align the individual service lines. Banner is an excellent example of integrating the service lines by coordination without placing the entire system at risk.

Integrating through synchronizing the service lines allows the institutions to remain financially independent while they agree to operate the service line in a distinct way, with set standards, treatment approaches, and even facility design. Synchronization is best used when markets are similar but not overly competitive, and no other compelling reasons to consolidate exist. Allina Health, a 13-hospital system in the Midwest, has 11 service lines. Each service line has a steering committee composed of senior clinical and administrative staff members who set strategic direction. Each line also has a program committee, which functions under the steering committee and is composed of physicians, data specialists, pharmacy representatives, performance improvement experts, nurses, and so on, that provides the tactical direction to the service line by setting performance standards and protocols. The decisions of the program committees are reflected in the way the care is provided and the outcomes are reported for that particular service line in all hospitals across the system. Allina has synchronized its service lines by directing the committees' strategy and operations across the system, with the service line leadership all reporting to a single, system-level executive team.

In healthcare enterprises, a formal decision to integrate the service lines by consolidation under a single entity ensures economies of scale, facilitates cost reduction, reduces duplication, and provides for a seamless system of care. It is best employed when the markets served by the system are similar or the same, and financial pressures are driving strategy. The Siteman Cancer Center at Barnes Jewish Hospital is a good example of consolidation as an integration strategy. Siteman is a joint venture between BJC HealthCare, a large, nonprofit, integrated delivery system, and Washington University School of Medicine, both in the St. Louis area. It has four separate service locations, all of which are staffed by Washington University faculty and run exclusively by that institution with funding and facility support from BJC. All services and staff are directed by Washington University but data are reported through the system.

Successfully operating a service line in a system requires a clear strategy set at the system level, clear roles and responsibilities for all organizations in the system, and a commitment to a common goal (which, in turn, requires agreement and support from the executive staffs of all the hospitals in the system). The structure and organization of the service line itself needs to be consistent with the market in which it operates and with the organizational culture of the system. Consistency can only be maintained when there is a single, system-level reporting structure.

What Is the Best Strategy?

Value-based care, or *population health* as it is commonly referred to today, has a focus on reallocating resources to those with the greatest need, driving interventions further upstream, and supporting wellness and coordinated care at all levels. In this new paradigm, acute care is only one component—population health, or accountable care, is not focused on acute care. Healthcare needs to understand and accept this vital fact to move forward.

The service line structure—which started out based in hospitals but really focuses a mix of resources on the care of a defined group of patients—positions the organization well to facilitate this change to a broader scope. Even now, the service line model positions those organizations to address the shifts of the changing environment. For example, because the service line is patient focused, organizations will experience less difficulty rating well in the Hospital Consumer Assessment of Healthcare Providers and Systems survey. Service lines have a strong quality focus, preparing organizations for pay for performance; their focus on financial performance and access lends itself well to the transition to bundled-payment contracts as well. All elements already exist in this model (see exhibit 7.2).

Exhibit 7.2: Service Line Model

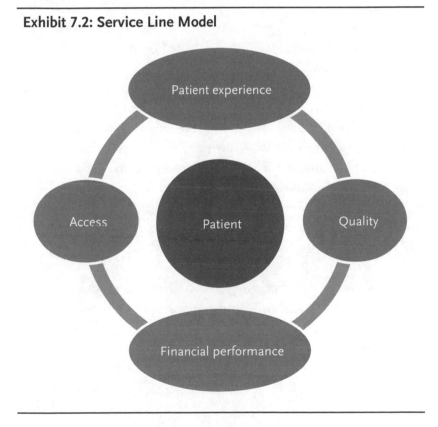

Service lines already use evidenced-based medicine to create clinical pathways, protocols, and even metrics that reduce unwanted variations in care, improve outcomes, and lower costs. The result is an increase in value, and that improvement becomes a strategic advantage when working toward future payment models. In fact, organizations must now expand the service line model beyond the hospital, including the continuum of care from prehospitalization to post-acute care. In the recent past, healthcare worked toward episodic efficiency, striving to reduce costs and improve quality. In the twenty-first century, the focus is on the total health of the patient. What can we do to prevent hospitalization? If hospitalization becomes necessary, how can we improve the patient's quality of life afterward? The focus must extend that broadly. The service line is no longer focused only on acute care, and efficiency is no longer sufficient.

How does the strategy change? If the service line is already well structured and performs to your anticipated goals, it needs to extend to include the continuum of care necessary to cover a post-acute recovery. This approach requires centralized planning and coordination, standardized processes, and decentralized decision-making down to the patient level. The transformation of the service line from an acute care focus to a health-enhancement focus must include more emphasis on the ambulatory care setting—a portfolio of services covering not only the continuum of care but also the geography of the population served. Extending across the continuum, regionalizing planning and control, and positioning to manage broad populations will require the organization to work toward the following goals:

- *Optimizing the leadership model.* Once the model is selected, the authority and responsibility of the leaders must be aligned to ensure attainment of the defined objectives.
- *Creating an inclusive physician alignment strategy.* This inclusion needs to be consistent across the system but

appropriate to the various specialties and primary care physicians.

- *Aligning the incentive compensation model.* The move to value-based payment models requires all incentive compensation models to change.
- *Enhancing data collection to provide for appropriate analytics.* While data will not solve any problems or improve care, they will help to find variations and compare performance across the multiple providers and sites of care. This goal requires a financial investment, but one that will pay dividends if well used.
- *Preparing to be flexible.* With the pace of change increasing and a wide variety of care sites involved, standards are necessary but cannot be impervious to changes made in response to fluctuation in the environment.
- *Working on matrix functions.* A matrix reporting structure is the norm in this type of process, and to be successful, that fact must be known and accepted by everyone in the system.

THE SERVICE LINE MODEL

Having settled on the strategy, the focus now must be on the right organizational model for leading and managing the service line. Several organizational and market characteristics should be considered in deciding on the appropriate model. I have observed the possibilities shown in exhibit 7.3.

To understand how best to organize a service line, we need to clearly understand the culture and the characteristics of our health system. By examining the organizational characteristics listed vertically in the leftmost column of the exhibit, one can determine what might be the best approach to leading the service line. Model types displayed horizontally across the top of the exhibit were selected

Exhibit 7.3: Selecting the Right Model

	Promoter Model	Leader Model	Executive Model	Organization Model
Culture	Entrenched in traditional culture	Focus on departments, not patient groups	Beginning to shift focus from internal depts. to market	Market-oriented culture; adapts easily to change
Strategic Orientation	Focus on revenues	Focus on growth, quality	Achieves dominance in key service lines; focus on growth, quality, cost	Population health management
Management Leadership	Equates service lines with packaging/ promotion	Recognizes service line value; remains organized around departments	Management team understands and "thinks" service lines	Very strong, visible, accountable
Physician Leadership	Medical staff not aligned	Good leadership potential but still new to "job"	Physician leadership focuses on quality and processes	Strong leadership; clinically integrated medical staff
Market Dynamics	Limited competition; visibility is primary need	Losing market share to "centers of excellence"	Strong competition; market sophistication rising	ACOs, bundled payments, VBP driving market
Information Systems	Limited ability to analyze service line performance	Basic financial and market performance available at service line level	Full profits and losses available by service line	Information systems must cross campuses, settings, and departments

Note: VBP = value-based payments

only to facilitate the discussion regarding the structure of the service line and the primary focus of the key leadership positions line; they are not intended to indicate in any way the status or positioning of the service line in the organization. I have found little contemporary use of the Promoter or Organization models, but I include them here to help the reader understand that those models can be, and have been, employed in other organizations with a certain level of success. Our discussion in this section will focus only on the differences and similarities of the Leader and the Executive models.

Once again, the starting point is a clear understanding of how the service line is currently organized before determining the changes necessary to change the service line for success in a value-based environment. The basic difference between the Leader model and the Executive model is that in the former, the leader has little or no authority over service line operations and is heavily reliant on matrixed relationships across the organization. The manager of the line bears responsibility for strategy, program development, growth, and quality, but she must accomplish all this while working through the typical hospital hierarchical organizational structure.

The person responsible in the Executive model, on the other hand, has responsibility not only for the strategy and program development but also for the growth and quality of the service line. She assumes responsibility for actively managing the daily performance of the staff in providing the care, the financial performance and the implementation of the programs and initiatives, and appropriate physician alignment. In short, she runs the service line as if it were a distinct organization. She assumes executive control.

To ensure that either model functions smoothly in the overall organization, a champion from the senior leadership team— sometimes called an *executive sponsor*—is required. The purpose of the sponsor is fairly straightforward: ensuring coordination with the other elements of the organization and medical staff, providing mentorship to the leader to facilitate professional growth and development, aligning the service line with organizational priorities and objectives, and facilitating organizational changes needed to support the service line. The service line will not succeed without support from the senior levels of the organization.

The Executive model flips the reporting structure typically found in healthcare organizations—and therein lie some of the stickiest problems the service line manager must overcome (see exhibit 7.4).

The primary reporting line now goes to the service line executive with a matrixed relationship with the functional managers. Role clarification and reporting structure for both the service line executive and the functional manager is the key. As you can see, the organization must have a specific type of culture to make this work correctly. Over time, the model will become clearer to all, but initiating it can cause confusion and take substantial effort from

Exhibit 7.4: Executive Model for Service Lines Flips Reporting Relationships

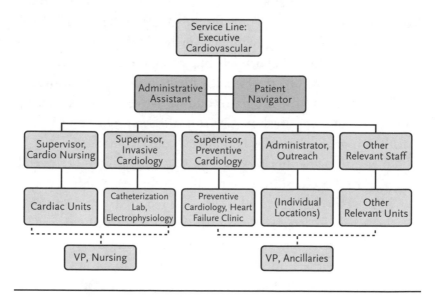

both the service line executive and the senior sponsor. Again, the senior sponsor is essential to the overall success of the service line.

Support must be evident from the highest levels of the organization regardless of whether it employs the Executive model or the Leader model. A realistic evaluation of the organizational characteristics, as discussed earlier in this section, is absolutely necessary before an appropriate model can be initiated. Some organizations have found success by starting with the least disruptive model possible and then working toward transforming to the Executive model. This tactic appears to have the greatest opportunity for success in the reformed environment; because it permits more flexibility, it allows the organization to establish the relationships with other providers that are necessary under population health.

The objectives of the service line should be consistent with the assigned responsibilities and authority of the executive. Knowing that the executive has both the accountability and the authority to move the service line to meet the objectives is key to its success. The characteristics and skill set needed under the Executive and Leader models are similar, in that the leader or the executive must be a resourceful, analytic strategic thinker, as well as a team builder. However, the executive must add to that list the skills of management and operations, coordination, and entrepreneurship, as well as the ability to work closely with the clinical and medical staff to reach the assigned objectives.

The administrative lead should not work alone. Dyads often lead service lines—typically a two-person administrative and medical team with a doctor and an administrator paired to ensure that all aspects of the service line are covered effectively (see exhibit 7.5). These partnerships have proven effective in both models. Pairing the right physician with the right administrator is always essential. They need shared values, aligned financial and nonfinancial incentives, responsibility for financial quality and cost targets, and team accountability. They must have a common view of the strategic plan and the management of the service line.

Exhibit 7.5: Dyad Management Responsibilities

Physician Partner
- Physician engagement
- Physician recruitment, retention, behavior
- Quality initiatives
- Evidence-based practices
- Compliance
- Utilization management

Administrative Partner
- Operations
- Performance reporting
- Revenue management
- Capital planning
- Service line metrics
- Staffing models
- Support systems and services

Organizations sometimes add a third person to service line leadership teams. The triad adds a clinical lead to the medical and administrative leads in the dyad. The clinical lead is typically a nurse. However, the bottom line responsibility ultimately rests with the administrative lead. The clinical lead assumes responsibility for such things as staffing ratios, standards of care, staff education and development, patient satisfaction initiatives, evidence-based clinical pathway development, and implementation, and he serves as a liaison between nursing leadership and the service line. I have found that this triad works best in larger, more diverse organizations.

Often, each service line will also have a multidisciplinary advisory team to facilitate organizational buy-in and operational alignment with the service line. Such an advisory team helps to keep the functional departments aligned and informed about the efforts of the service line and can assist with providing guidance and technical support when needed. Such a relationship, established through working groups or teams, can help address essential operational issues.

We could talk about all of the other possibilities in the structure of service lines, but, in essence, the leadership team (either dyad or triad), supported by an executive sponsor and a multidisciplinary advisory team, can make the organizational model work. Some service lines have augmented their teams with patient navigators, financial representatives, or planning support, but the absolute minimum needed is an acknowledged model, organizational support (a sponsor), a defined leadership team, and operational objectives and vision.

Service Line Reporting Structure

The reporting structure for the service line varies by organization as well. Some service lines report directly to a C-suite officer, while others report to a vice president–level position, not a direct C-suite officer. A few service lines also report to more than one person and are directed by a board or an executive committee. Each organization's structure is influenced by culture, size, and complexity. The only characteristic that every successful service line shares is a reporting relationship that is clear, known, and understood throughout the organization. In all structures, top-level leadership support is a must.

As we look to make the service line work in a value-based care environment, we find its structure growing more complex and more broad-based. Authority over or coordination with other providers affecting patient care—over the continuum of service necessary to enhance the health of the patient—becomes ever more essential. As a result, the leadership must have the capacity for added responsibility—a need extending to both the medical and the administrative leads, as well as the clinical lead, if present.

We will talk more about the added leadership requirements later in this chapter. At this point, we are assuring ourselves of just a few things: the strategy and vision of the service line, the organizational structure and authority under which the service line works, and the necessary leadership structure required to make it function. Now we can turn our attention to the need for appropriate physician integration and development for success of the service line.

PHYSICIAN RELATIONSHIP AND DEVELOPMENT

The single critical success factor that readers must understand about value-based care is that it is led by physicians and driven by primary care. While service lines have had physicians involved in various ways to address clinical issues, much of the leadership rested elsewhere. Moving from a system organized around individual physicians to a team-based approach focused on the patient will require elevating physicians to a new level of organizational leadership. How we engage and prepare physicians must change if health systems are to remain successful. The new service line must be professionally managed and clinically led.

In the past, the healthcare sector pursued advantages for the discharge-driven, often hierarchical organization that was the hospital by integrating physicians. Now, we need to align the physicians with the organization as we shift our focus from acute care, adjust financial and compensation incentives, and widely share the data needed to improve the health of a population. The next generation of physician leaders must be adept at driving change, not just helping with it. They must bring about physician engagement through consensus building and through creating a culture that values high quality, efficiency, and appropriate care. They need to be comfortable with continuous performance improvement and adept at evidenced-based practices, and they must bridge the gap between medical and surgical specialties.

The many required changes to the role of the physician will also transform the manner in which healthcare organizations collaborate with, pay, and incentivize their physician partners. Value creation, not income transfer, is required in a value-based care environment. Physicians must build collaborative relationships with providers in other environments, ensuring coordination of care across the continuum and within the system both vertically and horizontally. They must ensure coordinated transitions among primary, acute, post-acute, ambulatory, long-term, and restorative care. Prioritizing "my practice" is no longer sufficient. In value-based care, healthcare must be about "our patient" and "our practice." This series of facts boils down to one thing: the need to develop trusting relationships with the physicians (see exhibit 7.6).

The old methods of alignment, such as practice management support, professional service agreements, and comanagement arrangements are still necessary in legally appropriate ways, but they now need to be applied in a slightly different manner. One method will no longer suffice, because the sector is no longer dealing with a single subspecialty, but needs to incorporate physicians from across the continuum and from varying service providers.

The new healthcare environment will require new approaches to physician alignment. Driven by the fee-for-service system, many alignment models of the past were focused on admissions and procedures, with decision-making dispersed among the service lines. In

Exhibit 7.6: Developing Trust with Physicians

Physician-Perceived Degree of Control

	High	Low	
High	Healthy, productive relationship	Vendor relationship	Physicians must trust the hospital to look out for them, while the hospital must share control with physicians.
Low	Dictating relationship	Resentful relationship	

Physician Level of Trust in the System (vertical axis label)

the twenty-first century, we must become more flexible and tailored to local conditions and to the varying specialties. The effects of these various strategies should be centrally monitored to ensure fairness across the continuum and the organization.

The key principles of new alignment models should include the following:

- *Getting early buy-in from all physicians and agreement on the strategic objectives of the service line and the health system.* The best option is to include them in the planning process to ensure that they are aware of clinical capability needs, the payment models being considered, and other providers beyond those in the acute care setting who may be needed to make the vision work.
- *Identifying physician partners required to make the service line successful.* Different physician characteristics are required for different strategies.
- *Developing a full portfolio of alignment strategies to include a combination of mechanisms and models.* Employment does not always produce alignment. Leverage the loyal physicians who are capable of driving performance improvement.
- *Giving physicians a more powerful voice to help drive the changes necessary to reach the established objectives and metrics.* Physicians will be engaged if they are empowered to act.
- *Updating the incentive models to align with the complex nature of the service.* It is difficult but necessary to support full alignment. Remember, physician culture is often driven more by strong internal motivation and personal responsibility (Hamory, Smith, and Singh 2016).

To determine which alignment models best fit your particular situation, answer a few key questions:

1. What is needed to achieve your strategic goals? Poor physician performance will have direct financial consequences under accountable care and bundled-payment mechanisms. Understanding the desired goals will help determine your needed alignment model.

2. How much time and energy are the physicians willing to commit? The more risk physician performance places on the system, the tighter the alignment needed. However, this question is hard to judge without good physician leadership and input. Most physicians are driven by internal motivators, so full employment is not a guarantee for alignment.

3. How will the alignment model affect service line physicians' relationships with other physician groups? The accountable care organization relationships that are developed will drive the need to create different selection criteria and different models for the inclusion of varying specialties in the service line.

4. How much control is the system willing to give up, and how much are the physicians willing to assume? After overcoming the inherent issue with system culture, the predominant payment structures may help determine this. The varying models will require more control from one party or another, with risk-based arrangements requiring more physician control. As payment models change, however, this strategy will change as well.

5. How much are the physicians willing to invest financially in the system? This determinant requires careful consideration of market dynamics and relationship models. However, the physician payment models are changing and what works under the current payment structures may not be the best alternative in the future.

Physician alignment cannot be taken for granted. Changes in payment structures are driving more physicians to leave private practice and seek the financial security of larger groups, and many are seeking employment by health systems. However, full employment is not always necessary to create a lasting, trusting relationship. What is required for true collaboration is to secure mutual confidence in the credibility, reliability, and intimacy between the administrative leadership and physicians. Self-interest will quickly diminish this trust.

As a continuum of care is needed to secure population health, healthcare organizations should narrow their alignment relationships with valuable specialists. Medical/surgical specialists must be aligned to secure clinical improvements and reduce costs. Because accountable care is driven by primary care, however, primary care physicians also need to be involved in the planning efforts. All of these must be considered before an approach to physician integration and alignment can be selected. Creating a single contract and offering that to the network physicians is no longer sufficient. Much thought and a good strategic plan are necessary to even begin the process.

Even the traditional medical staff structure is coming under review and modification, given the changes in the field. There are some organizations that have mirrored their service line structure in the medical staff, with the traditional department replaced by organized, service-specific units that often match the operational service lines in the organization. This new structure facilitates a performance-driven clinical model, with physician leadership a critical component of improving quality and care integration. Where this type of restructuring has occurred, the majority of the typical work of the medical staff, such as credentialing, privileging, and peer review, is still provided through a committee structure that reports to a medical executive committee.

Engaging the physicians in this model requires a new level of physician leadership. However, not many organizations have formal programs to develop physician leaders. We need to enhance physician leaders' knowledge and understanding of financial and business methods and of the broader health system plans and programs. Formal fellowships are beginning to appear in several organizations.

Those programs aim to enhance physicians' understanding of the service line organization, strategic planning, healthcare finances, even corporate compliance regulations, and, most of all, the culture of the system. Such programs also include a concentration on performance improvement techniques and a general understanding of healthcare reform. Developing fellowships can take time, and it is expensive—from many perspectives. It is also necessary to prepare for the coming changes. The organization that is professionally managed and clinically led will succeed.

The organizational changes required to meet the needs of the value-based care environment will also require primary care and specialty physicians to be on the same team while discussing future plans, performance improvement, and care coordination. Medical/surgical specialties will have to serve together and help define clinical outcomes that will reduce unnecessary admissions and readmissions. Making use of evidence-based processes, physicians will aim to minimize variations and use predictive analysis to prioritize care and treatment when appropriate. They will work with other providers both upstream and downstream, engaging preventive health and wellness centers and post-acute care and rehabilitative facilities. Value-based care is not centered on acute care, and that fact itself will make transformation less difficult if the physicians are truly engaged and informed.

ORGANIZATIONAL PREPARATION AND LEADERSHIP

I have outlined the organizational and cultural changes inherent in employing a service line strategy. The overall organizational preparedness to embrace service lines will be challenged even more when we attempt to manage the service lines through this transformation to the healthcare model of the twenty-first century. That transformation will be dependent on a few key factors. The first is the issue of addressing the comfort of the organization in working with a matrixed environment. The ability to work effectively with the matrix will be especially important as we move to incorporate more providers to cover the continuum of care, enhance the health status of the patient, and accept risk responsibility for the total cost of care. The relationships that may have been established under a fee-for-service payment model will be further changed when healthcare organizations attempt to assume more risk. That transformation will require a shift in the way leaders manage. The field will see that as an organization transforms to accept more risk, it also becomes more complex. That complexity will require a different kind of management and leadership than we are accustomed to employing. That kind of leadership, charged with directing transformation in the matrix and across the continuum, will become the second major factor in successfully negotiating the transformation to a risk- and value-based payment model.

Managing the Matrix

Matrix relationships are inherent in the operating environment of a service line, and they are often the greatest omission as organizations move to further develop service lines. The reliance on the matrix requires strong senior leadership support. Without that support, there is a high potential for compromised results. The true success of the service line will depend on whether all leaders can work together cooperatively. Indeed, the organizational culture needs to be collaborative, and it needs to empower managers to work together more closely.

Regardless of which model is selected to operate the service line, it will challenge the culture of the organization. To make the matrix succeed, the healthcare enterprise must be able to break down traditional silos and interrupt traditional reporting structures. When faced with this type of change, it is important that allegiances be anticipated early and corrected through the use of a structured and consistent communication plan. In exhibit 7.7, the cardiac nurse needs to know to whom to take concerns when they are related to process and when they are related to clinical quality.

Anticipating all situations that could develop over time is impossible, but the creation of a plan for coordination and communication will certainly help relieve some of the stress of operating in a matrix organization. The effect on the culture of the organization cannot be overemphasized. This step is not to be taken lightly but rather with forethought and with a clear understanding by all leaders of the desired outcomes and the support that will be required. That support will take on many aspects: support to the frontline caregiver, the manager, the service line executive, and the medical staff. All stakeholders will need to understand the reasons for the new reporting structure and the responsibilities of the various parties involved. This change to the culture of the organization is probably the most significant that the staff will experience in their working lives there, and it needs to be done with a commensurate degree

Exhibit 7.7: The Matrix Under a Service Line Leader and Executive

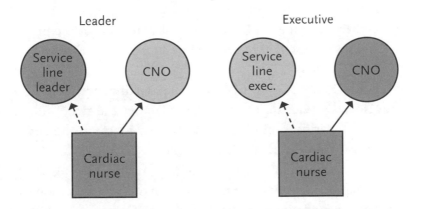

A service line leader is most dependent on strong matrix relationships. A service line executive role becomes more challenging as it shifts the balance of power.

of concern and care. It cannot be dictated; it must be deliberate, thoughtful, and clearly communicated to all stakeholders.

To further help forestall the inherent problems in a matrixed structure, plainly defining what is in the service line is necessary. As discussed earlier in this chapter, the reasons to include a particular area in the service line are many, but once decided, all parties must understand the appropriate working relationship. As shown in exhibit 7.7, those who are "in" have a direct line to the service line executive, while those not included but important to the functioning of the service line will have a dotted line to the service line executive and a direct line to the functional manager.

Employees must clearly understand the reasons behind inclusion in a direct reporting structure. Considerations such as the following will need to be openly discussed, explained, and formalized:

- Is the unit primarily used for service line activities, or does it conduct other business as well?
- Is the service large enough or important enough to warrant full-time administrative support?
- In the unit, how much time is spent on service line–related activities versus other activities?
- Is there special expertise needed solely for the service line?
- Is the unit essential to service line success?

Exhibit 7.8 is an example of how the reporting structure of a cardiovascular service line might change under the two models. The need for clarification of the reporting structure to the entire organization is obvious from this example.

Exhibit 7.9 illustrates the dual reporting relationship resulting from this matrix. For example, the director of the catheterization lab should have that relationship clearly outlined. That director reports to the chief nursing executive (CNO) for issues such as plans of care, staffing levels, and education but reports to the service line manager for financial performance, performance measures, and staffing schedules. The performance evaluation for the catheterization lab director

Exhibit 7.8: Cardiovascular Service Line Under Executive and Leader Models

Executive
- Direct Report
  - Planning analyst
  - Physician liaison
  - Catheterization lab
  - Cardiac care unit
  - Cardiac diagnostics
- Matrix Reporting
  - Cardiac surgery team
  - Marketing
  - Financial analyst

Leader
- Direct Report
  - Planning analyst
  - Physician liaison
- Matrix Reporting
  - Cardiac surgery team
  - Cardiac care unit
  - Cardiac diagnostics
  - Catheterization lab
  - Marketing
  - Financial analyst

should be a collaborative effort between the CNO and the service line manager, with one being directly responsible for submitting that report. In all cases, these reporting requirements and relationships should be handled in writing and monitored by the senior-level sponsor—in this case, the CEO or chief operating officer (COO).

Many organizations and scholars have made numerous attempts to clarify these matrixed relationships. One example involves conducting an RACI evaluation and report—that is, defining the person *Responsible* for working on the activity; the person *Accountable*, who has the final decision-making authority; the key stakeholders to be *Consulted*; and, finally, the people who need to know of the decision or action and therefore need to be *Informed*. A form of written partnership agreement between the service line and the functional department is also available as a tool to help manage the matrix. This agreement should clearly spell out the responsibilities and expectations of support and service between the department and service line. The matrix relationships need to work well in a very collaborative environment for the service line to succeed. Clarifying the standards and the expectations and communicating them

Exhibit 7.9: Cardiovascular Service Line Executive Matrix

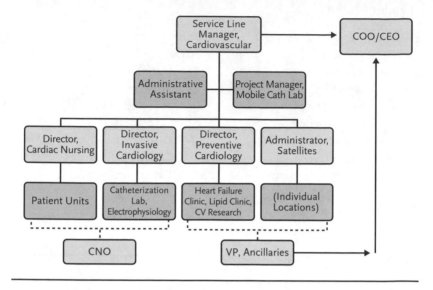

to the affected staff will make collaboration that much easier and more successful.

The matrix takes on a third dimension when there are multiple organizations involved in the service line. Depending on the management style of the system, the service line executive could be reporting to two or more sets of senior leaders and work with two or more sets of support staff. Once again, from the system level, the relationships must be clearly defined and understood throughout the organization to help tame the matrix.

Leadership

The presence of a dynamic leader is the most critical determinant of service line wins. Great managers have leadership skills, a quality that separates them from good managers. Successful leaders display a combination of strategic vision and tactical skills that can be the key to encouraging performance improvement efforts throughout the organization. In the past, service line leaders were often very good nurses or technicians who had a lot of clinical skills. That approach worked when the healthcare field operated on fee-for-service payments and needed efficiency and quality improvements. Currently, the leader needs an executive focus to increase the value of the care provided, not just the volume. The service line leader must have the skills necessary to coordinate across the continuum and the system (vertically and horizontally) and to achieve buy-in from all the stakeholders. Most important, she needs to respond to disruptive forces in other areas as well. Not only are payment methods changing, but the entire healthcare delivery environment is, too. Nontraditional clinics, urgent care centers, retail clinics, and telemedicine are all growing. Maintaining a hospital-based approach will not produce a successful service line in the payment structures on the horizon.

New leadership strategies are needed to meet the challenges of growing environmental complexity. While the healthcare sector conceptualized leadership dyads and triads in the past, it always assumed the administrative lead would handle areas other than clinical pathways and quality improvement. In tomorrow's healthcare organization, the service line executive will need expanded responsibility and the authority to act. That means budget control, sufficient full-time equivalents, and the expansion of clinical responsibilities across the continuum. Service line executives must be leaders with vision and presence, and to make the service line work, they must have senior executive support to ensure organization-wide understanding of their role, expanded responsibilities, and accountability.

The healthcare environment is moving from one that has always been complicated to one that is becoming increasingly complex. Systems that are merely complicated have many parts that are linked in discernable ways and operate in a predictable fashion. Given a set of starting conditions, it is possible to predict the outcome with some certainty, even in very complicated systems.

A complicated system becomes complex when there is an increase in the number of connections and interdependencies. In other words, the contemporary healthcare field has many more moving parts than it once did. When this happens, local events and interactions can cascade and reshape the entire system through a process called *emergence*. That new structure then influences the frontline agents, resulting in further changes to the system, and so on. The system therefore continues to evolve in hard-to-predict ways because it is changing from the bottom up in response to the environment. Examples exist in all forms of life—from business to biological.

The key takeaway is that, in complex systems, it is difficult to apply cause-and-effect assessments and thus difficult to predict outcomes with any certainty. In such an environment, efficiency is not enough. The key is to employ adaptability and resilience. The system needs to adjust to any change but maintain its general structure and remain focused on its goals—all while keeping in mind that the process may need to change. In complex systems, change is not episodic; it is almost continuous and creates many new interactions. (Thus, the term *emergence*, which happens when changes spread from the bottom up to affect the entire system, instead of emanating from the top.)

In twenty-first-century healthcare, unintended consequences unfolding after seemingly rare events have a major impact on the system. Using the same old top-down strategies will not work effectively. The field must be more realistic about what it can predict and control. We need to constantly expect the unexpected, remaining flexible and agile, able to roll with the punches. To succeed during a time of confusion, everyone in the organization must know and understand what is happening. Communication must be continuous so that employees can think and act as a unit, however diverse or remote they may be.

The new leaders in healthcare—and the service line executive— are no exception. They need to work outside of the traditional silos and develop greater feelings of trust and common purpose in all stakeholders. They must be comfortable working with teams of people to develop and employ. The coordination of those teams will be centralized with the common leader, but the execution and control of the team should be decentralized to the team leader and even to the individual team members themselves. As each team experiences the changes and reacts, it has to keep the other teams informed. That linkage—the communication between teams—creates the power to change the organization universally that the individual teams do not possess. To be effective, each team must trust the other teams to work toward a common goal, which gives all a common purpose. That trust and that purpose are the key ingredients, and they are bolstered by communication.

Effective leadership relies on communication. Rising levels of uncertainty caused by changes to the fundamental healthcare structure create anxiety in the organization. That anxiety engenders volatility. The need for clear and continuous communications increases with the level of volatility. Volatility within and uncertainty without—this is the complex environment in which we now work.

The good news is that when open communication becomes a fundamental part of the operations in an organization, it begins to break down silos and enhance flexibility and agility. This evolution is crucial to the new model of healthcare. Clear communication enables concentration of resources and reduces confusion, which in turn reduces anxiety.

This formula applies not only to the vision and strategies that should be translated into relevance for the average employee but also to the manner in which healthcare leaders share care-related information. We must include the clinical, medical, and managerial areas of our organizations in the transmission of continuous and clear care-related information. The method and form of communication healthcare organizations employ must include all clinician stakeholders and must remain compliant with privacy regulations. The ultimate goal must be to eliminate the barriers between management and medicine.

The service line needs good leadership to be successful—but that service line executive needs to be supported by a senior-level leader.

The senior-level leader drives transparency across the organization and ensures cross-functional cooperation. His goal should be to create a sense of "joint cognition" in the organization (that is, the ability, across all functions, to think and act as one unit). This dynamic creates an emphasis on the need to share actionable information, not just data—creating a culture of sharing. A truly transparent environment takes time, attention, and financial resources. However, to be successful in a complex environment, it is essential that healthcare develops and implements strong and open communication channels.

Over the past 30 years, authors have written many books about functioning in a more complex environment—and not just in healthcare. Society has seen an ever-increasing pace of change, most of it accelerated by the information technology revolution. Systems once separate are now interconnected and interdependent and therefore more complex. Recognizing that technological advances are coming faster than we can absorb requires us to change our management approach. For any organization to maintain effectiveness and viability, it needs to adapt and be resilient, to expect surprises and be redundant enough to provide protective checks and balances, and to create feedback loops and mechanisms that will foster trust.

The current trends in the healthcare sector—and beyond—have led healthcare leaders to the realization that the service line executive of the twenty-first century must have strategy in her skill set. She must have market insight, be adept at change management, and be comfortable in a cross-functional organization that spans the full continuum of care. She needs to be a team leader—customer-focused yet results-oriented. She must also be comfortable with ambiguity, be able to discover and react to problems on a daily or even hourly basis, and be a good communicator. In short, the service line executive will require many of the same skills and qualities as today's CEO.

THE ORGANIZATIONAL IMPACT

Moving to a value-based payment model involves a different set of processes and resources. Whether the model is pay for performance, shared savings, or bundled payments, each will necessitate different relationships with both providers and payers. The shift requires that the continuum of service be incorporated into the service line structure in some form. The current service line focus is acute care, with very limited attention to pre- or post-acute care services. Value-based payment models require that the hospital assume greater risk for all the care provided to the patient both upstream and downstream. That requires an expansion of the service line purview to include such things as preventive care and ambulatory clinics as well as post-acute care and home care.

Current healthcare delivery systems cannot meet the demands of the twenty-first century alone. Doing so entails outreach to an array of community and social services, and such relationships will vary by provider and payment model. The delivery system will need to decide if it should build the service from scratch, buy the service from another provider, or partner with a provider for the service. This decision to make, buy, or partner should start with considering the underlying strategy of the service line and assessing the inherent organizational expertise and the availability of facility space. Leaders must also consider the presence of a market leader already providing the service, the market demand that is anticipated for the service, and, of course, the existing culture of the organization. Furthermore, market conditions and geographic considerations will play a decision-making role. Regardless, a degree of alignment must be established to secure the service, and that alignment will vary by the type of payment model as well.

The changes, however, do not stop there. Moving from a volume-based business to a business based on value means satisfying the customer. Healthcare's concept of "the customer" is shifting from the sick patient to the healthy individual intent on maintaining his quality of life. Value cannot be reached by merely caring for the sick. Value for the population will come by working with the broader community to keep people well.

As we start to rethink service lines, we need to look first at strategy, rethink service line definitions, clearly outline the goals and objectives, and clarify the role of the service line in the overall organization. Next, healthcare organizations must look to their internal organizational structures to clarify reporting relationships and balance integration and consolidation as necessary. Determine the model that best fits with the culture and the needs of the organization. Define the alignment models to be employed with the full continuum of providers, with particular emphasis on primary care and related specialties. Work with your system to engage a physician champion and prepare that physician to lead the change.

Then, leaders must prepare the organization. They should work to create a dynamic leadership structure, identify the service line leadership team, and prepare its members for the tasks at hand. The team should look to the broader organization and prepare all departments to work within the redefined system by clarifying the matrix relationships. Be very clear in communicating the plans, vision, and objectives to all involved or affected. Engage not only the employees but also the senior leaders, the board, and the medical staff to maintain commitment and support for the overall plan. Leaders should facilitate, not dictate, the dramatic cultural change required to succeed. They must strive to communicate, at all levels, in a clear, concise, and transparent manner at all times. Communication helps build trust by defining purpose and making it relevant to all involved. Above all else, stay focused on the patient. The environment may become more complex by the day, but enhancing the health of the populations served requires that the healthcare field stay as resilient and flexible as possible while maintaining its focus.

REFERENCES

Gee, E. P. 2014. *The Service Line Solution: Consumer-Focused Strategies for the Accountable Care Era*. Danvers, MA: HealthLeaders Media.

Hamory, B., G. Smith, and R. Singh. 2016. "5 Practices That Can Help Health Systems Build Improved Relations with Doctors." Published May 26. http://health.oliverwyman.com/transform-care/2016/05/5_practices_thatcan.html.

HealthLeaders Media. 2013. *Service Line Optimization: Strategies to Drive Value Along the Care Continuum*. Published June. www.healthleadersmedia.com/report/intel/service-line-optimization-strategies-drive-value-along-care-continuum.

Health Information Management for the Twenty-First-Century Healthcare Enterprise

Lee Pierce
Mike Harmer
Brent Heaton
Lonny Northrup
Naveen Maram
Sid Thornton

THE DATA AND analytics revolution is in full swing, affecting all industries and companies of varying shapes and sizes and transforming the way they help run our businesses and deliver value to our customers. Healthcare has been a part of this revolution for many years, but recent times have seen a new focus on data management and analytics. Much of this surge comes as a result of the proliferation of electronic health records (EHRs), enterprise resource planning systems (ERPs), and other electronic transactional systems that support and automate business processes. The output of these systems is ones and zeros, commonly called *data*, stored in databases or file systems.

Data are an asset that is just as important and valuable as many of the assets listed on a typical balance sheet, but they are rarely treated as such in healthcare organizations. A balance sheet for a company generally includes a list of assets—things that the company owns that have future economic value, that can be measured. Balance sheet assets include accounts (such as cash), land, buildings, equipment, and supplies. In each company, there are departments, personnel, policies and procedures, and a tremendous amount of work that goes into understanding and managing each of these assets to the benefit of the company. Healthcare organizations need to devote just as much focus and management to data to achieve their full potential value.

Data are an asset that healthcare companies own. They have current and future values that can and should be measured. Value can be measured with the following equation:

$$\text{Value} = \text{Results} \div \text{Cost.}$$

Value can be measured in dollars and cents, by showing hard dollar savings as a result of reduced length of stay through data-based decision-making; it can be measured in clinical outcomes and results, such as improving the quality of care provided to cardiovascular patients; it can be measured by a caregiver's improved quality of life after receiving the tools and aides necessary to better care. Value can also be measured in lives saved.

However, data must be carefully managed to be leveraged fully for high-quality outcomes. Their management involves integrating disparate data sources, managing data quality, standardizing data, and defining stewardship and decision rights around data assets. We will talk about each of these data management activities throughout this chapter.

Leveraging data is where analytics come into play. The creation of analytics solutions includes reports and dashboards, statistical analysis, algorithm development, and new insights that can be applied

Exhibit 8.1: From Data to Value

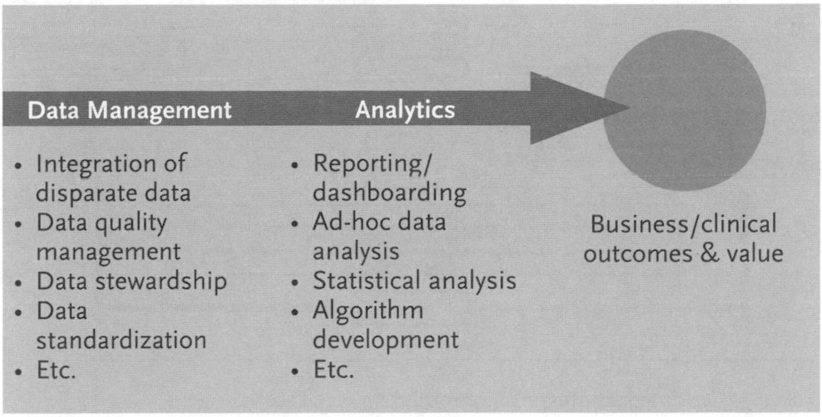

Data Management
- Integration of disparate data
- Data quality management
- Data stewardship
- Data standardization
- Etc.

Analytics
- Reporting/ dashboarding
- Ad-hoc data analysis
- Statistical analysis
- Algorithm development
- Etc.

Business/clinical outcomes & value

toward better decision-making. The goal of data management and analytics activities is to create value for all participants in the healthcare delivery ecosystem (see exhibit 8.1).

Data in healthcare follow a cycle that leads to business and clinical outcomes and value (see exhibit 8.2). The cycle starts with the process of patient care and delivery and the use of the electronic systems that support these processes. The data that are generated are drawn from many areas, including clinical, financial, claims, patient satisfaction, device data, and unstructured data. Data then need to be organized and integrated in order to support analytical processes. Insight is the result of analytical activities. But insight without action will provide little-to-no value—we must close the loop by applying a business or clinical process that results in the improvement of patient care or another process. Each of the data cycle steps will be reviewed in this chapter (see exhibit 8.2) and include the following:

- The input of data from disparate sources (e.g., claims, devices, patient satisfaction, nonclinical determinants)

Exhibit 8.2: Data Value Cycle

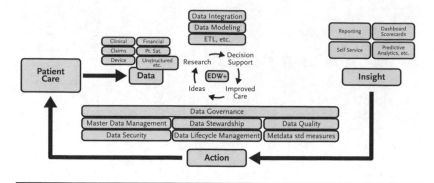

Source: Reprinted courtesy of Intermountain Healthcare.
Note: EDW = enterprise data warehouse

- The integration of data through data modeling and extraction, transfer, and loading (ETL) techniques
- Data governance, which includes security, stewardship, integrity, quality, and metrics
- Insight through role-based dashboards or scorecards that contribute to the optimal care of the patient

HEALTHCARE DATA ECOSYSTEM: SYSTEMS AND APPLICATIONS

A typical healthcare organization has a series of electronic systems and applications that make up its ecosystem. Data sources can be organized into the following categories: core and clinical systems, external data sources, research data sources, and devices and streaming data sources. Let's dive into each of these to better understand the systems and applications that make them up (see exhibit 8.3).

Exhibit 8.3: Data Sources

Core and Clinical Systems	External	Research	Devices and Streaming
• EHR—HELP 1 & 2, Cerner, Centricity • ERP/HR—Peoplesoft • Claims—Facets • Labs • Home health • Bio repository • Omics data • Etc.	• Partners/affiliates • HIE • Claims—Non-SelectHealth • Surveys • Registries • Social media • Environmental • Government—CMS, NIH, FDA • Etc.	• Research study sets • Clinical trials • Tissue and organ banks • Omics data (proteomics, epigenomics, metabolomics)	• Biometrics • Home health monitor streams • Wearable device output (e.g., Fitbit) • Clinical monitors • E-visit videos

Images Social EHR Mobile Text Biologics Cloud Biometrics Streaming Video

Core and Clinical Systems

Most healthcare organizations have invested in core data systems to help run their business and clinical functions. These include hospital EHRs, ambulatory EHRs, home health EHRs, laboratory systems, ERP systems, human resources software, claims processing software, and imaging systems. These systems consume significant financial and information technology (IT) resources to purchase, implement, and maintain. The data from these systems comprise the foundational building blocks that need to be managed and leveraged to achieve data's potential value.

External Data Sources

An inventory of data used by healthcare organizations is not complete without accounting for sources that exist outside of the core systems. These external sources include environmental data such as weather and pollution; affiliated health systems data; claims data from various payers; and data from the government, clinical registries, and social media. External sets augment internal sets to help researchers and analysts provide insights that would not have been possible using only internal information.

Research Data Sources

Clinical research produces valuable data that can also be integrated with internal and external data sources. Clinical trials, research study data sets, tissue and organ banks, and omics data (proteomics, epigenomics, metabolomics) are all useful. Research data sources are increasingly complete and rich, and both research and operational values are being derived from their use.

Devices and Streaming Data Sources

The world generates tremendous amounts of information from devices and associated streaming data. Examples of these sources include wearables such as FitBit and Apple watches, home health monitors, clinical monitors, and e-visit videos. Device data will continue to be used and integrated with data sources to derive novel insights.

DATA MANAGEMENT: DATA GOVERNANCE PRINCIPLES AND BEST PRACTICES

Data governance is the exercise and enforcement of decision-making authority over the management of data assets and the performance of data functions. According to the American Health Information Management Association (Empel 2018), it is "an organization-wide framework for managing information throughout its lifecycle and supporting the organization's strategy, operations, regulatory, legal, risk, and environmental requirements." Data governance requires the adoption and integration of principles, a framework, rules of the road, and managed processes. It accepts and assumes that the organization views and treats information as a mission-critical asset, that information has a life cycle, and that not all information is equal in value.

The adoption of correctly applied data governance principles enables the safe use of healthcare information technology (HIT) systems, ensuring that we identify the right patient, associate her with the correct information, increase the quality of care, lower costs, reduce information risk, elevate the reliability of performance measures, and ensure the appropriate and ethical use of information. Data governance enables the business to engage in the decision-making process for the organization's critical data assets.

For a healthcare organization to use data effectively in its effort to improve quality, those data must be trusted. The decision-making authority for the collection and use of data must reside with the business function that has accountability for the processes that produce the data. An enterprise must have tools and processes in place to ensure the data are of high quality, correctly defined, and protected appropriately, regardless of the information system (IS) that produces or consumes them.

The scope of data governance falls primarily into five functional areas: data stewardship, data quality, master data management, metadata management, and security and privacy.

Data Stewardship

Data stewardship is an approach to data governance that formalizes accountability for managing information resources for the best interests of the organization and the patient. This type of program represents the operational aspect of data governance. It consists of the people, organizations, and processes that ensure designated stewards are responsible for oversight of the governed data. Through data stewardship, all of the metadata for key business elements are collected and documented, data decisions are based on knowledge, fiduciary standards for the data are upheld, and the organization's data assets are improved in quality and used to drive business outcomes.

Stewards do the day-to-day work of administering enterprise data. They are aligned with a specific data-producing business function, and they are identified directly with the data elements for that function. Stewards own the definitions and quality issues; they are subject matter experts. A business data steward is assigned by and typically reports to the owner of the business function; she is typically the single point of contact for data on the function, and this exclusivity allows for consistent meaning and usage within and across departments, which result in streamlined decision-making and issue resolution.

Data Quality

Data governance can positively affect overall data quality and enable a culture where quality is considered in every data process. This is accomplished by developing systematic processes, providing frameworks for consistent and credible information, and implementing data quality tools that aid in the discovery and monitoring of issues.

Master Data Management

Master data are the high-value, core information used to support critical business processes in an organization. They are a subcategory for all data sources. In healthcare, master data are information about patients, members, providers, locations, organizations, employees, and even populations and communities. They are at the heart of every critical business transaction, application, and decision. According to the Gartner Master Data Report, master data management (MDM) is a discipline in which the business and the IT organization work together to ensure the uniformity, accuracy, semantic persistence, stewardship, and accountability for the organization's official, shared master data. Data governance provides the processes, people, working groups, and boards who create and manage master data to ensure their quality, accuracy, and value. Business owners and data stewards are assigned to master data domains to define and perform management activities under the direction of the governance processes. MDM software solutions can then be leveraged to automate, execute, and track master data content and activities.

Metadata Management

Metadata management is the discipline of capturing and maintaining both business and technical metadata to support the management of the organization's critical data. Key business data elements are identified and defined, and business rules are determined. These are then linked to physical data assets. This information is clearly documented and then published for interested parties. Business data stewards capture this information for the data elements for which they are accountable. Metadata management activities are supported by the data governance program. A business glossary and metadata repository are the preferred places for this information to be stored in an enterprise.

Security and Privacy

Most healthcare organizations have an IS security function and a privacy office. Data governance supports these functions by providing a framework for linking the process owners and stewards to the existing security and privacy policies and procedures.

DATA STANDARDIZATION IN HEALTHCARE

The optimization and potential value of healthcare data are predicated on the ability of health information systems, applications, and devices to be semantically interoperable; just being able to exchange the data alone will not be sufficient. Data being sent, received, stored, retrieved, or aggregated must be understood so that they are actionable and consumable from one computer or system to another. According to the Office of the National Coordinator for Health Information Technology (2018), "an interoperable health IT ecosystem makes the right data available to the right people at the right time across products and organizations in a way that can be relied upon and meaningfully used by recipients." Semantic interoperability is the ability to not only share data but also understand and interpret the data across systems—usually by using standards that establish the common framework, terminology, and structure for data. Data standards establish a universal definition, format, and context for data concepts and provide the capacity to meaningfully encode information that is captured (see Public Health Data Standards Consortium 2017).

Human communication is rife with ambiguity, especially in the realm of healthcare; data standards help to solve this issue. For example, think about the term *cold* in a health record. Does this indicate a patient has a cold (viral infection), that the patient feels cold to the touch, that the patient is experiencing the sensation of coldness, or that the patient's actions are rude and uncaring? Without data standards, the meaning or context of the term is impossible to understand. They provide definition, context, and disambiguation of clinical concepts.

Data standards for content include vocabularies, terminologies, and classification systems. Vocabulary and terminology systems provide the basic nomenclature of concepts or terms, their synonyms, and the associated universal codes. Classification systems are specific groups or domains of related concepts. Relationships to domains or other concepts help provide meaning. Concepts may have specific properties or attributes to clarify definition or context. As adoption and implementation of terminologies have evolved, collaborative efforts have worked toward integrating and reducing redundant terms, increasing content coverage, and forming sophisticated knowledge-based ontologies. In 1998, Dr. James Cimino outlined key guidelines for controlled medical vocabularies in the twenty-first century. Items, referred to as *desiderata* (desired essentials), included the following:

- Content
- Concept orientation
- Concept permanence
- Nonsemantic concept identifiers
- Polyhierarchies
- Concept definitions
- Rejection of "not elsewhere classified" terms
- Multiple granularity
- Consistent views
- Context
- Graceful evolution
- Recognized redundancy

The HIT field has made much progress, and newer terminologies are conforming to the desiderata and enhancing the overall quality of content. Following the guidelines of Cimino's desiderata, standard terminologies help solve the problem that comes with the term *cold* (see exhibit 8.4).

While there are numerous clinical terminologies, for the purpose of this discussion we will focus on the more commonly used ones, including Systematized Nomenclature of Medicine Clinical Terms (SNOMED CT); Logical Observation Identifiers Names and Codes (LOINC); RxNorm; International Classification of Diseases and Related Health Problems, Tenth Revision, Clinical Modification (ICD-10-CM); and International Classification of Diseases and Related Health Problems, Tenth Revision, Procedure

Exhibit 8.4: Standard Terminologies

Data Concept	Code	Definition
Cold	13542	A viral infection
Cold	679810	Feels cold; cold to touch
Cold	1144587	Feeling cold; subject is feeling cold
Cold	1459218	Perception of behavior that is rude

Coding System (ICD-10-PCS). Each of these is unique and has a specific purpose.

SNOMED CT is a comprehensive clinical terminology that provides an extensive range of unique clinical concepts within a poly-hierarchical structure that are defined by relationships, attributes, and synonyms. Each concept is given unique numerical identifiers. Available in multiple languages, and used in more than 50 countries, SNOMED CT is considered "a common global language for health terms" (SNOMED International 2017). Exhibit 8.5 shows an example of a SNOMED CT concept.

Think about all the various ways to say and represent medical concepts. If a physician compiles a problem list in a patient's health record and wants to share that information with reporting agencies, outside providers, or any other data repositories, the data need to have a standardized code for them to be understood by other systems. If the EHR lists deep-vein thrombosis, and this is connected to the associated SNOMED CT code, the physician can communicate the patient's problem with precision. Regardless of how another system represents the data (e.g., using the terms *DVT* or *deep venous thrombosis*, written in a different language), the data will have the same SNOMED CT code and be recognized as the same concept. The standard code enables disparate systems to share data in a way that is meaningful.

Exhibit 8.5: SNOMED CT Example

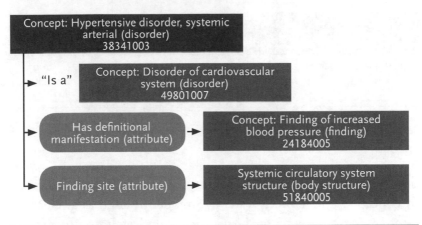

LOINC is a coding system that communicates information about laboratory tests, measurements, and clinical observations. Each unique LOINC code represents an individual concept and describes it using six attributes or *parts* (exhibit 8.6). These six parts are component, property, time, system (specimen), scale, and method. The *component* is what is being observed or measured; *property* is any characteristic; *time* represents when an observation was made or the interval of time; *system* identifies the body system or specimen; *scale* identifies how the value is expressed—either quantitative, ordinal, narrative, or nominal; and *method* is an optional part that is used to specify whether a specific technique or procedure was used to make the observation or measurement (Regenstrief Institute 2017).

For example, if a physician wants to see the lab results from a glucose test, the LOINC code provides the exact definition of the glucose test to get the correct results. (Did he want to view the glucometer result? The fasting glucose? One-hour postchallenge?) The LOINC code allows information exchange to occur between the lab and other systems to place the order and communicate the results.

RxNorm is a nomenclature used to represent brand name and generic clinical drugs by using the active ingredient, strength, and

Exhibit 8.6: Example of the Structure of LOINC Code 806-0

LOINC Code	Component	Property	Timing	System	Scale	Method
806-0	Leukocytes	NC (number concentration)	Pt (point in time)	CSF (cerebral spinal fluid)	QN	Manual count

dose form. A wide range of different types of relationships are linked to concepts. The naming system is frequently used as a reference terminology for transactional data, such as in the sale or dispensation of medications, in order to translate codes from proprietary drug nomenclatures.

Having a reference terminology for drug nomenclature is important for care coordination. Disparate systems must be able to exchange information and translate the data exactly as they were intended. For example, if a patient is discharging from a hospital to another provider that uses a different drug terminology, the medication list will be translated with RxNorm. The name, ingredient, strength, and route of all orders on a medication list can be exchanged and understood between the different systems, allowing for continuity of care.

The ICD is managed by the World Health Organization and used for statistical purposes related to epidemiology and mortality rates. It is a classification system that provides codes for diseases along with other associated findings, signs, symptoms, causes, and information related to the disorder. ICD-9-CM was based on the ICD, Ninth Revision (ICD-9) and was created by the US National Center for Health Statistics. This system provides codes for diagnoses for inpatient and outpatient settings and for inpatient procedures. Organizations use these codes to track healthcare utilization and morbidity rates in the Unites States. This classification system has continued to evolve into the current versions: ICD-10-CM for diagnoses and

ICD-10-PCS for procedures. These provide significantly expanded content and more granularity. The codes for these systems have letters, numbers, and characters. ICD-10-CM codes begin in a specific, categorized, three-digit code. As more specificity and granularity are present in the term, more digits are added to the three-digit code after a decimal. The final product can be as many as seven digits. The more digits present, the more detail is given. ICD-10-PCS has a similar structure. Categories of procedures are defined with characters representing specific meanings. Each additional character added to the base category supplements the description of the procedure (see exhibit 8.7) (World Health Organization 2018).

ICD-10 codes are used in many ways. Procedures and diagnoses from the providers are associated with these codes. They are used for reimbursement, epidemiology and disease surveillance, outcome and quality measures, and research. The standardized data allow for

---

Exhibit 8.7: Example of Additional Characters

ICD-10-CM: Open bite of right shoulder, initial encounter

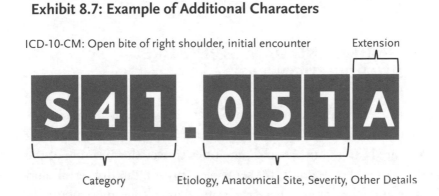

ICD-10-PCS: Insertion of infusion device into right brachial artery, open approach

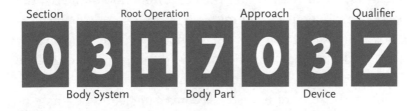

---

information to be shared, aggregated, and compared—all of which are important to healthcare advancement.

While individual terminologies have helped support individual business needs, such as billing or documentation, emerging uses related to health information exchange (HIE), MDM, and population health require rethinking the terminology and cultivating convergence. The organizations behind SNOMED CT and LOINC are currently collaborating and working on harmonizing certain portions of the terminologies. An extension of these efforts includes the addition of RxNorm. The combination is known as SOLOR (based on the names of SNOMED, LOINC, and RxNorm). The goal is to provide a sharable, logical model of postcoordinated expressions of clinical content (Raths 2016). After decades of ignorance regarding standards, the health community became aware and then more informed; it is now very standards driven. Coupled with this shift in terminology standardization, data structure standardization is also evolving.

MESSAGING AND DATA STRUCTURE STANDARDIZATION

Syntax and semantics are two important ideas in any discussion of the structure of clinical messages. Syntax is the way information is structured (its grammar), and semantics convey the meaning of the information. For example, the sentences "my son eats dry cereal" and "my son flies red water" have the same syntax; they are structurally (grammatically) the same. However, their semantics are completely different. One makes sense and the other does not. Similarly, the sentences "medication was administered for pain" and "pain medication was administered" have different syntax, but depending on how they are used, they may or may not have the same meaning. These examples are evidence of the difficulty of communicating information (not in the sense of individuals conversing, corresponding, or exchanging data but in the sense of one electronic system exchanging information with another). The way information is structured, stored, and presented to users varies so widely from system to system that simply transmitting it from one to another isn't enough (Parker et al. 2004). Terminology (the words or concepts and their symbolic representations) must be standardized to remove any definitional ambiguity, as previously discussed, but the way in which the terminology is put together to form messages (the syntax) must also be standardized. When placed in a standardized message structure, the sentence "pain medication was administered" becomes not only understandable but also computable for use in things such as clinical decision support, data mining, natural language processing, big data processing, and predictive modeling.

LOGICAL CLINICAL INFORMATION MODELS

To address these challenges, many efforts are underway to standardize the way in which clinical information is structured; the Clinical Information Modeling Initiative and OpenEHR projects are two examples. Both seek to create a set of detailed clinical information models that can be used and shared with all information systems. These models aspire to be a standard structure for the healthcare informatics industry for describing instances of data. A simple example is the structural description of a heart rate measurement. At its most basic, the structure consists of the measurement and the value of the measurement. For example,

- Key = Heart rate measurement
- Value = 72 beats/min

These elements constitute a simple syntax. However, additional information may be needed that adds meaning to the value of the measurement or adjusts how the value could be interpreted—for instance, the position of the body during measurement, any associated preexisting conditions, and the location on the body where the measurement was obtained. Provenance information may also need to be collected. Adding these would change the structure to look like the following:

- Key = Heart rate measurement
- Value = 72 beats/min
- Qualifier body position = Prone
- Qualifier body location = Right wrist
- Qualifier-associated precondition = Patient has pacemaker
- Attribution performer = Registered nurse
- Attribution performed date time = 201701151807

Note that these basic structures or data models, used as standards, do not prescribe how the basic structures and data models are to be used or implemented. They do not stipulate that the model be expressed in XML, JSON, UML, or any other programming or modeling language, nor do they stipulate that specific system data be captured as part of the structure. Such an approach allows the implementing entities to have the flexibility to determine the optimal path for individual systems to advance semantic interoperability and its resultant benefits. These standardized models are referred to as *logical models* or *reference models*, while those that are language specific (or include implementation data) are referred to as *implementation models*.

The ultimate goal behind creating logical clinical information models is to create semantic interoperability—that is, the ability for systems to share data without having to interpret, infer, or guess at meaning. This clarity is achieved when systems use the same logical structures to define clinical concepts.

Another powerful aspect of creating logical models as a standard is the ability to bind elements of the models to standard terminologies, increasing the semantic interoperability of the model. For example, a high degree of ambiguity is inherent if the key of the earlier heart rate model is left as simple text. If the only semantic need is for humans to be able to read it, then everything is fine. However, if it is bound to a specific concept and code (say, the LOINC code of 41920-0 Heart rate 1 hour mean), then there is no ambiguity; all systems can know exactly what kind of heart rate is being represented and be able to use it computationally. This binding of the key to a specific system and code greatly increases the degree of semantic interoperability. The same can be done for the other elements in the logical model (Richesson and Chute 2015).

FAST HEALTH INTEROPERABILITY RESOURCES: A BRIDGE BETWEEN LOGICAL CLINICAL INFORMATION MODELS AND IMPLEMENTATION MODELS

In 1987, the world was introduced to a messaging standard called Health Level 7 Version 2 (HL7 v2). It was developed as an application protocol for the electronic transference of data in healthcare systems. Since then, it has gone through several iterations; the current version is HL7 v2.7, released in 2011. Among healthcare organizations in the United States and more than 35 other countries throughout the world, 95 percent use a version of HL7 v2. Version 2 has done much to standardize HIT's exchange and sharing of data, at least syntactically (Mendes and Rodrigues 2013). However, it is far from being semantically interoperable. The standard allows for ad hoc interpretation of the message by either the sending or receiving institution. Different implementations of the standard require the use of specialized mapping software. It lacks a common information model, computational data-type specifications, the infrastructure for binding terminology values to message elements, and a top-down message development process (Mead 2006).

HL7's solution to these issues was the creation of the Version 3 Reference Information Model (RIM) and the tools to implement it. The RIM was designed as the cornerstone on which all messages were to be created. Like version 2, version 3 made great strides in moving the informatics world toward true interoperability. In spite of its well-thought-out design and its success at describing a complete information model, version 3 does have issues—it lacks usability in specialized domains and demonstrates problems in scope, technique, and antiquated methodologies (Smith and Ceusters 2006). These issues have led to a low rate of use in the healthcare sector. One part of the version 3 standard, however, has seen wide adoption: clinical document architecture (CDA) and its compressed version—consolidated clinical document architecture (C-CDA). But CDA and C-CDA messages are limited in their degree of interoperability (D'Amore et al. 2014).

HL7 recognized these difficulties with the v2 and v3 specifications and created a Fresh Look task force to research the best solutions (Benson and Grieve 2016). From this effort came Fast Healthcare Interoperability Resources (FHIR, pronounced "fire"), a new specification to exchange healthcare information. It is a collection of defined data structures called *resources*. These resources are like templates by which instances of data can be created, used in application programming interfaces, or even as data objects in object-driven databases. There are four aspects that make FHIR such a usable specification: the use of RESTful (representational state transfer) services, the use of basic information models as resources, flexibility within the resources to handle extensibility, and the ability for implementations to define the profiles of the resources.

The use of RESTful services is of particular interest. REST is a set of architectures, services, and design constraints for the purpose of creating scalable, reliable, and easy-to-use interfaces. The wide use of the RESTful paradigm across what seems to be all of IT makes its use in the exchange of healthcare information sensible.

Much like HL7 v2, FHIR is highly flexible. Each resource and each element in a resource has an "extension" element. The difference between the flexibility of HL7 v2 and FHIR is in how the extension is defined. FHIR requires that, to be compliant, the extension, along with its structure, must be registered with FHIR and readily obtainable by anyone. In addition, the extension must also use only the data types defined by FHIR. This alleviates the need for complex interfaces to interpret the extensions.

The basic information model aspect expressed by each resource also gives FHIR a great deal of interoperability. It seems that, even though they are not in strict adherence to the version 3 RIM, the resources are an implementation of it. The resources are grouped by type (administrative, clinical, financial, infrastructure, and conformance—these domains are highly defined in the RIM). They describe the basic structures of data in those domains: patient, organization, observation, condition, document, and so on.

The ability to create profiles of resources is where data standardization and FHIR come together. The FHIR resources are technically called *structure definitions*. FHIR allows them to be subtyped. The creation of a new structure definition is based on one of the base resources or another structure definition. This makes it possible to create profiles (subtypes) of the reference resources that have additional elements needed or desired by specific systems. The profile can then be used and shared with others, increasing interoperability.

Healthcare historically has been a data-intensive industry. With the proliferation of sensors, the Internet of Things, and patient-reported data, the impending information overload heightens the urgency of data standardization and of semantic interoperability that maximizes the clinical and business values of the data. Semantically interoperable data can spotlight inconsistencies and quality issues much earlier in the data life cycle, lowering the cost of recognizing and fixing the issues and increasing the quality of healthcare delivery. Data standards for content, messaging, and structure must be implemented. "Such an infrastructure will support more efficient and effective systems, scientific advancement, and lead to a continuously improving health system that empowers individuals, customizes treatment, and accelerates cure of disease" (Office of the National Coordinator for Health Information Technology 2018).

DATA SHARING

The goal of HIE is for all appropriate patient health data, regardless of originating source, to be available and included in an electronic workflow, in a timely manner, to support decision-making—in other words, the right data at the right place at the right time. Data interoperability provides the healthcare team, including the patient and patient advocates, with an uninterrupted digital experience with access to all relevant data, knowledge, and derived data tailored for the patient across the continuum of care and various organizations. The improved decisions lead to more efficient care with lower costs and less redundancy, while at the same time improving patient safety and decreasing time to intervention. The technical and policy mechanisms supporting HIE are necessary for healthcare to become truly patient-centric. The transformative initiatives for healthcare reform and innovation rely on data sharing and workflow automation.

The principal challenge of HIE is the complex web of data-sharing partnerships, with each contributing entity having autonomous legal, regulatory, and technical policies and practices. Data sharing requires interorganizational agreement, conventions, and standardization. An individual patient's care may traverse a variety of healthcare entities. No single entity in a patient's continuum of care can coordinate all the detailed data handling between organizations. The distributed nature of HIE necessitates an evolutionary approach that incrementally achieves the goal of having a patient-centered experience with complete data.

Recognizing this challenge, the Office of the National Coordinator for Health Information Technology, in conjunction with various standards development organizations, has put forward a national road map for interoperability and the adoption of standards supporting HIE. Incentives for incremental progress have fostered various solutions, including the emergence of third-party intermediaries supporting data transformation and aggregation. Ultimately, the efficiencies of more integrated data transmission, filtering, and incorporation will achieve the promised simplicity.

Getting patient healthcare data to the right place can be facilitated by the provider or the patient. Either method of data movement can be automated by local software solutions or through intermediary organizations. Sometimes, the intermediary organizations have been called HIEs, which has led to some confusion between the process of exchanging data and the organizations that facilitate the exchange of data.

Data can be transmitted and received through protocols grouped into categories of *push*, *pull* (query/respond), and *publish/subscribe*. The standards supporting the protocols have a basis in the HL7. Early efforts for organization-to-organization data exchange relied on individual HL7 connections that were individually configured and validated.

The current trend is toward network-based connectivity, where a single connection is established on the network, giving access to the other connection points in the network. The first network connections were available for users of the same EHR vendor. Currently, the EHR-agnostic network protocols achieving the most widespread adoption are the Direct protocol and the Healtheway specifications (formerly NwHIN). The widespread adoption of these protocols can be attributed to their inclusion in certified technology associated with the Centers for Medicare & Medicaid Services (CMS) Meaningful Use. The certification requires software solutions for both provider-initiated workflow and patient-initiated data transmissions. Current HIE solutions are internet based and use the data security platforms aligned with web-based solutions—specifically, the Security Assertion Markup Language and the public/private key standards.

Patient privacy rights are enforced by the releasing organization according to their local policies and regulations. Patient authorizations for release are frequently exchanged between the requesting organization and the releasing organization. However, progress is being made toward interoperable patient authorizations for release, which will standardize and automate the assurances and attestations. Some organizations have adopted the eXtensible Access Control

Markup Language standard for authorizations, but the standard is not in widespread use at this time. When data sharing is constrained for health treatment purposes only, many organizations leverage the legal interpretation of protections for a covered entity. Other instances of bulk data exchange are leveraging specific organization-to-organization data-sharing agreements.

A significant step toward widespread adoption has been the use of the Direct project transport protocol, as specified in the CMS Meaningful Use programs. Direct is based on secure email standards and allows providers to push (send) clinical summaries and other document types to recipients also participating in the protocol. Security is enabled through shared certificates that have been expedited by federations such as Direct Trust, which manage a network of security certificates for vendors and for certified participating organizations. The lack of a central, shared directory of eligible organizations and providers has limited the operational use of Direct. Individual states, organizations, and some national groups have started projects toward a national provider directory. The Direct protocol is seeing success in integrating many providers previously ineligible for the CMS Meaningful Use incentives, including skilled nursing facilities and behavioral health providers.

The query/response functionality of HIE holds several advantages over push only. First, the specificity of the patient identity is fully constrained in the protocols currently endorsed by the Sequoia Project, an independent advocate for the creation of a worldwide HIE. Second, the protocols support automation of computer-to-computer exchange with message triggers driven from process events such as patient scheduling. The infrastructure supporting query and response is complicated by the patient lookup requirements to establish identity. The lack of robust patient identity correlations across organizations results in significant missed data exchanges and has led to a series of projects to enhance the ecosystem for patient identity across organizations. In addition to clinical care coordination, other use cases leveraging the infrastructure for query and response include population health and value-based reimbursement contracts.

Care coordination has been a foundational use case for HIE. Early stages of care coordination have been enabled with admission and discharge notifications among participants in an exchange network. The provider or coordinator of patient care will receive notice of the patient's treatment, such as a discharge notice, and can query for the detailed data as appropriate.

Progress toward workflow automation for HIE includes standardization of the document-based exchanges, such as CCR, CDA, and C-CDA. In addition, early development projects are underway using semantically constrained data models such as FHIR. The healthcare industry is moving toward a future of highly interoperable discrete data centered on an individual patient, with the security and privacy needs handled in the background. The expectation of data availability follows a path similar to that in other consumer-focused industries.

ENTERPRISE DATA INTEGRATION

Data Warehousing

The concept and implementation of data warehousing arose from the need for enhanced integrated analytics in organizations. While many systems purchased by organizations have analytic tools and capabilities to report from those systems, few allow for robust, systemwide integration of the data for population-based reporting. For the most part, those reporting capabilities have focused on real-time or operational reporting. Any organization can have upward of hundreds of data systems in need of integration, and a data warehousing platform allows for the planning, standardization, customization, and integration of these disparate data sources to provide meaningful and standardized data reporting.

More recently, however, data warehousing has expanded to include a variety of tools and technologies that allow users to not only analyze data in the warehouse but to combine those data with outcomes of analysis from external sources, streaming data, and other sources not typically used in population analytics. Gartner has termed this architecture the *logical data warehouse* and introduced the concept of integrating operational, population-based, and big data platforms as an integrated architecture.

Big Data

There are three big data characteristics, known as the "three Vs of big data"—volume, velocity, and variety. Volume is the storage of large amounts of data. Variety refers to the diverse types of structured and unstructured data to be stored. Velocity pertains to the speed at which data are processed.

These characteristics require new techniques for storing and processing data. Traditionally, these large data sets have been stored on multiple disparate systems. To gain the most analytics value from data, they need to be stored and processed on a single system. *Data lake* is a term that is used to describe the storage and processing of data in a single location. Data lakes are commonly supported by two technologies, massively parallel processing (MPP) databases and Hadoop.

MPP databases are intended to support structured (tabular) data. MPP databases allow most of today's analytics and reporting tools to connect to them. MPP databases allow data to be loaded, modified, and queried at real-time speeds. They have very quick query performance.

Hadoop works best in the storage and processing of unstructured (document, log, genomics) data. It also allows for structured data to be stored. Hadoop provides access to its processing and data through custom programs written in languages such as Python or Java. However, updates of data are difficult. Hadoop is better suited for batch, not real-time, processing. The technologies share similar characteristics—for example, both are able to use hundreds or thousands of servers to store and process data. The two are often used in conjunction. Custom applications written in Hadoop feed data into an MPP database for further data blending and more "performant" analytics. As the two technologies mature, the differences between MPP databases and Hadoop continue to blur.

Relational Data Warehouse Design

While there are many different ways to design a warehouse and store data in it, many follow key concepts to provide users with an environment that is meaningful and easy to navigate. While a transactional system (a database that collects, stores, and commits data frequently) is designed for individual quick transactions, a data warehouse (OLAP) is designed to return large sets of data for population type analysis. OLAP design combines data from multiple source system tables into fewer tables by prejoining the tables for access.

Dimensional Data Warehouse Design

A dimension data warehouse differs slightly in its design and is often referred to as a *star schema* or *snowflake design*. This design consists of tables called *fact tables* and *dimension tables*. The fact table (often at the center of the design) consists of actual values and data that can be aggregated or summed. The dimension tables are sets of tables used to describe or label the fact table values. These dimension tables are used in analysis to group data on a report; they almost always contain a date dimension. Other examples of a dimension are entities or facilities, departments, general ledger (GL) codes, and persons. Dimensional models are great for preaggregating data, slicing and dicing, and seeing trends in a specific data set because the data are preloaded or cached in the database.

Data Marts

Because a data warehouse can consist of thousands of tables, both detail and summary levels, the data are often organized into libraries called *data marts* (see exhibit 8.8). Data marts can be very general in nature (raw data from a source system) or very detailed and specific (calculations, measures, cohorts). Typically, data marts at the detailed level represent and support a unique business or clinical program's initiatives. These subject data marts often integrate data from many source systems to measure and support ongoing business and clinical outcomes and operations, and they also provide data summarization for regulatory and external agencies that require data extracts on an ongoing basis. Because the business logic is represented so tightly in the technical development, it is important that the business analyst work closely with the data warehouse developer to ensure the requirements are represented and to guarantee that the representation of the data meets all criteria.

Extraction, Transformation, and Loading

The method to move data from a transactional system into the data warehouse is referred to as *ETL*. ETL development is an instrumental step in the data warehouse development process and probably the most technical in nature. The extraction of the data includes setting up the connections to the source database and defining the criteria for which data will be pulled. While this seems straightforward, the developer must have a good understanding of the source system architecture as well as how the system inserts and updates its data. The criteria and definition of what data to pull on a frequent basis can be quite complex, but its identification is also mandatory if the organization is to avoid bad data or data duplication in the data warehouse.

The transformation of the data is the stage in which the data scrubbing, manipulation, and cleansing occur before entering the

Exhibit 8.8: Data Mart

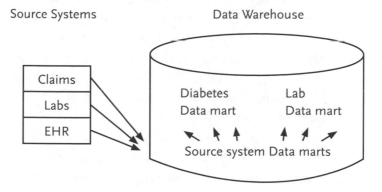

final tables of the data marts. While the transformation can be done using proprietary scripting or coding, there are many ETL applications on the market that offer the developer the ability to manipulate and program complex transformations using a graphical user interface. These applications help with both the standardization and the maintenance of ETL.

Loading the transformed data in the warehouse seems simple but requires a deep understanding of the database platform. Often, the volume of data being loaded into a data warehouse is quite large; the ETL and the database must be configured to handle large inserts without affecting end-user queries and reporting.

Reference and Master Data

Reference and master data are what enable the data warehouse to be integrated and often be enterprise-wide in nature. These data sets can be defined as the standardized definition and description of data throughout the enterprise. Without these master data, it would be very difficult to do comparative analytics across the data from various systems.

Master data in an organization are sets of data that are tightly managed by one master system and propagated to all other enterprise systems for management of their data. A master person or patient set (master person index) enables an organization to truly do enterprise analytics by propagating a unique person index throughout all systems in the organization. Thus, the patient or person can be identified in any enterprise system, and their data can be presented in a longitudinal manner.

Reference data are generally more standardized and can be defined within or outside the organization. Examples of internal reference data might include an organization's departmental structure, GL codes, or specific codes set up by a clinical program. External reference data include standardized definitions such as procedures, diagnosis, and current procedural terminologies that are maintained by outside entities. It is generally recommended that these reference sets be maintained by one master system and then burst or propagated to downstream systems to ensure consistency throughout the enterprise.

Metadata: Data About Data

Because the function of the data warehouse is data integration, it may become difficult to identify the original source or lineage of the data elements as they are propagated throughout data marts and tables in the data warehouse. In addition, because users often have specialized data knowledge related to their respective roles, it is necessary to have a robust data dictionary or metadata application to provide information, lineage, and descriptions of the data elements that reside in the data warehouse. This environment can also include information on the steward or owner of the data, when they were last updated, and any other particularities.

A healthcare enterprise analytics framework (see exhibit 8.9) is a helpful construct to consider how data and systems fit together in an architecture with the flexibility to accommodate the complex data environment that exists in healthcare today.

LEVERAGING DATA: ANALYTICS IN HEALTHCARE

Healthy pressures are creating a golden age for healthcare analytics. Enterprise systems have accumulated staggering amounts of data in the process of automating complex clinical and business workflows. Technology innovators have greatly advanced analysts' ability to mine, analyze, and leverage vast and growing data sets. As societal concerns over healthcare costs push back on healthcare costs, economics shift financial models away from a fee-for-service arrangement and into a fee-for-value model. Caregivers find that a disciplined application of analytics can improve clinical outcomes (and the health of populations) while reducing the overall cost of healthcare for the population.

Healthcare organizations use many strategies to advance analytics. The following are five best-practice initiatives and concepts you can use to more fully leverage analytics resources.

Conduct Change Readiness Conversations

In a perfect world, every analytical discovery, algorithm, and insight would be thoroughly implemented in a company. The reality is that operational change is difficult to implement.

Effective change readiness conversations with stakeholders, at a project's outset, can greatly increase an organization's ability to implement identified changes. In such a conversation, analysts and business leaders discuss the changes that will be required to implement the results of an analysis. Questions to discuss include the following:

- What changes will need to be made if this algorithm can be created?
- How will it affect workflows?
- What would be required to automate it?

Exhibit 8.9: Healthcare Enterprise Analytics Framework

Deliver

Information is delivered to internal and external lines of business in reports, visualizations, embedded applications, etc. Data are exchanged with other organizations. Analytics data may also be fed back into the collect layer for use in business applications.

Analyze

Methods are used to understand and find insights and patterns within the data to take action. Data may be further refined or filtered to meet the needs of a specific department or organization. The analyze layer prepares the data to be delivered through reports, visualizations, etc.

Organize (Enrich)

Data are integrated and aggregated through ETL, statistical processing, machine learning, federation, etc. The enriched data are then stored in new structures formatted for specific line of business analytics and reporting.

Acquire (Consolidate)

Data acquisition is the gathering of disparate sources of data into a single, consolidated location. When possible, data are gathered in near real time. Data are stored in their native format as found in the data source. Storing the data in one location allows data to be explored and discovered in a single system.

Collect (Data Source)

Data are collected and stored by applications such as ERP, EMR, or any system used to support business operations. These applications may reside onsite or in the cloud. Data may also be streamed by devices with no storage capabilities or collected from other external organizations.

Data architecture standards

Data acquisition and processing standards

Analytics standards

Data governance
- Quality
- Latency
- Persistence
- Lineage
- Terminology
- Metadata

Master data management
- Patient
- Provider
- Location
- Payer
- Drugs
- Personnel

Security

- How long will it take to get the required resources ready to implement the change?
- What obstacles do we expect to encounter, and how do we resolve them?

Often, these change-readiness conversations spur the organization to plan ahead and more successfully implement new findings and algorithms. When conducted effectively, intake conversations will occasionally result in a project being postponed or cancelled because the organization is not yet ready to implement the change. Although such postponements are disappointing, the organization is much better off investing its analytics resources in projects where success is more certain.

Measure Outcomes and Returns on Investment

Organizations do not invest in analytics for analytics' sake. Analytics investments must contribute to positive outcomes and returns. To do this, analysts, analytics leaders, and business leaders must develop a culture of accountability around analytics resources.

Following the conclusion of an analytics project (be it a new dashboard, an algorithm, or a recommended decision), the analysts should return and measure outcomes. Reviews may occur 6 or 12 months after the analysis was completed and implemented.

In many cases, the team will be able to measure the impact of the analysis on a change by measuring outcomes or other returns. For cases in which the outcomes were negative or not realized, analysts should reengage to determine whether refinements or further analyses are needed. This practice greatly assists the organization in maximizing returns, helps analyst teams sharpen their focus on business needs, and helps measure the value of analytics investments.

On occasion, analytics projects result in direct, hard-dollar returns that are easily measured and understood. More often, analytics returns are intertwined in the complexities of operations and may be measured in a number of more complex ways: decision support analysis may be measured by the difference between a higher cost proposal and a data-driven alternative decision. Analysts assisting clinicians on projects that affect patient experience, medical outcomes, or even mortality may measure results in terms of clinical outcomes. Some of these may yield a measurable return on investment or result in more noble, mission-based measures such as lives saved. Many operations-focused analysis projects result in operational efficiency improvements that require measuring the resulting freed-up capacity or resources.

Fully Analyze Paradoxes

Focusing on outcomes and return on investment in a complex healthcare organization can present unique challenges. Which variable to optimize must be carefully modeled to understand the inevitable unintended consequences on variables in other areas. Many such paradoxes are coming to light as the industry shifts payment models.

For example, in a fee-for-service model, companies are paid a set amount for every computed tomography (CT) scan performed. If optimizing for revenue, a company is incentivized to provide as many CT scans as possible. However, there were negative outcomes resulting from the long-term effects of increased radiation exposure and from the unintended incentive to provide unnecessary treatments. These paradoxes increase as healthcare organizations straddle the divide between population health—keeping populations healthy and not needing treatment—and traditional reimbursement models that pay more for more treatments.

Analytics can greatly assist healthcare leaders in navigating these complex paradoxes by focusing on mission. A mission statement gives clear direction to analysts and leaders who must sort out inevitable competing priorities as they seek to drive decisions on analytics.

To mitigate the impact of these paradoxes successfully, analysts should fully model a recommendation's impact and work with clinical and business partners to inform everyone who will be affected (whether positively or negatively). For example, consider the full effect on an organization that implements an algorithm to predict a respiratory disease outbreak:

- People are less likely to experience complications and may avoid problems altogether (targeted outcome)
- Community outreach teams will experience an increase in work as they use the algorithm to warn and engage the community
- Care managers will experience an increase in work as they connect with those identified in the risk cohorts
- Patient care employees will not be required to work as much overtime during outbreaks, which affects both employees' finances as well as operational expense
- The supply chain, with forewarning, will need to negotiate bulk purchase contracts while decreasing the needed supply delivery
- Inpatient volumes will decrease
- Financially, the organization will need to model decreases in both costs and revenues while increasing patient health

Modeling the impact of advanced analytics requires a coordinated, comprehensive look at all aspects of a given change. For the organization to leverage the change successfully, leaders in all affected areas should be informed of the forecasted changes in their respective areas of accountability. The organization's mission guides leaders' and analysts' decisions as they navigate the unintended consequences of change.

Implement Strategically Diverse Teams

In a rapidly evolving environment, such as the one healthcare is presently navigating, analytics teams must have access to diverse sets of resources. Changing business models, evolving legislation, new operating models, and the incredible pace of care innovations frequently require analytics teams to tap into widely varied resources. Analyst leaders must carefully and strategically plan for this diversity. The dimensions of diversity that organizations should consider in determining how to staff, grow, and connect teams of analysts include education, skills, experience, and management.

Education

Analyst strategic planning should include the acquisition of analysts with diverse educational backgrounds. Consider two hypothetical teams. Team A has five analysts, each with a statistics degree. Team B has five analysts with backgrounds in statistics, finance, applied mathematics, behavioral economics, and biostatistics. What type of solutions will each team produce?

Skills

Analytics skills are largely grouped into two general areas: statistical and mathematical skills or technical skills. Analyst teams that do not have access to both areas will struggle to deliver full value to the organization.

A team comprising primarily statisticians may excel in developing models and algorithms, but it may also spend an inordinate amount of time data wrangling, automating repetitive tasks, and manually processing ad hoc requests. Its members may not create solutions that are as fully operationalized as they could be if the team included stronger technical resources.

A team comprising primarily technically skilled analysts may excel in its visualizations and automation but struggle to move its services beyond descriptive or diagnostic levels. Its members can miss opportunities to create predictive algorithms and deliver needed sophisticated prescriptive solutions.

Experience

Analyst teams should be thoughtfully designed to include a healthy mix of both experienced and newer analysts. Teams with an appropriate mix of junior- and senior-level analysts enable project tasks to be divided more economically than a team with only senior analysts, allowing analysts to do what they do best and efficiently perform the tasks that best fit their experience. Teams with a good mix of new and experienced analysts also create environments with healthy succession plans and career opportunities, maximizing engagement and mitigating undesirable turnover.

Management

To get the full strength from diversity, analytics leaders must develop the ability to unite and lead diverse teams. Teams may be formal departments, or they may be ad hoc work teams challenged with a single project. Managers should also create long-term hiring and staffing strategies to ensure the right people are in place over time.

Cultivate Innovation and Collaboration

Analysts thrive in environments where innovation is supported. Innovation and collaboration can be fostered by carefully planning analytics events such as "hackathons" and analytics competitions.

In a hackathon, analysts work with interested business partners to self-identify unsolved business problems. The analysts form into ad hoc, cross-functional teams and are given a day or two to work together on their selected problem. These cross-functional teams allow analysts to get to know other analysts, be introduced to new skills, and experience collaboration in diverse teams. The hackathon culminates in project presentations and awards given to the winning teams. Successful projects may go on to be more fully developed and implemented in the organization.

Analytics competitions are another way to encourage innovation. Companies may create a data set around a known problem or perhaps an existing solution. Analysts may receive training on new skills or tools and are then given time to work on the problem or attempt improvements on an existing solution. The resulting solutions and improvements are presented to the group, and winning ideas are operationalized.

THE FUTURE OF HEALTHCARE ANALYTICS

Currently, analytics for the majority of healthcare providers is characterized by the analytics capabilities found in their electronic health record systems and by achieving reporting requirements mandated for reimbursements by CMS. Nearly 90 percent of the work performed by healthcare systems today is fee-for-service and not based on outcome. The progressive stages of Meaningful Use started with the creation of EHRs and are progressing toward reimbursement models that are outcomes-based rather than activity based (and the rest of the federal government and insurance providers are following suit). This progress includes assessing patient satisfaction through things such as Hospital Consumer Assessment of Healthcare Providers and Systems scores and continues with the Medicare Access and CHIP Reauthorization Act of 2015, which mandates that up to 25 percent of reimbursements be based on outcomes in the future.

The bottom line of this evolution is that analytics for the vast majority of healthcare providers are primarily driven by reporting requirements that change how they are reimbursed by the government and insurance companies. Furthermore, the ability to meet these requirements is primarily achieved by the capabilities of the EHR systems employed by a healthcare provider. In this section, we describe the progression of analytics to achieve these increasingly demanding regulatory and reimbursement requirements. We also discuss the movement beyond mandated measures and progress toward better health outcomes.

Progression of Analytics Capabilities

Analytics tend to experience the progression of maturity discussed in the following list and illustrated in exhibit 8.10.

- Descriptive stage (what has happened): Financial and operational reporting, cost analysis, quality and compliance, Meaningful Use, and so on
- Diagnostic stage (why things happened): Outcomes analysis, gaps in care, fraud detection, and so on
- Predictive stage (what will happen): Population health risk stratification, contract forecasting and modeling, diagnostic clinical decision support, and so on
- Prescriptive stage (what should happen): Care process models, prescriptive clinical decision support, precision medicine, and so on

For most healthcare systems today, the vast majority of reporting and analytics focus on descriptive analytics. Moving up the progression of maturity, diagnostic analytics provide insights that can lead to quality improvement activities and to clinical variation

Exhibit 8.10: Progression of Maturity

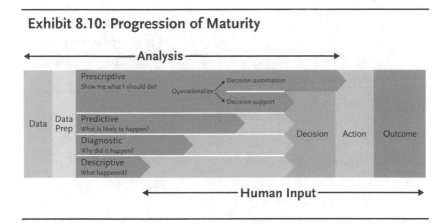

reduction. More advanced healthcare systems use predictive models to identify patients at risk for poor health as well as interventions for preventing adverse outcomes. Good examples of this are checklists administered prior to patient discharge to assess readmission risk, especially for high-cost conditions such as congestive heart failure. Early detection and intervention for serious infections such as sepsis have also been created and administered with significant success rates. The pinnacle of analytics maturity is the achievement of prescriptive analytics. Similar to a doctor's prescription of medications, population- and evidence-based care pathways or care processes are a great example of prescriptive analytics. Healthcare systems that have developed and that follow these evidence-based practices have been successful in delivering lower-cost, higher-quality clinical outcomes than systems that have not achieved this level of analytics sophistication and maturity.

Analytics Tools and Methods

The following are descriptions of various analytics tools and methods that also represent a progression toward higher levels of analytics maturity.

- *Delivered reports.* These are reports that are typically pushed out by email (and similar methods) to business and clinical users on a schedule. Examples are reports for financial performance, purchasing and supply chain, quality and patient safety, payroll, human resources, and clinical areas.
- *Self-service reports.* Self-service reports are similar in nature to delivered reports but allow the users to execute the report on demand and also control filter and selection criteria (e.g., date range, group of patients, selected facilities or geographic regions).

- *Self-service dashboards.* Dashboards are more complex than reports in that they provide users with a wide variety of options for selecting and filtering data and allow a variety of options for graphical viewing of the data and results. In addition, these dashboards will typically allow the users to save queries to be repeated in the future and export resultant data to be used in additional analyses.
- *Data discovery and data preparation.* These tools allow data to be interrogated in order to discover patterns, formatting, and data quality. More capable solutions allow the data to be transformed and standardized for more advanced analysis. Feature engineering in preparation for advanced statistical analysis is also typically performed by these tools.
- *Statistical analysis.* Statistical analytics tools allow statistical analysts and actuaries to use advanced analytics methods, such as linear and logical regression, random forest, K-means, Bayesian networks, gradient boosted trees, and decision trees, to perform correlation and outlier analysis leading to the development of predictive algorithms.
- *Analytics applications.* Once algorithms have been developed that need to be applied to a clinical or business workflow, teams can deploy purpose-built analytics, custom alerts, and embedded analytics as stand-alone applications. They can also be embedded in existing operational systems, such as EHRs or financial systems.
- *Machine learning (cognitive computing, artificial intelligence, deep learning).* These more advanced analytics tools employ iterative execution of statistical methods combined with "learning" from the data themselves. Supervised and unsupervised methods are employed to achieve algorithms that are superior to those achieved with traditional statistical methods alone.

Current Electronic Health Record Systems and Commercial Analytics Capabilities

Most EHR systems provide basic operational reporting capabilities related to assessing the cost and quality associated with delivering inpatient and ambulatory care. This information includes a progression of clinical decision support; clinical registry reporting; quality measures reporting; and progress toward care coordination, patient engagement, population health, HIE data management functionality, and reporting capabilities. For healthcare systems using a variety of EHR systems, purchasing commercial reporting systems has generally become a necessity. Larger healthcare systems have moved in the direction of creating enterprise data warehouses that are supported by data and reporting professionals to acquire these complex data management and data reporting capabilities.

The most advanced healthcare systems have been using aggregated data for many years, drawing on sources ranging in number from the dozens to the hundreds. These more mature organizations have tens of thousands of employees and typically produce thousands of reports and hundreds of self-service dashboards addressing every aspect of running a healthcare business, from supply chain, financial systems, human resources, to all inpatient and ambulatory clinical areas. Integrated payer and providers go a step farther by combining both clinical and claims data to achieve even more sophisticated capabilities.

Predictive Analytics in Healthcare Today

Many healthcare systems use a wide range of risk-scoring algorithms and disease state–specific risk-prediction algorithms. These algorithms include stratification for patients at risk for high utilization; readmissions; mortality; and clinical conditions such as congestive heart failure, chronic obstructive pulmonary disease, coronary artery disease, diabetes, preterm birth, chronic kidney disease, end-stage renal disease, and sepsis. The website MDcalc.com lists more than 300 scoring and prediction methods and algorithms. More recently, genomic testing has been producing treatment and clinical trials matching for precision medicine in oncology, pharmacogenomics, neonatal conditions, and cardiology. Most of these algorithms and methods have been developed using traditional statistical methods like those discussed earlier.

Machine Learning Solutions Today

While machine learning is considered an emerging analytics field in healthcare, here are some examples of what machine learning has accomplished so far:

- Deriving optimal care delivery for specific procedures such as total knee replacement
- Predicting preterm births using genomic data
- Improving colon cancer screening using data from simple historical lab tests
- Improving diagnosis of heart conditions from echocardiogram results
- Detecting disease states from medical imaging
- Other conditions improved through machine learning insights include, but are not limited to, Alzheimer's disease, multiple myeloma, rheumatoid arthritis, and Parkinson's disease

These examples of success with machine learning are being achieved by fewer than 5 percent of healthcare systems today, but the breadth of use cases points to the high probability that these successes will multiply at an accelerating pace.

PERSONALIZED DIAGNOSIS AND TREATMENT RECOMMENDATIONS

The emergence of a few platforms that have spent years developing continuously learning healthcare knowledge bases is a relatively new but extremely significant development. These bases have been trained in the following manner:

- Integrating clinical, claims, socioeconomic, consumer, environmental, and other data for millions of people
- Capturing thousands of patient-level data dimensions from structured and unstructured data sources
- Incorporating hundreds of healthcare risk and prediction models
- Augmenting available information with findings from thousands of published and peer-reviewed research studies
- Producing patient similarity algorithms

From all of this training, a nominal amount of data about an individual can be fed into these engines to produce patient-level diagnosis and treatment recommendations. These recommendations are given to clinicians to be shared with patients based on their clinical knowledge and experience. These systems are beginning to incorporate additional insights from a growing understanding of genomic markers as further predictors of disease propensity.

THE FUTURE OF ADVANCED ANALYTICS

The future of advanced analytics is most likely to be based on helping more people avoid diseases by better enabling them to follow healthy lifestyles. Prevention helps address many of the conditions we are currently treating at growing rates, such as diabetes, anxiety and depression, circulatory diseases, and cancers. The trends described in the machine learning section continue to expand, making the following use cases the norm rather than the exception in most healthcare systems:

- *Predicting high-cost patients.* Five percent of patients account for 50–60 percent of all healthcare costs; each year, this group churns between 50 and 80 percent of available resources.
- *Engaging highest-value patients (health activation).* Achieving 90 percent patient engagement and more than 95 percent patient satisfaction will be transformational.
- *Managing highest-value patients (optimized care process models).* Optimizing evidence-based care process models with highly engaged patients and minimum variance will maximize the impact of population health management.
- *Personalizing population-based care process models.* Aligning population-based care processes with precision medicine and personalized medicine will further enhance the quality of individual health outcomes while reducing cost.
- Augmenting diagnosis and treatment insights and recommendations with genomic data.
- Optimizing clinical operations for continuous improvement.

REFERENCES

Benson, T., and G. Grieve. 2016. *Principles of Health Interoperability: SNOMED CT, HL7 and FHIR.* New York: Springer.

Cimino, J. J. 1998. "Desiderata for Controlled Medical Vocabularies in the Twenty-First Century." *Methods of Information in Medicine* 37 (4–5): 394–403.

D'Amore, J. D., J. C. Mandel, D. A. Kreda, A. Swain, G. A. Koromia, S. Sundareswaran, L. Alschuler, R. H. Dolin, K. D. Mandl, I. S.

Kohane, and R. B. Ramoni. 2014. "Are Meaningful Use Stage 2 Certified EHRs Ready for Interoperability? Findings from the SMART C-CDA Collaborative." *Journal of the American Medical Informatics Association* 21 (6): 1060–68.

Empel, S. 2018. "Way Forward: AHIMA Develops Information Governance Principles to Lead Healthcare Toward Better Data Management." AHIMA. Accessed May 8. http://library.ahima .org/doc?oid=107468#.

Mead, C. N. 2006. "Data Interchange Standards in Healthcare IT—Computable Semantic Interoperability: Now Possible but Still Difficult, Do We Really Need a Better Mousetrap?" *Journal of Healthcare Information Management* 20 (1): 71–78.

Mendes, D., and I. P. Rodrigues. 2013. "A Semantic Web Pragmatic Approach to Develop Clinical Ontologies, and Thus Semantic Interoperability, Based in HL7 v2.XML Messaging." In *Information Systems and Technologies for Enhancing Health and Social Care*, edited by R. Martinho, R. Rijo, M. Cruz-Cunha, and J. Varajao, 205–14. Hershey, PA: IGI Global.

Office of the National Coordinator for Health Information Technology. 2018. *Connecting Health and Care for the Nation: A 10-Year Vision to Achieve an Interoperable Health IT Infrastructure.* Accessed May 3. www.healthit.gov/sites/default/files /ONC10yearInteroperabilityConceptPaper.pdf.

Parker, C. G., R. A. Rocha, J. R. Campbell, S. W. Tu, and S. M. Huff. 2004. "Detailed Clinical Models for Sharable, Executable Guidelines." *Studies in Health Technology and Informatics* 107: 145–48.

Public Health Data Standards Consortium. 2017. "Data Standards." Accessed February 7. www.phdsc.org/standards/health -information/D_Standards.asp.

Raths, D. 2016. "Can SOLOR (SnOmed LOinc, Rxnor) Project Create Terminology Foundation for Interoperability?" *Healthcare Informatics.* Published July 22. www.healthcare-informatics

.com/blogs/david-raths/interoperability/can-solor-snomed-loinc-rxnorm-project-create-terminology.

Regenstrief Institute. 2017. "Get Started." Accessed February 9. http://loinc.org/get-started.

Richesson, R. L., and C. G. Chute. 2015. *Health Information Technology Data Standards Get Down to Business: Maturation Within Domains and the Emergence of Interoperability*. New York: Oxford University Press.

Smith, B., and W. Ceusters. 2006. "HL7 RIM: An Incoherent Standard." In *Ubiquity: Technologies for Better Health in Aging Societies*, edited by A. Hasman, R. Haux, J. van der Lei, E. De Clerq, and F. H. Roger France. Lansdale, PA: IOS Press.

SNOMED International. 2017. "SNOMED CT: The Global Language of Healthcare." Accessed February 9. www.snomed.org/snomed-ct.

World Health Organization. 2018. "Classifications." Accessed May 8. www.who.int/classifications/icd/en/.

CHAPTER 9

Managing Actuarial Risk

Steven Johnson

A PROVIDER-SPONSORED HEALTH plan (PSHP) is a licensed insurance entity owned by a provider (e.g., hospital, health system, medical group). It receives direct premium payments for its assumption of first-dollar risk (e.g., without a deductible) for the total cost of the care delivered to insured individuals or populations, as consistent with the coverage purchased.

A PSHP owned by a hospital or health system but not operated in the context of an integrated delivery network (IDN)—that is, integrated with clinical operations—is simply an operating asset, as is a hospital, an ambulatory surgery center, or any other clinical enterprise. The greatest leveraging value from a PSHP is not in its financial performance as a stand-alone entity. Rather, it is as a means for the provider to hold first-dollar risk in a clinical enterprise and serve as a catalyzing agent toward the realization of population health management.

In addition to touching on the many operational and regulatory intricacies that come with owning and operating a PSHP (they are substantial and demanding), this chapter describes the experiences of Health First, a health system based in Rockledge, Florida, and its Health First Health Plans. Based on my experience as president and CEO, I will discuss aspects of our chosen strategy and the struggles we encountered, as well as lessons learned, in our quest to enhance value for the people we serve. Health First's objective: to deliver illness prevention and health restoration services through a customer-centric experience at the lowest possible price.

One purpose of this chapter is to describe how a PSHP can play a role in creating the economic structure that supports the Institute for Healthcare Improvement's Quadruple Aim. PSHPs are not the only way to achieve these goals; such an approach represents only one way to begin to do so. In addition, this chapter provides some description of calculation, pricing, selling, and servicing of actuarial risk in the form of health insurance products.

Health system leaders are accustomed to extraordinary regulation. Rules; inspections; accreditations by local, state, and federal agencies; and other processes meant to regulate our activity are commonplace. We accommodate the oversight while recognizing the burdens inherent in operating in such a complex environment.

Health plans are no less complex and no less regulated. Regulatory synergies between the clinical delivery world and insurance plans would be highly advantageous—but few synergies exist. While many agencies regulating operation of the clinical delivery components and insurance plans are the same (e.g., the state-level agencies regulating healthcare in general, the Centers for Medicare & Medicaid Services [CMS] at the federal level), the sections or functions within those agencies that perform the regulating are not the same. Generally, the rules and personnel differ significantly. In addition, other agencies with which clinical organizations do not have experience come into play. Most notably, a licensed health plan is subject to significant state-level oversight by the department of insurance (in our case, the Office of Insurance Regulation in Florida).

Over the past year, external auditors in our health plan have performed audits required by regulatory agencies on approximately 75 percent of business days. The audits are mandated by statute and regulations, sometimes in response to real or perceived issues of the health insurance industry (e.g., complaints, claims patterns). The process involves production of data and documents and participation in numerous interviews. Issues of varying importance are typically found, requiring plans of correction; reporting; and, of course, follow-up audits, which repeat and extend the process.

In addition to regulatory activities, special business-related actions, such as the recent conversion of one of our health plan companies from for-profit to not-for-profit status, can be complex and time-consuming. That change alone took 18 months of concerted work led by the chief financial officer (CFO) of our IDN and thousands of staff, consultant, and attorney hours spent working through a complex, iterative process that involved CMS, the Internal Revenue Service, and the Florida Office of Insurance Regulation and Agency for Health Care Administration (both state agencies).

A PROVIDER-SPONSORED HEALTH PLAN IN AN INTEGRATED DELIVERY NETWORK

PSHPs pose material operational challenges as well, particularly if the organization intends to operate that plan as an organizing asset for an IDN, as we do. The following questions, while not all-inclusive, offer some indication of the matters that an IDN must address:

- How should care be managed? Should it be managed differently for health plan members than for other customers of the clinical delivery platform?
- How do high-risk, high-cost members get treated?
- Does the healthcare system create focused, condition-specific services to mitigate disease (e.g., extensivist approaches or specialized clinics for patients with diabetes, chronic obstructive pulmonary disease, or congestive heart failure)?
- Are such services available to customers outside the PSHP, to members of other health plans and insurers? If so, how is the healthcare system paid for them?

For Health First, the answers are mixed and evolving. For example, we recently combined our quality and care management functions IDN-wide and house them through the health plan. The care managers work to coordinate services for the right care, in the right place, and at the right time, irrespective of payer source. We have, however, decided to restrict *extensivist care* (care coordinators or physicians who focus on high-risk, complex patients throughout the continuum of care) to our health plan members, whereby we reduce cost and improve health—creating an attractive clinical feature that differentiates our health plan. In addition, this feature allows us to avoid the challenge of finding suitable reimbursement for such services for patients with other payers. Our current approach is far from ideal, as all people we serve should have access to the same care, but the economic realities cannot be ignored.

With the economic realities of contemporary healthcare delivery and the emergence and increasing prevalence of value-based purchasing, bundled payments, and other forms of pay-for-performance methodologies, achieving the Quadruple Aim has never been more of an imperative. The key rationale for using a PSHP as a central and coordinating principle of an IDN is in its ability to offer two foundational advantages. The PSHP provides the IDN with the requisite (1) economic means and (2) population health tools to support the achievement of that lofty goal. For Health First, our health plan was and is our key asset for achieving both of our high-level strategic goals: to operate an IDN on a local basis and to achieve a scale that is self-sustaining.

Health First is located on Florida's Space Coast, an area largely dominated by the aerospace and defense industries. The organization has annual revenues of approximately $1.8 billion and currently includes four hospitals (three general community, one tertiary); a health plan with approximately 160,000 members in all typical lines of business; a 350-provider medical group; and a well-diversified array of ambulatory and wellness services, from home care to hospice—including three fitness centers. All of these components form and operate an IDN.

The PSHP sits at the center of the IDN. It is the integrating force and the financial vehicle through which old fee-for-service payment incentives can be transformed to incentivize the promotion of population health. However, what is an IDN? Unless a term (such as *accountable care organization*) is defined by a regulatory body, a definitive explanation often is not possible. The definition of IDN offered here is derived from many sources and provided for context.

An IDN generally has the following characteristics:

1. Integrates services and brings them to market as a whole through or with a risk-holding vehicle (in our case, Health First Health Plans); manages the health of a population, in part or in full
2. Links preventive, pre-acute, acute, and post-acute care services into a continuum: right care, right time, right place—no more, no less
3. Engages physicians and other clinicians in the ongoing refinement of evidence-based care and prevention
4. Designs and integrates its clinical and insurance systems and services to be customer-centric as it strives to deliver a unified experience for customers
5. Achieves and sustains superior performance in safety, clinical quality, experience, and cost—the value equation for customers
6. Moves steadily toward prevention and wellness promotion while continuing to provide disease- and condition-specific services

Like many health systems, Health First had been significantly hospital-centric. That is, our nonhospital assets functioned in large measure to meet the needs of the hospitals. Each clinical entity operated mostly autonomously, and many had redundant, or at least overlapping, support functions (e.g., finance, information technology, decision support). Each leader's job was to optimize the performance of her individual business, not that of the entire system—a classic example of siloed management. This is not to suggest that the previous leaders of our system were underperforming or somehow missing the mark. The individual businesses operated well under the old model of healthcare economics, and the aggregated performance of the whole reasonably supported its constituent parts. But it was not integrated; one part could not talk easily to another, and our customers experienced each piece as unique and unrelated to our other capabilities.

The charge given to me by the Health First board of directors on my hiring was to create an integrated healthcare solution that would improve the value equation for the individuals, companies, and government entities we serve. Looking at systems that had successfully navigated toward this goal, we selected the development of an IDN as our central local strategy. It also appeared likely that, at $1.8 billion in revenue, our scale might not be sufficient to operationalize that goal fully. To address this issue, we developed a complementary scaling strategy using the health plan as our principal asset to enhance our scale.

Historically, we had been structured in a traditional fashion around a budget with a strong emphasis on business unit–level operating profitability. Despite our emphasis on and continuous conversation about behaving like an IDN, we often experienced siloed business advocacy and behavior. Let me provide a couple of examples that highlight how our previous approach affected the operation of Health First Health Plans.

First, the chief medical officers of our health plan and our hospital division sometimes debated and then engaged an outside party to determine whether a Health First Health Plans member should be designated as inpatient or observation. The financial difference in the outcome was minimal, as we were paying ourselves, but each executive was accountable for a different bottom line. Another example is in how our health plan related to our ambulatory pharmacy. The pharmacy leaders had turned that business unit from a net financial loser to one generating an operating margin of more than $3 million annually—on its face, a good situation. However, more than

90 percent of the pharmacy's customers were Health First Health Plans members. The pharmacy was not really an independent profit center but rather a cost center of the health plan. With business unit–centric profitability as the measure, was the pharmacy missing opportunities to move members to less costly generic drugs? These would create lower margins for the pharmacy but higher margins for the health plan, and they would lower cost for our health plan members. Were other cost-reduction opportunities for the health plan and its members being missed?

Similar circumstances led us to change our reporting and incentives framework from one driven by a divisional bottom line and budget methodology to one that measures key performance indicators (KPIs) and uses performance-forecasting methodology. Our key metrics for profitability now rest at the aggregate IDN level rather than the divisional level; each division and business unit has goals that drive and support overall IDN performance. For example, we monitor cost per variable unit of service in most operating units and often break that down by labor or nonlabor expense. Many divisions also include measures of their growth known to be associated with profitability. For example, one KPI in the pharmacy is the percentage of its revenue that is derived from non–Health First Health Plans customers; other KPIs target the percentage of health plan members it serves, its cost per unit, and member satisfaction. The focus for all KPIs is on ultimately driving the performance of the entire IDN rather than individual units in isolation, with the affordability of the health plan as Health First's lead and organizing business goal.

Our IDN forecast is updated on a quarterly basis. Using the current forecast as a predictive baseline, we work toward creating the future state necessary to achieve or exceed the annual forecast and commitments we have made to ourselves and the board. KPI forecasts include measures for each of our commitments. For Health First, these are the general categories of quality/no harm, stewardship, and customer experience. For example, for Health First Health Plans, we forecast performance in member satisfaction, medical loss ratio, revenue per member per month, and Healthcare

Effectiveness Data and Information Set measures (i.e., key health plan metrics for Medicare Advantage that affect the dollar rate). With a forecasting approach, the overall intention is to understand any variance, but we also focus on how shortfalls will be overcome to affect subsequent forecasts and how performance over forecast can be replicated and advanced.

While KPIs and performance forecasting with at-risk compensation tied to metrics are certainly not new practices in healthcare, they were new to us. By all indications, these changes are supporting substantially more IDN-centric behavior and outcomes. For example, the focus on KPIs pointed to the lack of internal coordination in care management, as evidenced by internal denial rates and related metrics. These KPIs led us to change the structure of the IDN-wide care management function such that both it and our quality function report directly to the health plan and operate as IDN-wide functions. Similarly, as we tracked KPIs reflecting the health plan transaction costs, it became clear that the traditional processing of claims from our health plan to our care delivery platform was not adding value, just cost and complexity. We are now moving to internal prepayment with simplified tracking of encounters. The value of such changes became apparent through the tracking of KPIs when they are designed to be IDN-centric.

Health First Health Plans has developed over a 20-year period, beginning as a very small plan and a narrow network under capitation. Our health plan team consisted predominantly of professionals from our care delivery platform, largely our hospitals. The health plan stayed relatively small—around 60,000 members—and had grown slowly to that size. The plan appeared to run well, but it was small enough that a group of dedicated and smart people could "muscle" it into performance.

As we began to grow fairly rapidly, it became clear that we lacked the skills and experience of a major health plan. We came to recognize that there were simply things we did not know or possess. We have, therefore, recruited highly experienced health plan executives, including a chief operating officer (COO) with more than 25 years of health plan experience (most recently as the COO of an 800,000-member plan). We also recruited a health plan CFO with similar experience. These professionals brought a rich understanding of health plan operations that we had not even known to look for. They are developing their teams internally and by recruitment, and the health plan's operations are improving rapidly.

Health First is in pursuit of two primary strategies: to become an IDN on the local level and to achieve additional scale to sustain our operations. Both of these goals rely on Health First Health Plans as a critical asset.

A means to hold financial risk is an important characteristic for an integrated system to function optimally. For Health First, that vehicle is our health plan. It is increasingly serving as a principal organizing structure of clinical care and wellness services.

Significant effort has been applied to increase the size of the health plan and the number of lives under risk. The higher the proportion of our total revenue that is derived from lives under first-dollar risk, the more rational and easier is the pivot from a traditional volume-based care delivery system to one more focused on population health. In an ideal world, the health plan would be the sole profit center of Health First, with all care delivery components functioning as cost centers. In such a scenario, the financial performance of the IDN is enhanced as the health and well-being of its members improve. We are, not surprisingly, far from such a full transition.

Currently, Health First Health Plans represents more than 25 percent of the revenue of our delivery system. The largest share of our revenue is derived from traditional arrangements with other payers, commercial and governmental, which will likely continue into the foreseeable future. The conundrum is clear: How do we pivot to population health for our health plan to have maximum impact and continue to live in a fee-for-service world for the majority of our clinical revenues? For us, the answer is to apply population health and disease state–specific strategies to many of our customers, not just our health plan members. Doing so means that competing health plans benefit from our efforts, but it is difficult to function ethically in worlds with competing incentives.

We have made and will continue to make a significant investment in our health plan's capabilities (e.g., analytic IT capabilities for population health) and some in the delivery platform (e.g., extensivist clinics and related resources, consumer-oriented access enhancements) to better serve the population health risk we now hold through the health plan. We intend to compete in the marketplace with other health plans, as we have to date, and to deliver a product with a superior value proposition. Health First will offer the greatest customer experience and quality (in both restorative and preventive services) at the lowest possible cost.

ACHIEVING IDN SCALE THROUGH THE HEALTH PLAN

In addition to serving as the integrating vehicle and public face of our IDN, our health plan is also the principal means by which we are working to enhance our scale. With revenues of approximately $1.8 billion, Health First is of insufficient size to generate all of the resources we believe will be needed to pivot fully and successfully to a customer-centric IDN world, even with the sustained, respectable 4 to 5 percent operating margins we produce. At a certain point in our development, the question for us, then, became, How can we best achieve the scale we believe necessary while supporting (or, at a minimum, not competing with) our principal local strategy of creating that customer-centric IDN we aspire to be?

We considered whether we could accomplish significant growth in our health plan organically by expanding into new geographic markets. It was quickly evident that pursuing such a goal was economically unreasonable. While our brand is measurably strong and well regarded in our market, it has no equity in other markets in our state or region. Establishing a brand that can succeed in the highly competitive health plan space is a very expensive and a far-from-certain endeavor.

Having concluded that health plan growth by organic geographic expansion was both impractical and unlikely to be successful, we considered other means to achieve scale using the health plan. We discussed full or partial sale to an existing health plan but concluded that our brand would be diluted and that we would run the risk of strengthening a competitor, competing with ourselves, or both. We also considered selling third-party administrator or other back-of-shop services to health systems working on population health strategies with vehicles such as accountable care organizations or clinically integrated networks that typically lack robust means to manage the financial risk. We discovered, however, that our health plan systems were not sufficiently robust to serve such clients in the numbers that would be needed (hundreds of thousands of members) to achieve scale given the relatively modest payment available for such services.

We next considered partnering with a like-minded not-for-profit system (or systems) to provide private-label health plan products in their markets under our license and administration. We required a partner health system with a strong reputation and hearty brand, a clinical footprint that would facilitate significant growth of our health plan, and a leadership team committed to moving toward population health management.

One might ask why a health system with a strong brand and operations, as well as a broad footprint, wouldn't just start its own health plan. Although entirely new health plans are started by health systems, the limitations to such a greenfield approach are significant and involve time, money, and personnel, all of which interact and may involve overreach for many healthcare organizations and systems.

Capitalizing a health plan to normal operations and breakeven performance is likely to require at least $30–$50 million. While many systems can afford such an investment, it is substantial enough to make them reconsider. In addition, the talent to operate a health plan must be recruited and teams must be built; these individuals are in high demand and have many opportunities. It is difficult to discern which candidates have the "right stuff" to both operate a health plan and to do so in the context of an IDN. Finally, systems must factor in the speed to market. Considering the regulatory requirements, as well as the necessary systems building, recruitment, licensing, and learnings, taking a greenfield health plan from conception to enrollment can take three to five years. With the growing imperative to hold and manage financial risk for populations, the healthcare marketplace may look very different in five years, and there may be diminished or little room for start-up health plans. For these reasons, it appears reasonable for health systems desiring to manage population health to preserve capital and significantly enhance speed to market by finding an existing PSHP with which to partner.

We found a partner system with these attributes and goals and are entering our fourth year of that relationship. We are providing health plan products initially in Medicare Advantage, individual (on and off the Health Insurance Marketplace), and employer (insured and self-funded) market segments in four of our partner organization's counties and have doubled our membership to approximately 160,000, about half of which is full risk. The relationship is working well for both parties, and we plan to continue our expansion across our partner organization's markets. By full maturity, our jointly owned health plan will likely have 400,000–500,000 members. Such growth will not fully realize our need for enhanced scale but will advance progress toward that goal.

The unsustainability of our historic economic model and the emergence of forces, such as the Quadruple Aim, have stimulated much-needed change in healthcare, the type and pace of which are nearly revolutionary. For Health First, the road toward that lofty yet imperative goal has been through the creation, or perhaps evolution, of an IDN with a PSHP at its center. The following sections present a description of the calculation, pricing, selling, and servicing of actuarial risk in the form of health insurance products.

As we review Health First's need for, and learnings from, a journey to understand and manage actuarial risk, particularly as it applies to Health First Health Plans's product development and sales functions, some historical perspective adds context.

BURNING PLATFORM

In March 2012, the leadership team of the Health First Health Plan had a mandate: to reverse our recent trend of enrollment decline and begin to increase health plan membership. At that time, the health plan was data challenged. A historical enrollment report was difficult to obtain; however, one was developed that listed health plan membership for each of the previous six years. The results were uncomfortable. Health First Health Plans had been bleeding enrollment, losing membership in five of the six most recent years. As a result of data limitations, health plan and IDN leadership had not been aware that enrollment and market share were shrinking for this length of time or to this extent.

I labeled this information Health First's *burning platform*. As the relatively new system CEO, I hoped that from that moment, a heightened level of attention would empower the entire IDN to support the need for immediate action to turn around the health plan's decline.

The *burning platform*, a term that became very familiar to my team in 2012 and 2013, provided a clarity of vision and offered a way to start afresh (see exhibit 9.1). However, we did not know at that time that the health plan's consistent pattern of profitability would be challenged beginning in 2014. This rupture was, in large part, the corresponding result of the challenges of shrinking enrollment; adverse selection; actuarial naiveté; a smaller revenue base over which to spread fixed costs; and the data challenges that plagued sales and enrollment, as well as all functional areas throughout the organization.

Exhibit 9.1: Burning Platform (Enrollments by Year)

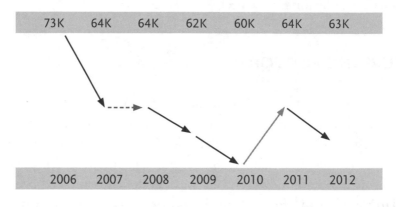

Market Challenge

| 73K | 64K | 64K | 62K | 60K | 64K | 63K |

| 2006 | 2007 | 2008 | 2009 | 2010 | 2011 | 2012 |

The Plan

With that inauspicious introduction to Health First Health Plans, the health plan's vice president (VP) of sales and business development was commissioned to develop a strategic growth plan. This sales executive, hired within the previous month, had been selected because he brought two decades of health plan sales leadership, much of it with provider-sponsored and IDN health plans, including the healthcare sector's largest. That executive drafted and presented a five-point strategic sales plan with the intention to build a foundation to turn and eventually reverse the enrollment decline.

At the time of the plan's introduction in May 2012, we used a cliché to underscore our situation: turning a battleship. The first step to turn a large ship would be, of course, to stop sailing in the wrong direction. That seems obvious, even trite, but the underlying point is that we would not grow just by simply selling harder or because we wished to. We needed to understand the underlying causes of enrollment decline, face painful realities, and then, to put it simply, do things differently. The following sections outline the health plan's blueprint for growth.

Product

As with many smaller health plans with less nimble technology, the company had convinced itself that it was acceptable to have fewer benefit options and that we should not pursue the newest trends of higher-deductible or lower-benefit plans because of competing internal priorities. We were not researching or attempting to learn from our competitions' actions. Reversing these trends constituted the first step because it was completely within our control and, at least in part, could be quickly addressed.

In 2012, the health plan introduced less-rich benefit plans to the employer market, and group terminations almost immediately began to decline. We adapted some effective product concepts from our competitors and introduced a few wrinkles of our own. We realized, after the fact, that prior to these benefit adjustments, the health plan had been subject to adverse selection of its own making. We had been offering fewer options and richer, costlier levels of benefits than our competition, a recipe for both adverse selection and membership decline. As we began to market and sell the lower benefit options that employers and brokers were demanding, we found that we could simultaneously improve risk competitiveness.

We continued to advance our product development efforts, building broader product choices and more rational plan designs for additional market segments. In 2013, we introduced individual coverage, the last year before the Affordable Care Act launched, and continued into the new landscape of "Obamacare" in 2014. Also, in 2014, we realigned our three Medicare Advantage Plan D options to follow a more rational high-mid-low benefit design, which spread risk and premium in a way that balanced that risk and supported growth. In more recent years, we have retired unprofitable preferred provider organization, Medicare supplement, and prescription drug plan coverage lines and added a more stable point-of-service product.

Promotion

Historically, the health plan housed a small marketing and communications unit in its sales department that practiced budgetary marketing. Once the marketing budget was determined, it would be spent. There was little science and no focus on return on investment (ROI).

A separate, larger marketing and communications department also existed in the IDN. This department managed marketing and communications strategies for the balance of the IDN using a more scientific approach to marketing: impression ratio (see exhibit 9.2). With impression ratio marketing, the budget is determined by a series of calculations; for instance, they consider the click-through

Exhibit 9.2: Impression Ratio Marketing

Elements	Methods of Development or Calculation
Business goal	Receive from internal client
Close ratio (10%)	Standard unless historical data indicate otherwise
CTAs (calls to action—marketing goal)	Divide business goal by close ratio
CTA ratio (.5%)	Standard unless historical data indicate otherwise
Impressions	Divide CTA by CTA ratio
Cost/CTA	Depends on several factors, including audience, budget, and tactics

ratio = number of clicks ÷ impressions (number of times a marketing item is shown). The impression ratio has provided the IDN with measurements of marketing spending, which has led to repeated successes and, ultimately, demonstrable ROI for its marketing money.

In 2013, a decision was made to merge the health plan's marketing unit with the IDN marketing and communications department. The combined department assumed responsibility for health plan advertising, communications, public relations, and marketing services. This adjustment allowed each department, such as sales and marketing, to follow its expertise, an approach that over time created a working partnership between the departments.

The partnership led to an ROI approach to health plan marketing. The sales and marketing teams found immediate growth and retention improvement, which has continued with each subsequent year.

People

People and Structure

If the revenue of a health plan is not growing, neither is its staff. Health First Health Plans had not invested in additional sales staffing resources for a number of years. We employed few among our sales management team with extensive experience in the healthcare sector. Furthermore, the structure of the sales department mirrored that of a health maintenance organization circa 1990: not market facing; inaccessible to customers, members, and brokers; and out of step with most competitors.

Health First essentially wagered on the future. We began to invest by hiring additional sales resources and greater levels of expertise in advance of expected growth. Concurrent with increasing sales resources, the VP of sales implemented a market-facing structure that was well received by external customer stakeholders in each market segment. To define it in direct terms, the VP restructured the sales department to be organized by market segment rather than by function.

Culture

Following years of decline, the sales department had developed a defensive, passive culture. What began as a reaction evolved over time into one of the causes of ongoing enrollment decline. By combining denial with passive acceptance, this culture, this symptom, had essentially become its own cause.

The new sales leadership team took immediate steps. They addressed denial with data, sharing the results of the past six years and their debilitating effects with the sales associates. Acceptance was addressed by presentation of a vision centered on the five-step strategic growth plan.

This step represents the traditional sales management aspects of the plan—what some might refer to as the "soft elements." It was built, however, on a firm foundation of organizational and product change. This is worth noting because stronger sales efforts by themselves might generate more prospects but not necessarily more sales. By changing both reality and perception, the health plan ended its annual string of membership losses.

Beginning in October 2012, the battleship began to turn. After 22 consecutive months without net membership gain, the health plan began a string of monthly enrollment growth that stretched more than six months and generally has continued since.

Place

As with many locally developed PSHPs, ours was geographically landlocked. Health First Health Plans naturally wrapped around the physicians and facilities employed or operated by Health First. The service area looked a bit like a fourteenth-century map of the world—it was flat and small, and the edges fell off from view at the end of our known world.

In 2012, we began to expand our service area. What started as a small, one-county expansion evolved into a significant journey, the breadth of which we did not initially foresee. After spreading the health plan service area beyond our home county, with only moderately successful expansion in a small neighboring county, we began discussions with Florida Hospital, a division of Adventist Health System, in 2013. Florida Hospital is a large healthcare system in contiguous but not competitive regions of central Florida. Its geographic footprint stretches through 12 counties and the most populous Florida regions outside southern Florida, including Orlando, Daytona Beach, and Tampa Bay.

After several unsuccessful attempts to build or collaborate with other health plans, Florida Hospital sought a relationship more permanent than a traditional insurer–provider contract with an experienced IDN to create an ability to hold and manage risk, expand its portfolio, and enhance population management skill sets. In other words, it sought to become an IDN in a similar fashion as Health First, but by using Health First Health Plans as the integrating force with its provider system rather than pursuing the expensive, arduous, and high-risk task of building and managing its own health plan.

Health First believes that to hold risk, scale matters. And scale is exactly what Health First sought from the relationship with Florida Hospital—the opportunity to scale in a way that would have been impossible for a formerly landlocked, local health plan.

With the dramatic changes to the reimbursement models for facilities and insurers in the past decade, it is simply more feasible to scale a health plan than it is to scale hospitals. Healthcare reimbursement of today, and what we envision for the future, points Health First on a path of insurance expansion. Opportunities for both growth and margin are simply greater for a PSHP within an IDN that uses its health plan as a core strategic focus and as the integrating force in the IDN.

At its low point during the recent years of membership decline, Health First Health Plans enrollment had fallen to roughly 62,000 members from an earlier apex of 73,000. By 2017, just three years after the first Florida Hospital health plan members began to enroll, Health First Health Plans's enrollment had grown nearly 150 percent, to 160,000. Yet at that point, neither of Florida Hospital's largest consumer markets, Orlando or Tampa Bay, had been tapped. Expectations are that these markets will increase the scale of membership to 400,000 or more in the following decade.

Price

In 2012, we found that the health plan's employer premium rates were no lower than those charged by Blue Cross Blue Shield, United, Cigna, and Aetna, commonly referred to as the BUCAs. Complicating the challenge, Health First facilities and physicians held commercial provider contracts with the BUCAs. Therefore, our insurance competitors were offering employer groups a network that included Health First providers, with equivalent or occasionally lower premium pricing than that of Health First Health Plans. The health plan is an exclusive provider network (EPO) with, by definition, a more limited local provider network than its competitors. In addition, it did not offer a national network, a perceived competitive advantage of national insurers.

We were not initially in a position to address premium pricing. At that time, the underlying cost structure of our health system did not support adding lower "related party" contractual pricing to its own health plan. The underlying cost structure, to put it plainly, was too high. An adjustment of employer group premium pricing in 2012 essentially would have entailed adopting a buy (as opposed to sell) business strategy, which would not have been sustainable.

Simultaneous to the health plan's enrollment turnaround efforts, Health First engaged in an effort to carve out more than $100 million in costs from its health system. In 2014 and 2015, the provider elements of Health First were in a position to address the EPO pricing inequity. Health First began to offer Health First Health Plans, its only insurance contract that marketed an exclusive Health First provider network—lower contractual provider pricing that rewarded exclusivity.

The health plan passed along the cost reduction to its customers. Its commercial premium pricing began to reflect a competitive advantage by 2015. Not coincidentally, employer group voluntary retention began to exceed 90 percent and increased to 94 percent in 2017.

However, these pricing adjustments were not feasible in 2012. The strategic plan's initial four steps generated significant growth for the Medicare and individual market segments, yet only incremental progress in the employer market, before Health First was in a position to address employer pricing.

As we began to grow, we were met with an unexpected challenge. We were about to learn that growth alone did not provide the actuarial risk management and protection that Health First Health Plans would later develop.

One Step Forward, Two Steps Back

During the second half of 2013, Health First Health Plans, a historically profitable division of Health First, began to miss monthly and quarterly financial budgets. Although still profitable, the gap to budget was growing and a number of months were unprofitable. The trend continued to decline. As troubling as the numbers were, the inability to predict even short-term results may have been the most telling signal of the tsunami the health plan was to encounter. In January and February of 2014, the wave hit. Despite hitting our January growth targets, the health plan division now projected a financial loss for the 2014 fiscal year. The most disconcerting factor was that we did not know why.

This chapter in Health First's development became an organization-changing moment. Eventually, we would perceive it as an organization-defining moment. However, for the ensuing year, we experienced all the pain, difficult questions, and hard choices that normally occur during challenging times.

Twelve months passed before the health plan was stabilized. The division, in fact, did not lose money that year. The hard work and focused attention of that period improved what might otherwise have been a year of loss. Yet despite some short-term improvement, we realized that our ability to predict and manage risk was compromised.

WHAT WE LEARNED AND WHAT WE DID

This chapter is not about a financial turnaround, but rather what Health First learned about holding actuarial risk and how we have since put these learnings in place. By 2015, our risk consciousness had dramatically expanded. At this point, we began to understand how to hold and manage actuarial risk, an understanding that continued to grow in subsequent years.

As we drilled into actuarial risk, we realized that we were not managing risk, or at least not well. We were approaching it solely through mathematics. We had already employed an actuary. We also contracted with an independent actuarial consulting firm. But these were viewed as exercises in arithmetic required for purposes of state and CMS annual rate filings.

We also employed an underwriting unit, under different management from that of the actuarial team. This divided structure had existed for years, likely following a theory of providing greater financial control. What it did, in fact, was create barriers between those evaluating and those managing risk. We learned to integrate risk management factors into sales and product development to create a more sustainable program.

Yet in 2013, no other departments of the organization beyond the actuarial unit—certainly not the sales department—gave more than a passing thought to managing actuarial risk. By 2015, it was top of mind. We turned these learnings into actions, which fall into two categories.

Engage the Community

Most business writers include some version of "begin with the customer in mind" in their advice. We are joining their ranks. Historically, we found that our product was designed in a black box and presented in final form, fully wrapped, to both the sales department and the customer. We learned that customers expect a say in the products they purchase. We discovered an effective method to accomplish this: task sales department leadership with playing a lead role in product design and innovation.

The Sales Department, by its nature and in its daily tasks, communicates with the customer, the member, the prospective member, the insurance broker, and the benefit consultant. The Sales Department, also by its nature and in its daily tasks, reviews what competing organizations have designed in their effort to address customer requirements.

If product design is created in an actuarial model, divorced from the customer, the math will always be correct, but the assumptions may not. Health First Health Plans has redesigned its end-to-end product development process to begin with an innovation phase led by sales. This structure introduces the voice of the customer and the view of the competitive market. Beyond design, as a practical matter, customer engagement enables an organization to educate a community and create a greater sense of collaboration between the insurance-buying community and the health plan.

From the earliest point of product innovation, the health plan has the opportunity to educate the community about the unique nature of Health First as an IDN. In other words, why purchase a health plan from an IDN rather than from the nationals? This early stage is the key. Moving in front of the sales cycle by engaging customer constituencies in a collaborative manner—before a proposal is requested by the customer or annual benefit programs are designed by the insurer—creates a community relationship.

Beyond relationship building, concrete outcomes resulted. As we built a product design relationship with customer constituencies, we found that the purchasing community developed a sense of ownership in the outcome. The meaning and value of this quickly became clear: The community was more likely to buy, retain, or recommend what it had an opportunity to influence.

This customer-centric design process takes discipline. In difficult financial times, it is tempting for an organization to turn over product design to its financial leadership. If an organization's business processes are not operating efficiently, it may be tempting to turn over design to its operational leadership. As for Health First, in earlier years, our actuaries had worked out much of the design without the voice of the customer. Recall our burning platform: the customer was not buying.

Engage Ourselves

In retrospect, we divided our actuarial and underwriting resources under separate leadership in a well-intentioned, but ineffective, effort to provide control. We have since combined the leadership of these units.

Our most critical internal engagement, however, was one created between the leadership of the Sales Department and the actuarial underwriting teams. The group renewal process, annual pricing and rate filings, product design, and other elements that touch both units are now, in large part, developed together by these teams.

Workflow creates habits, and habits develop a culture. These teams now expect to work together. Many health plans would report that their sales and actuarial underwriting units have a healthy, or sometimes less than healthy, push–pull relationship. These Health First Health Plans teams, on the other hand, see their interests served by coordination of effort. We are now beginning to link incentive compensation between sales and actuarial underwriting to ensure that mutual objectives are rewarded.

At times, pricing decisions are made via role reversal. It is not uncommon to attend an internal employer renewal planning meeting between account managers and underwriters in which the account manager advocates for a higher rate increase than the underwriter initially suggests or the reverse by the underwriter. Our sales associates are engaged as we build sustainable products, and they recommend benefit changes for each successive year in a bottom-up fashion. These are just several of many examples of a healthy organization that coordinates, rather than manages, risk and does so throughout its organization. The business is not about risk from just a predictive, mathematical perspective; rather, it is about building ownership and expertise throughout the organization.

Any health plan can contract with actuarial firms. In fact, all do. But that in itself does not adequately manage risk and ensure growth. Our organization created cross-functional teams of sales, product, underwriting, and actuarial staff to help us manage and understand actuarial risk. What began as a reaction to a financial challenge became something burned into our DNA.

We view our insurance risk—and manage it—far differently from how we once did. We have a model that we believe is both scalable and transferable. As of January 2018, Health First Health Plans, which was once shrinking to 62,000 members, had surpassed 160,000. Geographic expansion planned for 2017–2020 puts 200,000 in the foreground and 400,000 in sight for several years and beyond—growth that we are confident is financially sustainable.

Best-Practice, Evidence-Based Management That Minimizes Costs and Optimizes Outcomes

Jon Burroughs
Steve Berger

HEALTHCARE MANAGEMENT PRESSURES

Although most healthcare leaders are familiar with evidence-based and precision medicine clinical approaches based on standardized policies, most are less familiar with evidence-based management approaches to optimizing clinical, operational, and business outcomes. Some are deservedly cautious of such a method, recognizing the inherent complexity of healthcare and the need to customize managerial approaches to specific situations. However, the industry now recognizes the significant role that non-value-added variation plays in the creation of unnecessary cost in such areas as labor and supply chain. In the same vein, thoughtful leaders are increasingly using an evidence-based philosophy to solve tough questions arising from an increasingly value-based business model.

Though this approach seems reasonable, it is often met with resistance stemming from what scholars Jeffrey Pfeffer and Robert Sutton (2006) identify as clinicians' and executives' most common intellectual traps: legacy and conventional wisdom, experience, tradition, and benchmarked comparisons with other organizations and practitioners. "Evidence-based management, like evidence-based medicine, entails a distinct mind-set that clashes with the way many managers and companies operate. It features a willingness to put aside belief and conventional wisdom—the dangerous half-truths that many embrace—and replace these with an unrelenting commitment to gather the necessary facts to make more informed and intelligent decisions" (Pfeffer and Sutton 2006).

Globalization amid Growing National and International Competition

Healthcare is going the way of the world economy—though many providers still focus on their primary and secondary service areas, the sector is globalizing. According to author Josef Woodman (2015), approximately 1.7 million Americans left the United States to seek affordable healthcare services in 2016, particularly for life-threatening conditions such as cancer. The ever-increasing cost of healthcare has given rise to high-deductible policies, which entail significant out-of-pocket expenses that may lead to personal bankruptcy. Cost savings overseas can be as high as 90 percent, meaning the difference between solvency and insolvency. The international medical tourism market is worth between $45 billion and $75 billion and is projected to double every two years. This phenomenon introduces national and global entrants into the strategic mix of every healthcare organization and requires that healthcare leaders work to optimize their clinical *and* business outcomes as soon as feasible through the use of evidence-based approaches.

Commoditization, Necessitating Lower Cost

As all industries mature, they experience a "race to the bottom," whereby lowering cost structure effectively without sacrificing quality or service (and even improving on it) becomes a significant competitive advantage. The shift from volume-based to value-based contracting is only the beginning for healthcare, as value-starved consumers, employers, and payers offer increasingly significant incentives (and loyalty) to healthcare brands that provide quality and service at a fraction of the price.

For example, consider e-health, which provides around-the-clock care for people with low-risk conditions for as little as $59. Although these services may be seen as inferior to the traditional care provision they disrupt, their cost structure and ease of access are highly appealing for many consumers. In fact, there were more than 100 million e-health visits in the United States alone in 2016. E-health exemplifies the sort of commoditization that requires management to drive down operating costs through the implementation of clinical and business analytics, effective cost accounting, and the development of new delivery models. Management must do so to compete and even to survive.

HEALTHCARE'S NEW APPROACHES

In the clinical world, evidence-based approaches were introduced in the 1980s by The Joint Commission as ORYX measures, later developing into Centers for Medicare & Medicaid Services core measures. The measures revolve around the treatment of people who suffer from the top three causes of death, disability, and cost in the United States: congestive heart failure (CHF), community-acquired pneumonia (CAP), and acute myocardial infarction (AMI). Management is taking the same approach with labor and supply chain management, which account for an average of 56 percent and 17 percent of total operating costs, respectively.

Unfortunately, the majority of healthcare organizations make insufficient efforts to significantly lower cost structure through the standardization and optimization of clinical and managerial practices. According to a report based on a survey of 150 hospitals and healthcare systems, the majority of healthcare organizations (51 percent) have minimal or nonexistent cost accounting measures in place; half of these organization have no plans to do so for the next five years (Daly 2017). This pattern is troublesome because experts predict that organizations will need to cut their cost structures by at least 25–35 percent to compete for a place in a narrow or tiered network and become a provider of choice. However, organizations engaged in cost-reducing initiatives tend to focus on the traditional areas of labor and supply chain, such as Lean and Six Sigma, but few look at clinical variation or overall cost accounting, where the most significant savings are found.

Like every other sector, healthcare is going through transformational changes that require more rigorous and evidence-based approaches to managerial decisions. The following sections outline many of the most notable, including digitization, value-analysis process, continuous improvement for supply chain management, and standardization of key clinical and operational areas.

Digitization of Healthcare Information (Clinical and Managerial)

It has been less than a decade since meaningful use requirements gave rise to the widespread adoption of electronic health records (EHRs) and the software and analytics necessary to support them. Healthcare was late to digitization because of the sector's complexity and cost. However, the field is now fully committed to digitization through significant economic incentives (e.g., the Medicare Access and CHIP Reauthorization Act [MACRA]) and value-based contracts that require monitoring of key performance indicators (KPIs), which include clinical and business outcomes. In addition, digitization now permits the rapid expansion of key clinical and business delivery models that were not possible before, including patient portals, wearable health monitors, predictive analysis, telehealth or e-health, genomics and genetic engineering, big data, enterprise data warehouses, and artificial intelligence.

With this new technology comes opportunity but also the responsibility for greater precision, specificity, and timeliness in decision-making. These will likely render forecasting and retrospective data gathering largely obsolete. EHRs are a major part of the healthcare field's push to apply evidence-based approaches to managerial decisions.

Standardization of Labor Management

Labor is healthcare organizations' largest expense, thereby offering the greatest opportunity to address costs. The remarkable fact is that labor costs vary by as much as 20 percent across the nation with little impact on clinical outcomes.

Labor decisions are often made on the basis of traditional political, economic, regulatory, and legal thinking that confuses trends with facts. One example is the ratio of full-time equivalents (FTEs) to adjusted patient days, which focuses on days and not costs and has little to do with acuity, complexity, severity, and resource-dependent labor demands. Another is the common notion that physicians should manage patients of low risk and low complexity or should spend half of their time performing clinical documentation. Mismanaging physicians' time in this way generates no revenue and often results in inadequate documentation, a below-average case-mix index (CMI), and lower-than-expected quality ratings stemming from an inappropriately low risk-adjustment score. Focusing on labor costs in a more objective, rigorous, and analytical fashion provides a significant opportunity to reduce operating costs and even optimize clinical outcomes by ensuring that the right level of expertise (and cost) is available for the right level of acuity.

The foundation of a more evidence-based management approach to labor is the labor ratio, which is defined as

Labor ratio = Total labor costs ÷ Total operating revenue.

Such a calculation includes salaries and wages, benefits, and contract labor, including physicians and external resources (e.g., locum tenens practitioners, traveling nurses). Many organizations create a false lower ratio by excluding the contract labor costs. As mentioned earlier, the remarkable feature of this ratio is that most healthcare organizations don't measure it consistently—the ratio shows a great deal of national variation. In fact, Fitch, one of the big three bond-rating agencies, publishes annual information on acute care–hospital labor compensation ratios and factors them into its rating methodology.

Why is there so much variation throughout the country? Many organizations still manage labor based on many of the following factors:

- Average patient days, rather than resources required by degree of complexity or acuity
- Assignment to a department and shift, not to areas in which resources are required
- Monitoring of resources by shift, rather than by hour
- Static staffing plans based on average demand, rather than dynamic staffing plans that fluctuate with demand and times of day or days of the week
- Lack of job analysis to determine the lowest-cost worker able to fulfill job requirements successfully
- Lack of real-time information through labor analytics so that all information is retrospective and variances cannot be immediately corrected

Achieving a best-practice labor ratio requires a multipronged approach. As you would with any type of budget, work backward from the budgetary and ratio goals set by the leadership. The organization must calculate the labor ratio and consistently track it over time. Divide all FTEs into care delivery (direct) costs or overhead (indirect) costs so that the organization can maximize hands-on care and minimize overheads. Examples of direct costs include nurses, physicians, unit clerks, and lab technologists. Indirect costs include administrators, controllers, and overhead.

Another best practice is separating all direct and indirect costs into fixed or variable costs. Fixed costs have labor standards established per FTE, and variable costs have labor standards established per workload unit (productivity). Labor costs equal hours paid (both hours paid at work and hours paid during time off) multiplied by pay rate.

Healthcare organizations make an effort to establish productivity measures and standards. Leadership can do this by weighting procedures or volume by the level of acuity or complexity to fairly measure the work an individual is doing. There are two techniques for this process: (1) weighting procedures or (2) creating severity-adjusted patient days by incorporating severity adjustments or relative value units (RVUs) to determine complexity and acuity. That way, total units of service are calculated by adding the specific units after they are multiplied by a relative value factor (acuity or complexity) and a unit of time to determine what the total productivity is for any given time frame. For example, a technologist performs three procedures in one hour and accomplishes a rate of 1.10 units of service per hour according to the following calculations:

First procedure × 0.25 hour × Weight of 1.2 = 0.3,
Second procedure × 0.25 hour × Weight of 1.0 = 0.25, and
Third procedure × 0.5 hour × Weight of 1.1 = 0.55, so
0.3 + 0.25 + 0.55 = 1.10.

This calculation is aggregated by performing an inventory of all procedures in a department by volume and multiplied by weighting factor to achieve a sum of weighted volumes. Common workload units include adjusted or severity-adjusted patient days; severity-adjusted admissions, discharges, and transfers; RVUs; severity-adjusted cases; and minutes per case.

Organizations also determine targeted inputs per unit of output. This figure is divided into variable and fixed labor costs as follows:

- Variable costs = Budgeted worked hours ÷ Budgeted units of service
- Fixed costs = Budgeted worked hours ÷ Number of pay periods per year (typically 26)

The productivity target is calculated by dividing the number of budgeted hours by the total weighted units of service. If budgeted hours equal 3,864 and budgeted weighted units of service equal 60,000, then the productivity target equals 3,864 ÷ 60,000, or 0.0644.

Another best practice in the healthcare field is to track productivity using the productivity target and total worked hour targets as benchmarks per pay period over time. This technique might look like the following table:

	Pay Period 1	Pay Period 2	Pay Period 3
Total weighted units of service × Productivity target (0.0644)	62,000	60,000	58,000
Target worked hours	3,992.8	3,864	3,735.2
Total actual worked hours	3,880	3,900	4,100
Productivity index (%)	102.9	99.1	91.1

Obviously, this institution's figures are not going in a good direction. Its leadership must determine whether the culprit is high costs (e.g., contract labor), decreased productivity (fewer or less-complex procedures), or too many personnel. The key is to automate this tracking mechanism with labor analytics, coupled with decision support tools that notify managers (and those with a need to know) of variances that should be addressed in real time. Such measures prevent this kind of situation from taking everyone by surprise.

If you want to improve your labor ratio, optimize the pay rate by matching each task to the least costly individual qualified to perform it. For instance, does a physician need to enter documentation data into an EHR, or are there better-qualified and less costly clinicians available? Does a registered nurse need to enter the nursing care plan or progress notes into the nursing record, or are there nursing assistants who are qualified? These considerations reduce the labor cost per weighted unit significantly and support the morale of professionals trained (and paid) to perform more complex tasks.

Many healthcare organizations save money by creating a staffing plan with incremental increases or decreases based on a predefined range of activity or units of service provided. This methodology represents a breakdown of all personnel in a department as required by units of service, typically in increments that separate numbers of FTEs required. For instance, consider the following table:

Units of Service	Supervisors	Technologists	Technologist Assistants	Administrative Staff
0–10,000	1	3	2	1
10,001–20,000	2	5	3	1
20,001–30,000	2	6	4	1

Another way to save money on labor is to create a staffing performance report based on actual and expected paid hours and labor expense with a variance analysis. Once the plan and budget are laid out, it is helpful to track actual performance against these objectives by comparing predicted and actual performance. Variances may result from mismanagement of resources; however, they may also result from overly optimistic or overly pessimistic projections that did not take all operational exigencies into account. Such a report may look like the following table:

Work Group	Paid Hours			Labor Expense		
	Actual	Expected	Variance (%)	Actual ($)	Expected ($)	Variance (%)
Variable						
Supervisors	235	210	11	16,200	14,300	13
Technologists	1,543	1,299	19	56,755	44,322	28
Aides	520	490	6	8,111	6,000	35
Nonvariable						
Managers	120	110	9	4,411	3,699	19
Administrative staff	221	201	10	2,211	1,999	11

Variances can be based on rate differences (skill levels) or on efficiency (number of labor hours that differ from those planned). It is also helpful to examine variances closely to determine weaknesses that may contribute to the majority of outlier costs.

Generally, variances with volume-based budgets that are within 2 percent can be considered in range, and variances within 10 percent should be addressed promptly to determine whether the issue relates to managerial misjudgments or unrealistic forecasting.

Ideally, organizations are putting into place labor analytics that enable this kind of monitoring in real time, with decision alerts to notify all relevant leaders and managers when there are (or are predicted to be) significant variances that require immediate adjustment. Some organizations report this information every one to two hours, around the clock. The industry as a whole is slowly moving in this direction (Daly 2017).

Certain components of labor expenses, such as overtime and contract labor (travelers), cause significant variance outliers in a surprisingly short time; ideally, these are addressed before they occur. The analytics should differentiate between efficiency (hours worked) and rate (amount paid per time unit) variances, as the steps necessary to address these variances are significantly different.

Finally, remember that the labor ratio should be one of your key operating metrics, and your organization's goal should be to lower it continually toward a best practice as you monitor the results over time.

Standardization of Supply Chain Management

Like the labor ratio, the supply chain ratio is an operating metric essential to proper management. It exemplifies the rigorous and evidence-based approaches to managerial decisions essential in today's increasingly challenging market. It is calculated as follows:

Supply chain ratio = Total supply chain costs ÷ Total operating revenue

Note that the total supply chain costs exclude depreciation, interest, and bad debts and typically include office supplies, pharmaceuticals, food, and medical supplies. They exclude purchased services, professional and management fees, and operation of the physical plant.

As for the labor ratio, observers find significant national variation in performance. Best-practice institutions achieve a 12–13 percent ratio, the median is 17 percent, and 26 percent constitutes poor performance.

Why the significant national variation in the performance of this key operating metric? Reasons include the following:

- Lack of standardization of the supply chain process
- Lack of automation of the supply chain process (e.g., no automated inventory management with radio-frequency identification [RFID] codes)
- Excess inventory with excess shelf life
- Too many vendors, with resultant excess margins
- Too many physician preference items (PPIs), particularly those contributing to non-value-added variation in physician setups, equipment, and diagnostic or operative technology

Most executives understand that the healthcare supply chain is complex and often includes the following components:

- Purchasing
- Receiving
- Warehousing
- Sterile processing
- Facilities management
- Accounts payable
- Every department, and its staff, that interfaces with the supply chain

Most managers only understand the piece of the supply chain that they directly touch. Even for executives who manage the entire system (e.g., chief financial officer [CFO], chief operating officer [COO], director of materials management), it is useful to walk through the supply chain periodically to understand how the complete system operates. In larger organizations, the supply chain manager is an essential executive who reports to the COO and oversees all of the operating components of the supply chain. She often chairs (or cochairs, with a physician executive such as the chief medical officer) the value analysis committee, which plays a key role in standardizing physician preference items and vets new technologies and clinical paradigms.

The authors recommend the following tactics to standardize, and thus optimize, the supply chain: establish performance standards and measures, determine group purchasing organization participation, determine capitalization policies, and determine warehouse usage.

Establish Performance Standards and Measures

The ideal approach to the supply chain is to establish performance standards and measures in comparison to nationally established benchmarks. Look to percentile metrics as a guide, aiming for a level of efficiency in the ninetieth percentile. Current statistics are obtained from either of two proprietary hospital benchmarking services. In addition, many top-performing organizations are generous in sharing their best practices, and industry analysts expect the variation from highest performers to lowest performers to narrow over time.

In a time of squeezed margins and the "race to the bottom" in cost structure, it is in the self-interest of every organization to work toward the top decile performance. Most COOs want to establish a risk- and severity-adjusted supply cost per adjusted admission—one that is both organization-wide and specific to departments, service lines, and clinical institutes to take into account both inpatient and outpatient components.

Determine Group Purchasing Organization Participation

There are both upsides and downsides to working with large group-purchasing organizations (GPOs). Upsides include greater purchasing power, easier access to goods and services (often through e-commerce), and automation through the use of RFID units that trigger automatic purchasing orders.

On the other hand, GPOs have at least three major downsides. First, contractual obligations limit access to suppliers who do not contract directly with a specific GPO. Second, specific contractual requirements may inadvertently add cost or inefficiencies to the system, including minimum volumes and minimum percentage usage that create excess inventory and additional costs. Specific legal or regulatory compliance requirements may also add overhead requirements and costs. Third, contract terms may interfere with mergers, acquisitions, or restructuring of corporate entities. They may also inadvertently trigger noncompete clauses and other restrictive covenants. Given these pros and cons, potential GPO alignment is a significant decision.

Determine Capitalization Policies

In the quest to apply rigorous and evidence-based approaches to managerial decisions, it is important to delineate the difference between capital (supply chain) expenses and operating expenses for budgeting purposes. Therefore, it is helpful to create specific definitions of items belonging to either category. Many organizations differentiate the two based on expected life of the item and cost benchmarks. Typically, capital expense items have a longer expected life, higher cost, and longer depreciation period than typical operating expense items. Differentiating between the two makes defining responsibilities and assigning accountability easier.

Determine Warehousing Needs and Usage

The traditional approach to managing inventory is to create a warehouse (external or internal) to store, inventory, and use supplies and equipment over time. Increasingly, organizations use just-in-time (JIT) inventory management approaches by outsourcing the inventory storage process to externally contracted logistical entities that provide materials on an as-needed basis. JIT makes it easier to manage through variations in demand and unanticipated emergencies or disasters through which the usual inventory management system is inadequate. Some GPOs and JIT companies agree to deliver goods and services on an accelerated or on-demand basis within a 24-hour period.

Advantages of a JIT inventory system include lower inventory management costs, more efficient supply chain management, less shrinkage (avoidance of theft), less frequent expiration of supplies, adequate storage capacity, and elimination of unnecessary staff.

Disadvantages include the extra payments required for JIT delivery, greater need for more generously sized staging areas, possible lack of immediate on-site access, and the par levels that would ensure instant availability. Thus, JIT inventory management service may both add cost (through the creation of a premium service) and reduce cost (through lower inventory management expenses). Healthcare organizations considering the system write business plans based on volume, need, and clinical or operational demands to determine which approach is best.

Employing a Value-Analysis Process

Many larger organizations implement a value-analysis process to vet new technologies and new clinical paradigms, choose or eliminate vendors, and add new items requiring significant capital investment. This evaluation involves the creation of a multidisciplinary committee made up of key administrative and physician leaders. It typically includes the members of the C-suite, the corporate compliance officer, in-house counsel, the director of supply chain management, and the directors of important clinical departments or service lines.

It is helpful to establish specific criteria for the issues or items that come before this committee based on cost, paradigm shift (e.g., required new infrastructure, technology, personnel, technical competencies), and consistency with the organization's mission or strategic priorities. The decision to introduce new clinical paradigms is complex and includes clinical issues (quality, safety, cost-effectiveness, service); business potential (projected operational and human resource infrastructure required); and considerations related to legal, regulatory, and accreditation requirements.

Dr. Burroughs recalls his involvement in the consideration of a new joint-resurfacing program, only to find out that the new approach had not been approved by the Federal Drug Administration, had no payment established by Medicare, and had not demonstrated any clinical advantages at that time. Obviously, these are essential considerations when vetting new, more complex, or more expensive modalities that may or may not add clinical or business value.

Whenever a new modality or paradigm is introduced to the committee, the first consideration is whether the new service should be introduced to the organization at all. If not, there is nothing further to discuss. However, if the members are in agreement to move forward, the clinicians need to develop eligibility criteria for any new clinical privileges, as well as quality parameters and metrics, while management must develop an operational and business plan for implementation that includes a modification of the existing infrastructure and collaboration with human resources over new personnel requirements or training. Any legal, regulatory, or accreditation concerns are worked through with legal counsel, corporate compliance, and relevant clinical administrative leadership.

Continuous Improvement Opportunities for Supply Chain Management

One of the most remarkable examples of supply chain improvement is Memorial Hermann Houston's Integrated Physician Network. According to Keith Fernandez, the former president of the Physicians Integrated ACO, by standardizing the supply chain and working with physicians to simplify the supply chain system and reduce vendors, particularly for PPIs, the organization was able to reduce supply chain costs over a three-year period by $150 million per year (out of a total operating budget of $2.8 billion), for a total savings of more than $450 million.

Healthcare organizations can, however, pursue improvement in multiple additional ways. Other effective examples include the following:

- Recruit nurses from key departments. These employees can work with materials management to understand the supply chain better and work directly with physicians regarding PPIs.
- Create approved gainsharing agreements for physicians— such arrangements incentivize them to work with management for continual supply chain cost reductions.
- Standardize and simplify the supply chain long term through collaboration with physicians, nurses, technical staff, and the executive team.
- Create systemwide metrics with benchmarks that are widely disseminated and integrated into both physician and staff contracts and employment agreements. These benchmarks are shared with the medical executive committee and every clinical leadership team.
- Work with physicians to create standardized clinical, cost, and operational algorithms for their 20 most common diagnosis-related groups (DRGs), working toward a single setup for each major procedure or clinical treatment.
- Standardize and simplify the systemwide formulary with specific medication choices embedded in the computerized physician order–entry system.
- Perform periodic audits to look for redundant products and services; billing and invoicing errors; lower-cost alternatives to high-margin supplies; excess unused inventory; theft; inefficient processes; effectiveness of supply chain leadership; and alternative contractors, vendors, and GPOs.
- Create a clinical executive leadership role focusing on the supply chain for larger systems. This person can champion cost-effective savings based on a robust value-analysis, audit, and management process.

Standardization of Cost Accounting

Despite the importance of managing costs and margin, throughout the twenty-first century, most healthcare organizations managed costs retrospectively and without adequate cost accounting systems. With the emergence of increasingly at-risk pay-for-value contracts and other reimbursement methodologies, this situation is rapidly changing. Organizations are scrambling to add clinical and cost analytics to their burgeoning information technology infrastructure. Cost accounting and profitability analysis are now essential core competencies in healthcare organizations and systems. In addition, a rapidly growing number of healthcare organizations create aligned compensation agreements with executives, managers, physicians, and staff so that everyone collaborates to reduce operating costs and optimize clinical outcomes and margins. Robust cost accounting systems break down variable costs, contribution margin, and net income by department, service line, DRG, managed care company, health plan, and individual practitioner. They can reasonably calculate the margins of payer contracts to enable management to have the same information that the payers have had for decades and thus negotiate contracts on a level playing field and in a more dynamic and transparent way.

Although precise total healthcare costs are almost impossible to measure, reasonable costs can be assigned to any episode of care that approximates the true expenses generated. Activity-based costing recognizes both direct costs (generated by providing a service) and indirect costs (generated by allocating overhead costs to a given service or department), as well as variable costs (varying with the volume of services provided) and fixed costs (independent of the volume of services provided). Robust cost accounting takes all of these component costs into account to approximate total costs for any defined episode or aggregate of care.

The ratio of cost to charges has been used by Medicare since the agency was created as a proxy to determine total costs; however, for obvious reasons (e.g., charges are almost always unrelated to true costs), this methodology is extremely inaccurate. A more accurate approach is through micro-based costing, or as it has recently been called, *time-driven activity-based costing* (TDABC). The method was refined by Robert Kaplan and his associates at Harvard Business School (Kaplan et al. 2014).

TDABC follows a specific procedure over the continuum of care. First, the organization chooses a clinical process or episode of care to analyze and creates a process map, taking into account every step throughout the continuum of care (inpatient and outpatient). Then, it estimates the amount of time that each step in the process will take, as well as a dollar-per-minute capacity cost for each step. This second phase is done by factoring the life expectancy (including depreciation) of a piece of equipment, adding up the total costs for that equipment, and dividing by total minutes during that time frame. It is also done for professional services by adding up the total costs (including overhead indirect costs) of that service per unit of time. Finally, the organization multiplies the estimated time of each step by the dollar-per-minute capacity cost and adds them all up throughout the process. This procedure will generate the TDABC total cost estimate. However, the organization must take into account nonprocess costs such as overhead (allocated indirect costs not factored in), bad debts, building depreciation, and so on.

The Kaplan and colleagues (2014) article gives several examples of how to calculate total costs using this methodology, with examples of actual episodes of care provided by hospitals in the greater Boston area. It also emphasizes the importance of weighting (or risk adjusting) the steps when performing the initial calculations to take into account acuity and complexity.

Allocating for indirect costs is a bit of an art—each cost requires a cost driver, and not everyone agrees on the ideal cost driver for each. Some of the most obvious are building depreciation (square feet), human resources (FTEs), administration (total expenses), laundry (laundry weight), and central transportation (number of admissions).

However, when choosing cost drivers for accounts receivable or accounting, what makes a unit of service inpatient or outpatient? Do you factor in all expenses across the continuum of care when the patient is no longer in your facility? As hospitals transition into integrated delivery systems, the allocation of indirect (or even direct) costs becomes increasingly problematic, particularly when costs are shared among different or even competing organizations. That being said, the alternative option of not calculating total costs for defined episodes of care is no longer an option.

Non-revenue-producing services, such as administration, food service, or materials management, can undergo expense analysis from benchmarking organizations such as Premier or IBM-Truven, and these services are allocated, through cost drivers, into the total cost equation. Thus, in the case of these indirect (overhead) costs, many organizations use the same step-down methodology defined by the 1966 Medicare cost report.

These calculations are performed automatically through cost accounting analytics programs that access the data, drive them through an enterprise data warehouse, and produce profitability analyses broken down by department or section as follows:

- Department, service line, or clinical institute
- Charges
- Contractual adjustments
- Expected payment
- Direct contribution costs
- Direct contribution margin
- Indirect costs
- Fixed costs
- Net margin (income)

This report is sorted by size, order, and positive or negative margin so that executives can now access the projected and actual profitability of each unit in real time, supported by a cost analysis of each. Such a report combines microlevel cost information into a macrolevel summary, allowing managers to spot trends and outliers quickly and easily. This agility enables adjustment, through portfolio management, of multiple clinical services.

Once an outlier is identified, a more comprehensive cost analysis is performed by looking at past, present, and projected numbers for each line item, with identification of line items that demonstrate variance above the threshold. Ideally, decision supports are embedded in the analytics so that variances are addressed by all relevant managers and leaders as they occur.

One of the most significant causes of cost variance is non-value-added clinical and operational variation that can be measured and reported by cost accounting analytics programs. For instance, most healthcare organizations that begin measuring physician-related direct variable costs for any given DRG are amazed to discover the variation to be as great as 1,000 percent. Physicians are generally responsive to credible data and information, particularly when they are compared to peers both locally and nationally. Modern cost accounting analytics report various data points by service line or clinical department: number of cases, CMI, average length of stay (ALOS), total charges, actual payment, variable cost, fixed cost, contribution margin, or net income.

If the cost accounting analytics program reports that a service line or department is a significant outlier, the user clicks on it, and a comprehensive list of DRGs treated by that service line or department is reported. Each DRG is broken down into these same nine categories. If a DRG with an unusually low or negative net income is identified, the program provides a list of all physicians and practitioners treating patients with that specific DRG. Each practitioner has information for that specific DRG that includes these categories as well, with the exception of CMI.

From this information, a medical director or chief medical officer works directly with clinicians to understand the reason for the clinical variation (by clicking on variable costs in the analytics program, all of the relevant costs used to calculate this number are identified). Often, this information alone has a profound impact on clinical performance, particularly if the physician is permitted to see the information of peers who are able to achieve excellent quality outcomes at a fraction of the cost. Physicians generally adapt their practices quickly when they realize that their performance is perceived as different by peers, and this awareness can have a significant impact on overall quality and margin, particularly if the most significant outliers are managed first.

For instance, in an actual cost and profitability report of DRG 89 (simple pneumonia, severity 1), the following represents the variation discovered in one report taken from a well-respected healthcare organization:

	Actual Payment ($)	Variable Cost ($)	Contribution ($) (Negative Value)	Net Income ($) (Negative Value)
Physician 1	5,780	6,121	(341)	(6,133)
Physician 2	27,686	5,663	22,023	15,974
Physician 3	31,837	4,618	27,220	22,288
Physician 4	5,780	7,256	(1,476)	(10,061)

In both authors' personal experience, this magnitude of variation is common, and most medical staffs are split between physicians and practitioners who drive a positive margin and those who drive a negative margin. Obviously, the reduction of clinical variation, which drives differences in both cost and clinical outcomes, is a necessary competency for healthcare leaders in the contemporary healthcare field—particularly when embarking on pay-for-value contracts. All payer contracts (public and private) should undergo both profitability and cost analysis to determine those same nine data points (number of cases, CMI, ALOS, total charges, actual payment, variable cost, fixed cost, contribution margin, net income) plus discount percentages.

Using this approach to standardized cost accounting supports a more rational and transparent negotiation of payer contracts, with shared information (which the payer already has) and a more dynamic method based on mutually agreed-on benchmarks (e.g., margin, indirect costs, medical loss ratio) that modulate over time.

Standardization of High-Risk, High-Cost Processes

As any accountant and physician knows, the majority of costs and clinical risks can be attributed to a surprisingly small number of patients. This tendency follows a pattern in business identified by management consultant Joseph M. Juran in the early twentieth century and named the Pareto Principle after the Italian economist Vilfredo Pareto. Thus, both clinicians and healthcare executives recognize the necessity of gaining greater control over those few elements and decisions that have a disproportionate and profound impact on the clinical and business outcomes for both individuals and organizations. As a result, the field has observed a rapidly growing trend toward standardization of critical business and clinical processes. Successes in this area have had significant impact based on evidence-based approaches.

Standardization of Quality Metrics Throughout the Enterprise

Until recently, quality was assumed to be what all clinicians aimed for, while collecting quality data and reporting them to accreditors and regulators was considered an overhead cost with little, if any, direct financial value. That attitude has changed with value-based purchasing for Medicare Part A and MACRA for Medicare Part B. Many innovative reimbursement models (e.g., bundled payments, shared savings, risk-based capitation, global budgets) significantly alter that paradigm, as quality now has a calculable monetary value for both clinicians and the enterprise at large (particularly with the growing number of employed clinicians). Thus, most healthcare organizations create a quality plan equal in scope and importance to the organization's financial plan. Many larger organizations have a chief quality officer to complement the chief medical officer and chief nursing officer, who typically take on responsibilities that are operational in nature.

A quality plan typically divides initiatives into regulatory quality (defined as quality required by payers to optimize reimbursement) and strategic quality (which focuses on the most important and so-called vital few). Examples of regulatory quality metrics include the following:

- Hospital Consumer Assessment of Healthcare Providers and Systems (HCAHPS)
- Safety metrics as a requirement of value-based purchasing
- Outcomes for CHF, CAP, and AMI (value-based purchasing)
- Hospital-acquired infections
- Healthcare Effectiveness Data and Information Set (required for National Committee for Quality Assurance accreditation)
- Surgical Quality Improvement Program measures (American College of Surgeons)
- Merit-based Incentive Payment System (MACRA)

The best approach is to combine all of the regulatory measures and hardwire them into operational processes to enable full compliance (unless there is a clinical reason to create an exception). Strategic quality, on the other hand, is formulated by combining all important quality measures from every clinical department, service line, and institute, and both monetizing them and looking at each metric's qualitative importance to the mission of the enterprise.

Many organizations now calculate return on investment (ROI) for competing strategic quality goals and objectives to determine which should be prioritized. With pay-for-value contracts, such metrics as CMI, top-box HCAHPS, adjusted cost per case, and ALOS now have specific financial value to organizations. With bundled-payment contracts, up to 50 percent of potential reimbursement is based on quality outcomes and cost reports of specific episodes of care (e.g., knee or hip replacement). Thus, competing priorities are quantified with a Pareto diagram or chart plotted to determine which key quality targets have the greatest financial and clinical impact on the organization.

Some quality targets, on the other hand, are essential because of their importance to the mission of the organization. For instance, if an organization is building a neuroscience institute with a national or even international brand, achieving top-decile performance for risk-adjusted morbidity and mortality outcomes may be considered an organizational priority that requires significant resources to achieve and maintain. These plans are independent of the monetary value such metrics have on the organization (or even market share) as a result of mission-critical importance.

Like other dashboards and scorecards, quality should be reported in an easy-to-interpret format with explanations of each metric, both in terms of financial value and qualitative value to the organization. Categories in a quality report include the following:

- Risk- and severity-adjusted clinical outcomes
- Safety (never events)
- Service (all stakeholders)
- Access
- Efficiency (throughput)
- Effectiveness (appropriateness of care)
- Cost-effectiveness

Each category of the report contains the most important strategic quality measures that have the greatest impact on the organization or that have the greatest strategic value. Ideally, once a metric is given a financial value based on an ROI calculation, the actual impact of the metric on the organization should be calculated retrospectively at the conclusion of a fiscal year to reprioritize quality goals for the subsequent year.

Standardization of Financial and Clinical Reports Throughout the Enterprise as Part of the Strategic Planning Process

The strategic plan and financial, operating, and quality metrics should be directly linked. These can be made available in the standardized format of a dashboard.

Everything begins with a strategic plan that spawns operational, financial, and quality plans that, in turn, support overarching strategic goals and objectives derived by key stakeholders. The stakeholders may include the following:

- Patients and consumers
- Physicians and other practitioners
- Executives and other managers
- Large employers
- Payers (public and private)
- Health plans
- Community organizations and members
- Legal, regulatory, and accreditation organizations

Thus, the development of the strategic plan should be collaborative to ensure that the most important objectives and goals, with the greatest impact on clinical and business performance, are represented. The plan itself is based on a careful analysis of the external environment (local, regional, national, international), internal environment (the organization, its operational components), and the organized medical staff (strategic medical staff development planning). A strategic gap is identified by the variance between current and future state based on available resources, and the organization develops the competencies necessary to fill these gaps. Each strategic initiative requires resources and competencies to support it, including the capital investment and defined expertise necessary to bridge the gaps.

Once key performance goals and objectives are established, KPI and metrics are developed to monitor and follow them over time. The organization creates tactics (or operating steps) to activate and promote the desired strategic outcomes. The KPIs and metrics are used to support accountability for desired outcomes.

Operational plans prioritize up to a dozen areas that have high impact, volume, cost, and potential revenue. Plans help focus on improvement targets and may include the following:

- Physician-related operations (e.g., operating room, service line)
- Throughput
- Labor
- Nonlabor (supply chain)
- Human resources initiatives
- Utilization
- Pharmacy
- Volume
- Revenue cycle

An operational steering committee then prioritizes each of these to calculate the projects' potential impact on mission and vision, revenue growth, market growth, savings, efficiency, service, and brand. This careful consideration permits the prioritization and delegation of resources to each key area of focus. Within each area, tactics (specific process initiatives) are developed. For example, if revenue and volume growth are key initiatives, specific tactics may include the following:

- Strategic growth of medical staff
- Pursuit of market expansion opportunities
- Ambulatory expansion (e.g., retail medicine, e-health)
- Population health initiatives
- Patient throughput and ALOS
- Potential new services or expansion of legacy services

Each of these tactics would be assigned a team responsible for planning and implementation.

Thus, there should be a direct link between the strategic plan and the creation of financial, operating, and quality metrics with benchmarks to guide a data-driven approach. These metrics, benchmarks, and data can be augmented by analytics to provide key role-based information in real time. For instance, a clinical leader's dashboard is significantly different from that of the CFO or COO. This variation engenders the necessity for data governance to reduce all of the metrics to key performance analytics and to work with all parties to ensure that each member of the organization has the specific information necessary to do his job.

In addition to role-specific dashboards, organizations should produce enterprise-wide dashboards. These documents include traditional financial statements such as balance sheets, statements of operations or income statements, statements of changes in net assets, statements of cash flows, footnotes to financial statements, and key financial ratios (e.g., profitability, liquidity, capital structure, asset efficiency). Dashboards also comprise traditional operating statements, such as volume statistics and indicators, price indicators, and efficiency indicators. Key operating ratios are also included, such as total labor costs as a percentage of total revenues; adjusted patient days; adjusted discharges; ALOS; FTEs per adjusted patient days; expenses per adjusted patient day; expenses per adjusted discharge; and revenues per FTE, labor, and nonlabor (supply chain).

The enterprise then creates a balanced dashboard or scorecard to summarize each of the key areas, which may include finance, service, internal processes, learning and growth, and operations. Once these are aggregated, each area is individually scored—ideally based on national benchmarks—and then weighted to provide the enterprise with an average score that indicates whether it is ahead of, on a par with, or behind benchmarked predictions and expectations.

CONCLUSION

In the same way that clinical practice is increasingly oriented toward evidence-based medicine, operational, financial, and quality managers are adopting similar best practices to optimize both clinical and business outcomes. Healthcare is increasingly guided by clinical and business analytics that provide both executives and managers with the information needed to make real-time and predictive decisions throughout the continuum of care. Retrospective reports alone no longer support top-tier performance, and both clinical and business healthcare executives are expected to modify their courses of action in shorter periods to guide their organizations to ever-rising levels of performance.

REFERENCES

Daly, R. 2017. "Majority of Hospitals Lack Robust Cost-Control Efforts: Survey." Healthcare Financial Management Association. Published September 18. www.hfma.org/Content .aspx?id=56057.

Kaplan, R., M. Witkowski, M. Abbott, A. B. Guzman, L. D. Higgins, J. G. Meara, E. Padden, A. P. Shah, P. Waters, M. Weidemeier, S. Wertheimer, and T. W. Feely. 2014. "Using Time-Driven Activity-Based Costing to Identify Value Improvement Activities in Healthcare." *Journal of Healthcare Management* 59 (6): 399–413.

Pfeffer, J., and R. Sutton. 2006. "Evidence-Based Management." *Harvard Business Review*. Published January. https://hbr.org/2006/01/evidence-based-management.

Woodman, J. 2015. *Patients Beyond Borders: Everybody's Guide to Affordable, World-Class Medical Travel*, 3rd ed. Chapel Hill, NC: Healthy Travel Media.

Operational Building Blocks and Success Factors for Population Health

Jon Burroughs

WHY IS HEALTHCARE moving from a sickness model to a health model, using a population health approach? It turns out that the vast majority of attributes that influence human health, well-being, and longevity have little to do with what we traditionally consider clinical practices. Nonclinical determinants such as genetics (30 percent), socioeconomic factors (28 percent), healthy behaviors (21 percent), and the safety of the environment in which patients live (7 percent) have, in aggregate, a vastly greater impact on the sum total of clinical interventions than what we consider to be traditional "healthcare" (14 percent). In fact, the single greatest determinant of life expectancy is zip code. For examples, in cities such as Washington, DC, and New Orleans, average life expectancy can vary by as much as 20 years, depending on a person's zip code. Thus, any serious consideration of health needs to take these determinants into account, if not center them. If healthcare organizations are going to be placed at risk for both clinical and business outcomes, they will have to reconsider ways in which they can leverage and influence factors that are not part of a traditional hospital or even healthcare setting.

From an academic perspective, population health represents a combination of clinical and public health competencies intended to influence, in David Kindig and David Stoddart's (2013, 380) words, "the distribution of health outcomes within a population, the determinants that influence this distribution, and the policies and interventions that impact these determinants." Although this is a comprehensive definition, it does not answer the simple and often elusive question, How do we do that? The purpose of this chapter is to explain population health from a pragmatic and operational perspective so that healthcare leaders understand not only the rationale for moving from a sickness model to a health model but also, even more important, how to redistribute and redirect scarce resources toward areas in which they are most needed and will have the greatest impact on both healthcare outcomes and costs.

THE FOUNDATION OF POPULATION HEALTH

In any group of covered lives (e.g., Medicare, Medicaid, commercial payers), there is a remarkably similar pyramidal distribution in terms of both risk and cost of beneficiaries that looks something like exhibit 11.1. This predictable distribution represents not only the foundation for operationalizing population health but also the imperative for doing so. Why?

The twentieth-century model of healthcare aggregated these groups together into a single approach. If you were sick, you went to the physician's office, and if you were very sick you went to the emergency department (ED), then perhaps you were admitted to the hospital. If you were well, you either saw a physician on an ongoing basis or you didn't, and most healthy individuals remained healthy over time. In other words, whether you were sick or well, there was a single system that determined how your health would be managed both short-term and long-term.

The challenge with this one-size-fits-all approach was that the sickest (the so-called vital few) received too little care too late and the healthy

Exhibit 11.1: Distribution of Risk and Cost in Covered Lives for a Typical Medicare Population

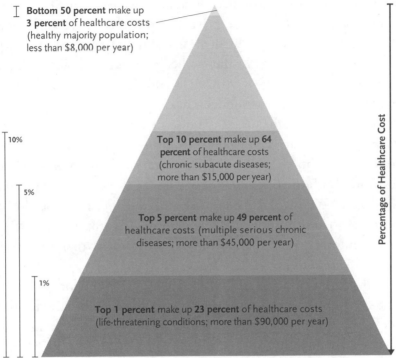

Percentage of Population

Bottom 50 percent make up 3 percent of healthcare costs (healthy majority population; less than $8,000 per year)

Top 10 percent make up 64 percent of healthcare costs (chronic subacute diseases; more than $15,000 per year)

Top 5 percent make up 49 percent of healthcare costs (multiple serious chronic diseases; more than $45,000 per year)

Top 1 percent make up 23 percent of healthcare costs (life-threatening conditions; more than $90,000 per year)

10% 5% 1%

Percentage of Healthcare Cost

majority received excessive and cost-ineffective care. The sickest minority make up more than half of all healthcare costs, and research has shown that early and proactive team-based interventions have a significant impact on not only the cost of care but also the long-term outcomes through the assessment of quality-adjusted life years (QALYs, or years lived without disability). A more comprehensive approach for these individuals reduces the cost of healthcare to the entire system, thus reducing insurance premiums for everyone. This shift makes healthcare more affordable and accessible, as those with the greatest need will receive the necessary care. Healthy people, on the other hand, don't necessarily require the ongoing services of a physician but can often manage their own care with the help of decision support tools (analytics), e-health, and retail medicine, as well as with the availability of care coordinators or navigators for input and guidance when necessary.

This pyramidal phenomenon also illustrates the necessity for both a public and private insurance-based healthcare system. The sickest among us can seldom afford private commercial coverage without the support of healthy individuals investing into a system that will eventually provide care for them when they enter a higher risk category unexpectedly or over time. In addition, commercial payers may not find a business model that can accommodate the sickest among us—hence, the necessity for some form of publicly financed managed Medicare and Medicaid. Thus, at its root, population health represents the redistribution or rationalization of resources to reduce both the risk and cost of care for those with the greatest need, greatest cost, and greatest risk and to reduce the allocation of resources to healthy individuals who, through disruptive innovation and technology, can be empowered to self-manage their care while they remain both low risk and low cost.

To create a rational care and clinical model to support each layer of the pyramid, key operational components must be assembled to provide the flexibility and scope to care for both the sick minority and healthy majority.

THE ORGANIZATIONAL AND OPERATIONAL BUILDING BLOCKS OF POPULATION HEALTH

Population health has four fundamental building blocks: (1) facilities and providers that are completely aligned with at-risk contracts; (2) integrated healthcare networks (IHNs); (3) health information exchanges (HIEs) and enterprise data warehouses (EDWs) with clinical and business analytics; and (4) appropriate population health infrastructure, including palliative care, disease management, post-acute care, retail medicine, and e-health.

The first three building blocks represent the foundation necessary to support the fourth. All four will be covered individually in this chapter to emphasize the importance and function of their operational contributions.

Facilities and Providers That Are Completely Aligned with At-Risk Contracts

As discussed in chapter 4, an organization that is unaligned cannot compete in today's increasingly global healthcare environment. All leadership groups (governance, management, physicians, other healthcare providers) must work together toward common strategic goals and objectives, both clinical and financial. This cooperation requires all facilities and providers to have at-risk contracts linking participants to work toward mutually agreed-on clinical and business goals and objectives. The great paradigm shift is that systems will need to align with outside organizations that may be beyond normal operational control—and with whom they may have, under past circumstances, competed. Furthermore, alignment will need to be achieved through common payer contracts in which healthcare organizations and systems can be held accountable for clearly defined metrics, with each unit affecting the payment for all. Thus, traditionally separate entities will need to come together to coordinate both contracts and care.

The health system should establish the new patterns of coordination in a particular sequence. First, contracts are developed that create both clinical and business outcome expectations and that require organizations to work with disparate organizations and providers. Alongside these contracts, alignment agreements are established between all organizations and providers that place a part of each agreement at risk for contractual metrics. This alignment transcends employment by involving all key organizations and individuals through some form of comanagement agreement.

Next, specific at-risk components or amounts are collaboratively negotiated between parties to ensure commitment. Over the term of the contract, at-risk agreements will modulate according to results. In general, contracts will vary based on the amount of risk organizations are willing to assume, quality ratings and cost reports, and the ability of organizations to meet payer and beneficiary expectations.

Many organizations create management oversight committees of administrative and clinical leaders who design and negotiate payment models with payers, outside organizations (e.g., skilled nursing facilities, nursing homes, rehabilitation facilities), and physicians and then oversee management of these contracts through shared clinical and business analytics. It is essential that all information is shared so that all parties can work toward common goals and hold each other accountable in a fair and transparent manner.

Methodology for Contracting for Population Health Services

One common methodology for contracting for population health services has five phases: identifying a population of covered lives; developing clinical and business analytics to assess clinical and financial risk; risk-stratifying all covered lives into functional subpopulations; developing cost-effective care and business models for each identified subpopulation; and monitoring, measuring, and modifying plans.

Your specific payer mix will determine which population of beneficiaries you will use to contract for population health. Most organizations start with their captive employee health plans to develop competence in managing population health and then expand to existing payer contracts. Once the employee health plan is managed well for population health services, organizations may expand into Medicare Advantage, managed Medicare plans, or managed Medicaid, as those groups typically represent both the greatest expenditures and the greatest opportunities for cost savings. Many commercial payers are now entering at-risk agreements, and these can often be negotiated separately with regional payers and health plans. Remember, each payer represents a population of covered lives that may either be managed separately or in aggregate with other payers.

Clinical and business analytics have been described in chapter 8 and will be further described in the next section; however, suffice to say that without predictive analytics to risk-stratify covered lives into relevant subpopulations, population health management is not possible. Strategically, it is necessary to develop role-based analytics or specific actionable information from both a clinical and business perspective that enables each member of the organization to manage and work with beneficiaries to optimize both clinical and business outcomes. Clinical and business analytics break down as follows:

- Clinical: health risk assessments, clinical data, pharmacy usage, QALYs, compliance with evidence-based recommendations, national-level quality measures, clinical outcomes, readmission rates, and similar data points
- Business: length of stay (LOS), adjusted cost per case, total cost per episode of care, case-mix index, shared savings, direct variable cost per episode of care, per member per month cost, and similar data points

Once a general population of covered lives is identified and all risk-related data on each beneficiary (particularly nonclinical determinants) are entered into an EDW, the typical pyramidal pattern will emerge, with seriously ill and potentially ill people making up the vast majority of potential costs (see exhibit 11.2).

Once this information is analyzed, cost-effective and appropriate clinical and business plans should be made for each of these risk-stratified groups (see exhibit 11.3).

Each group may be monitored through clinical and business analytics to optimize outcomes and to share information with providers, payers, and patients through customized and encrypted portals. Based on the measures of each subpopulation, adjustments can be made to both the clinical and business plans and to the

Exhibit 11.2: Healthcare Costs in a Defined Subpopulation (Employee Health Program) at Hospital X

Subpopulation	% of the Population	% of Cost	Cost ($)
Advanced illness	3	29	54,444
Multiple chronic illnesses	7	23	14,232
At risk	10	19	7,728
Stable	30	22	3,168
Healthy	50	7	660

Exhibit 11.3: Sample Clinical Plan

Subpopulation	Strategy
Advanced illness	Palliative care with intensive disease management, a team-based approach to care (e.g., care coordinator, physician, nurse, pharmacist, care manager, home health agency with wireless monitoring), disease registry with navigator
Multiple chronic illnesses	Disease management with team-based approach, patient-centered medical home or coordinated network of care, disease registry with navigator
At risk	Predictive analytics with decision support tools, disease registry with navigator, patient-centered medical home or wireless technology for periodic screening
Stable	E-health platforms with personalized applications, retail medicine for minor acute conditions, personalized health maintenance programs
Healthy	E-health platforms with personalized applications, retail medicine for minor acute conditions, personalized health maintenance programs

agreements themselves through the creation of dynamic and transparent contracts.

For example, the actual contract between St. Luke's Health System, (Boise, Idaho) and Select Health, a not-for-profit health plan subsidiary of Intermountain Health (Salt Lake City), operates on the following equation:

Premium = Total cost of care + 10% indirect costs
+ Insurance margin (87% medical loss ratio)
+ 2% to 3% margin (capped)

The medical loss ratio is the percentage of premium dollar that is directed to the care of the beneficiary. In addition, the book of business guarantees a six-year exclusive arrangement and an option to renew.

Integrated Healthcare Networks

Every IHN will, of necessity, be different as a result of differing markets, payer mix, clinical prevalence, demographics, and local financial and socioeconomic factors. However, many common elements may be found in a well-conceived network that will enable the provision of comprehensive healthcare services.

There are four generic principles that must be taken into account whenever building such a network: (1) The network must make clinical and business sense, (2) the network must be created by those with specialized expertise and good generalized leadership oversight, (3) the network should be able to manage an individual throughout the continuum of care, and (4) the network must be completely aligned.

What does it mean that the network must make clinical and business sense? In essence, it means that the structures and processes created, irrespective of their specific form or content, must lead to improved clinical outcomes, greater operational simplification, and better margins. Unfortunately, many organizations start beneficial initiatives by layering the new policies and structures onto old policies and structures. Every new layer, whether it is clinical or operational, requires some reconception of the entity as a whole so that there is a concurrent simplification or aggregation process that coincides with the addition of greater complexity. Innovation should not lead to non-value-added complexity that detracts from and undermines outcomes.

The IHN must be created by those with specialized expertise and good generalized leadership oversight. In other words, whether the operational entities include skilled nursing facilities, inpatient facilities, or outpatient rehabilitation, those with specialized expertise must participate in design decisions that have an impact on the system as a whole. This involvement requires a paradigm shift toward collaborative governance, matrix management (from both a clinical and an operational perspective), and care provision so that services can be seamlessly developed throughout the network. The purpose of generalist executive oversight is to ensure that the system works as a whole and that its component parts exist and function in proper proportion to their ultimate value for desired outcomes.

The IHN should ideally be able to manage a patient throughout the continuum of care. This capability requires a sufficiently comprehensive approach to system building so that if a person develops a complex cancer or chronic disease, her care can be carried out in an efficient and effective manner throughout the system. This coverage requires quaternary, tertiary, secondary, and primary healthcare facilities supported by information technology (IT), information-sharing agreements, and a comprehensive array of services and practitioners to support the full spectrum of resources and expertise throughout the continuum of care.

The final principle of building an IHN is that the network must be completely aligned. Many networks have "insiders" as well as "outsiders" who may not be party to at-risk agreements, and this dynamic will not work as effectively as a system in which providers and entities share agreements that align clinical and business outcomes. Again, the challenge is that healthcare organizations must contract with organizations of which they have no asset or operational control, and that situation requires a different kind of collaborative leadership.

What does a typical IHN look like? It often has the components and characteristics illustrated by St. Luke's Healthcare System (exhibit 11.4). Note that as a patient's healthcare condition shifts in acuity, there is a facility or entity that is appropriate for his care throughout time.

As exhibit 11.4 shows, a clinically integrated network begins and ends with a patient's home. Many experts believe that in the twenty-first century, most healthcare services for routine, easy-to-manage, or stable and chronic conditions will be accessed from a patient's home through wireless technology via the smartphone. These health problems represent the majority of healthcare services that the average individual requires throughout her life.

Schools, while not intuitively obvious sites for healthcare, are, in fact, where most children gain lifelong dietary and physical knowledge and habits. Thus, if healthcare organizations assume increasing

Exhibit 11.4: Example of Clinically Integrated Network

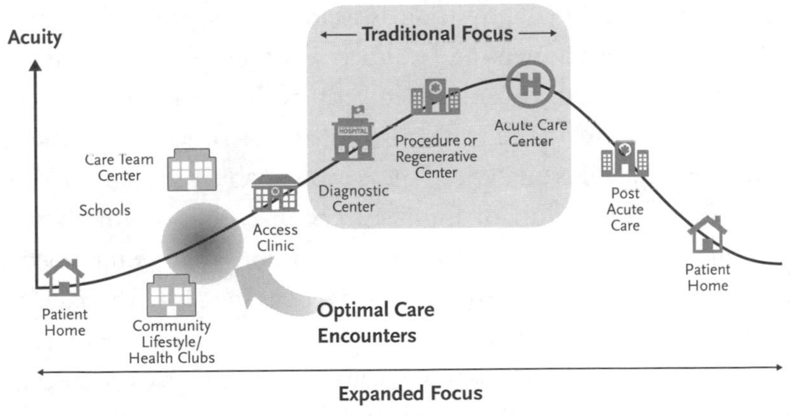

Source: Courtesy St. Luke's Healthcare System.

Chapter 11: Building Blocks and Success Factors for Population Health 339

risk for the overall healthcare costs of dependents of their contracted employees and beneficiaries, the foundational habits of children and young adults will have a significant impact on resultant outcomes and costs. For instance, according to the US Centers for Disease Control and Prevention, approximately 17 percent of American children aged 2 to 19 are obese, with a higher prevalence in the Southeast (Ogden et al. 2015). Thus, healthcare organizations increasingly find themselves working with schools to align their approaches with better long-term healthcare outcomes.

Another nontraditional concern of clinically integrated networks is the recreational facilities that adults use for sports, social activities, or meaningful hobbies. For example, some healthcare organizations work with golf clubs to encourage their members to walk rather than ride golf carts. Obviously, this requires some kind of aligned incentive, given that golf courses earn more on a volume basis by the use of carts—all aligned agreements must be win-win. Scholars have demonstrated that those who exercise regularly typically have lower healthcare costs, so many employers provide discount or copayment incentives for employees to regularly participate in exercise at a health club or other recreational facilities.

A care team center is another important element of St. Luke's network. Healthcare is increasingly a team effort led by a physician and care coordinator, with members who might include advanced-practice nurses (APNs), physician assistants, pharmacists, navigators, home health practitioners, and a variety of other specialists. They are increasingly located in centralized centers through which wireless technology supports the transmission of real-time and predictive clinical and business analytics. These tools enable the team to locate areas of concentration of high-risk, high-cost individuals with relapsing or newly developing clinical conditions that require specific interventions, a phenomenon known as *hot spotting*. The facilities can then develop interventional strategies to prioritize resources for these groups, starting with home visits and leading to a physician's office, retail medicine clinic, or ED only if necessary. Such centers are an integral part of any population health agreement.

Access clinics represent the entry point for most people to St. Luke's network. Traditionally, it has been a physician's office, but it now may also be a nurse practitioner's office, a local health center, an ambulatory clinic, a federally qualified health center (FQHC), or some form of retail clinic. These facilities are generally used by healthy people with minor, acute problems but can also be used by those with preexisting subacute chronic conditions that may require ongoing or intermittent interventions for minor, acute conditions.

When St. Luke's patients need further testing, they proceed to a diagnostic center. Most ancillary testing (e.g., X-rays, electrocardiograms, laboratory) takes place in lower-cost ambulatory facilities that may be owned and operated by a healthcare organization, physicians, nonhealthcare entities, or a combination of these. Those who can provide services at a low cost and with high reliability will outcompete traditional facilities.

Most routine elective procedures are performed in ambulatory procedure centers, and most post-acute care that requires skilled nursing is provided in ambulatory facilities with lower cost structures than hospitals. In the IHN of the future, it is essential to align with organizations that may or may not be within the traditional healthcare system.

Hospitals (or acute care centers) were the hub of the twentieth-century healthcare system; in IHNs, they become cost centers that will care only for those with the most complex and acute conditions. Payers will provide significant incentives to avoid hospital and critical care if possible. Many analysts believe that traditional inpatient capacity will fall by at least 40 percent over the next seven years, as an increasing number of ambulatory facilities are constructed and people choose to spend their final days at home rather than in acute care or critical care settings. Acute care will become increasingly regionalized, as particularly complex, high-risk care and procedures are concentrated in major regional centers to optimize both cost and outcome.

One of the greatest areas of improvement in healthcare outcomes and costs occurs following hospitalization, through low-cost, post-acute ambulatory, and home health services. St. Luke's monitors patients who are at high risk for relapse and readmission through wireless technology, using predictive analytics that identify those persons who require acute home or ambulatory interventions. These techniques enable the avoidance of unnecessary or preventable ED care or acute care admissions and readmissions.

These specific venues are illustrative of the facilities that are incorporated into well-conceived integrated networks in the twenty-first century. IHNs will include other essential facilities as each healthcare system's demographics, geography, and region allow, supporting its mission to provide high-quality services to defined populations.

Health Information Exchanges and Enterprise Data Warehouses with Clinical and Business Analytics

Population health is not possible without a completely aligned HIE, in which all key facilities and constituents are linked through compatible systems to enable aligned, at-risk agreements. Another essential element is an EDW, which can be used to convert undifferentiated data into actionable information. Though many of these issues have been discussed in chapter 8 from a technical perspective, the following section describes how this essential technology will be applied in necessary ways.

Health Information Exchanges

The healthcare industry is experiencing what the banking industry began in 1967, when the first automatic teller machine was created by John Shepherd-Barron and installed by Barclays in London. Older readers will recall a time in which it was necessary to enter the local branch of a bank during regular banking hours with a bank book and see a personal banker to make deposits and withdrawals. This old-fashioned process is akin to obtaining personal protected health information (PHI) at a healthcare facility today. In the not-too-distant future, people will be able to obtain PHI from the cloud, around the clock, through an encrypted and encoded process. This information will no longer be the exclusive property of the health-care organization. Only then will patients have unlimited ability to obtain healthcare services with complete documentation support worldwide around the clock, which will enable optimal medical care and accountability for both providers and patients.

Currently, most healthcare systems are working toward a unified IT platform to enable real-time, shared data. These platforms have appropriate information-sharing agreements to permit the transmission of protected peer reviews and health information to those with a need to know. The challenges obstructing this goal include the investment costs to build such a system, proprietary boundaries that prevent interoperability, the lack of standardized legal and regulatory guidance across state and national borders, and the variation among healthcare systems nationally and internationally that inhibits information sharing and interoperability. However, a global HIE will occur, and it will constitute a necessary and important transition that will support a globalized population health system.

As discussed in chapter 6, the EDW is the mechanism by which data are converted to actionable information through the process illustrated in exhibit 8.2.

The basis of an HIE is data. Organizations must acquire a variety of information, including nonclinical determinants (e.g., demographics, zip code, sex, risk factors). They can also use the data reported by medical devices (e.g., sensors, defibrillators, monitors, wireless technology from implantable devices such as pacemakers). The data are then synthesized through integration; modeling; and extraction, transfer, and loading processes so that the EDW can create a comprehensive profile of an individual's care from both clinical and business perspectives.

Once fully processed, the information emerges onto preprogrammed dashboards or scorecards that are specific to both role and function. For instance, each physician, member of the C-suite, payer, and patient requires unique sets of information that support good decision-making in real time and proactive planning through the creation of predictive analytics.

One of the key leadership functions while establishing an HIE is data governance through a multidisciplinary team of leaders, clinicians, payers, and key stakeholders. This group must oversee the essential attributes of data and information: integrity, credibility, security, stewardship, and privacy. This committee is of increasingly strategic importance as the system determines what pieces of information are necessary to support key strategic initiatives.

The ultimate goal of developing an HIE is optimized and cost-effective patient care, as determined by patients, providers, payers, and systems. This distinction is important, as each stakeholder has a unique perspective on what an optimized outcome represents and thus must be taken into account. The results of this final step inform subsequent cyclical iterations of information management and underlie how these tools are used going forward.

Clinical and Business Analytics

For a system to truly realize the potential of the population health model, real-time, actionable information must be role based according to need. Many kinds of data can be available; the following list covers a few:

- Revenue cycle management: accounts receivable days, net accounts receivable, late charges, denials, adjustments
- Enterprise quality: morbidity and mortality indexes, safety, adjusted LOS, employee injury, value-based purchasing data
- Cost accounting: total costs; direct variable costs per provider; labor chain and supply chain costs per hour, shift, day, week, month, or year
- Supply chain: costs by manufacturer, provider, and procedure; savings
- Clinical access: schedule fill rates, no shows, cancellations, timely appointments, copayments

- General operations: volume and revenue by cost center, observation and bed days, average daily census
- Population management: per member per month data, claims data, information on high-risk patients, hierarchical condition categories risk scores, chronic disease registries
- Provider performance: quality, cost, satisfaction, and safety metrics; work relative value units; coding and charge profiles; cost efficiency index
- Patient: customized health maintenance metrics with decision support tools

The ultimate purpose of analytics is to support timely and accurate decision-making as a means of achieving excellent clinical and business outcomes.

Population Health Infrastructure

Each element of the population health infrastructure is essential to providing comprehensive services to subpopulations: palliative care, disease management, post-acute care, retail medicine, and e-health. The purpose of each element is to optimize quality outcomes while having the same impact on cost of care for each subpopulation to enable the redistribution of resources in the most rational and appropriate way.

Palliative Care

Unfortunately, palliative care is inappropriately associated with end-of-life care. Palliative care goes far beyond hospice care through the comprehensive treatment of individuals with life-threatening conditions from the time of initial diagnosis. The World Health Organization (2018) defines palliative care as "an approach that improves the quality of life of patients and their families facing the problems associated with life-threatening illness, through the prevention and relief of suffering by means of early identification and impeccable assessment and treatment of pain and other problems, physical, psychosocial, and spiritual." Palliative care is an interdisciplinary, team-based approach that includes professionals such as the following:

- Care coordinators
- Physicians
- APNs or physician assistants
- Nurses
- Counselors
- Home health
- Chaplains or spiritual advisers
- Pharmacists
- Pain specialists
- Physiatrists
- Social workers
- Volunteers
- Public health specialists

The members of the palliative care team work together to provide comprehensive and customized interventions (as determined by predictive clinical and business analytics). The approach is comprehensive, with a focus on pain management, symptom management, functional management (i.e., optimizing activities of daily living), and emotional or spiritual management through the use of both customized and evidence-based practices. The team works with patients and their families to determine personal and life goals to optimize QALYs and healthy life expectancy. In addition, these goals are reconciled with personal and family values (e.g., autonomy, mobility, freedom), as well as the family's personal and material resources. Such discrepancies are at the root of noncompliance, which should be more accurately portrayed as unaligned recommendations.

Scholars have provided excellent evidence that the earlier palliative care is implemented, the greater the cost savings. In one of many studies illustrating the impact of palliative care on the direct costs of patients with life-threatening conditions, R. Sean Morrison and his team (2008) demonstrated that there is an immediate and almost 50 percent reduction in cost with the implementation of effective, team-based palliative care. Exhibit 11.5 shows one palliative care team's data, comparing it to the direct cost for patients who were discharged and those who died while inpatients.

Notice that the greatest difference between palliative and regular care is with laboratory, pharmacy, and intensive care unit (ICU) costs (particularly among those who died) and that significantly fewer deaths occur in the ICU with palliative care. Even more important, patients and their families had better acceptance and understanding of prognosis and potential for a good quality of life and did not feel that care was being denied or withdrawn for financial reasons. These discussions and interventions take time and require a deep understanding of the personal goals and values of the patient and each supporting family member.

Exhibit 11.5: Costs of Regular Care and Palliative Care: A Comparison

Costs	Live Discharges ($)		Difference (%)	Deaths ($)		Difference (%)
	Palliative	Regular		Palliative	Regular	
Per day	684	867	21	1,069	1,515	29
Per admission	9,992	11,498	13	16,831	23,521	28
Lab	833	1,160	28	1,772	2,805	37
Pharmacy	2,037	2,223	8	3,622	6,063	40
ICU care	1,726	6,974	75	7,755	15,531	50
Died in ICU (%)				4	18	78

While the advantages of this strategy seem apparent to most healthcare leaders, there are many pitfalls that undermine the ability to launch and support widespread palliative care services in the United States, including the following:

- Palliative care is thought of as a contemporary approach to hospice care; if care is not initiated until the end of life, QALYs and cost savings are never realized.
- Palliative care is viewed as the purview of several full-time equivalents rather than a systemic implementation of a full team to care for all of the eligible persons in the top 1 percent of covered lives in terms of risk and cost.
- The need for palliative care should be determined (with the approval and support of physicians) by predictive analytics, not by individual practitioners' referrals. Most physicians do not have access to properly integrated nonclinical determinants of care to accurately predict those with the greatest need.
- A culture supporting a standardized and customized approach to those with life-threatening conditions must replace the traditional cottage industry culture of complete customization and individualization.

Palliative care improves both the cost and quality of people's experiences with life-threatening conditions. It shrinks cost by reducing futile and non-value-added care and by fostering seamless communication and coordination between caregivers. Palliative care teams improve quality of life by optimizing personal control, autonomy, and self-actualization; optimally extending life without disability and in keeping with an individual's deepest values; effectively managing pain, symptoms, and functionality; and most important, achieving the goals set by patients and their families.

Palliative care assumes an even greater importance with the extension of human longevity, as most individuals will experience a relatively brief period of disability of two to three years toward the end of life, likely suffering from frailty, dementia, organ failure, or cancer. The creation of a cost-effective approach to optimizing functionality and quality of life—while minimizing costs—is essential.

Disease Management

Almost half of humans worldwide have some form of chronic disease, and management of these diseases makes up more than 75 percent of total healthcare costs in the United States. The numbers are enormous, with more than one-third of Americans suffering from either obesity or hypertension, and approximately one-quarter have some form of heart disease. Sixty million Americans suffer from a behavioral disorder for which they may be stigmatized, receiving little financial or social support, and 23.6 million have some form of diabetes. Each of these chronic diseases costs between $60 billion and $240 billion annually. Perhaps most astonishing are the costs of cancer, which affects approximately 11.1 million Americans but costs a staggering $1.6 trillion annually to the US economy (Nash et al. 2010).

More than 50 percent of chronic diseases have an underlying behavioral component, such as depression, bipolar disorder, anxiety, or addictive personality disorder, that the care team must address to achieve an optimal outcome. Thus, many disease management programs include a mandatory behavioral health component. In addition, more than 50 percent of chronic diseases have some significant socioeconomic factor, such as lack of adequate food, shelter, access to healthcare, or personal safety, that either perpetuates or exacerbates a disease. Social workers and care coordinators have a significant role to play in disease management in conjunction with the traditional healthcare team.

Disease management has at least four important elements. First, an approach that is centered around patients and families is vital, particularly when supported and facilitated by physicians and healthcare organizations. Second, effective disease management focuses on empowerment and self-motivation—it demonstrates the underlying behavior or root cause of affective or emotional issues in addition to treatment of the primary disease. Third, disease management requires an interdisciplinary team, evidence-based clinical and business practices, and clinical and business analytics monitored in real time. Finally, it is built on an approach that focuses on those few interventions that will have the greatest impact on the overall cost and quality of care.

As in palliative care, individuals eligible for disease management are identified through predictive analytics as part of the top 5 percent of risk in a typical population of covered lives. Also, as in palliative care, these people should be identified systemically, not based on individual physician referral, and the emphasis should be on early intervention to achieve the greatest optimization of quality of life and cost savings.

The IT component of disease management works as follows:

1. Payer contracts and predictive analytics determine key clinical and business performance indicators that are of strategic importance.
2. Covered lives for each payer undergo predictive analytics to identify and risk-stratify those who represent the top 5 percent of risk and cost to the system.
3. Patients in the top 5 percent are sorted based on diagnosis to determine the services required (e.g., primary care, care coordinator, ambulatory imaging or procedure center, home health) based on which evidence-based pathways are triggered.
4. Rule-based clinical and process approaches are derived from the specific combination of clinical pathways so that a customized approach for each individual may be derived from the standardized catalog.
5. Dashboards and scorecards demonstrate the specific interventions required for each person based on these rules. An example of a dashboard for a patient with diabetes is illustrated in exhibit 11.6.

To see how disease management works in day-to-day operations, it is useful to look at a specific initiative from St. Luke's, Project Zero. St. Luke's 1.3 percent surgical-site infection (SSI) rate was lower than the national average of 1.9 percent, but its staff chose to reduce it even more. SSIs constitute the single greatest risk and cost of routine surgery at the health system, generally resulting in a 106 percent cost increase ($16,051 above the normal cost of $15,131). Moreover, these complications were significant at St. Luke's as a result of the high volume of surgical cases (2,000 spine surgeries and 2,000 total joint replacements annually). SSIs represent the number-one cause of postoperative sepsis, a dangerous and potentially lethal complication of surgery.

The physicians did research and realized that four factors were largely responsible for their SSI rate. First was excessive traffic in the OR as carts were moved in and out throughout the surgery. Second, excessive particulate matter was present in the ventilation system

Exhibit 11.6: Example of Evidence-Based Rule-Generated Dashboard

Endocrine Events

HgbA1c:	25%	(8 weeks ago)	5.0%	(4 months ago)	
BP:	140/86 mmHg	(6 days ago)	111/59 mmHg	(11 days ago)	
LDL:	91 mg/dL	(8 weeks ago)	H 138 mg/dL	(4 months ago)	
Tobacco Use/Currently Using:	No	(6 weeks ago)	No	(6 weeks ago)	
Foot Exam:	08/12/10	(3 weeks ago)	07/28/10	(5 weeks ago)	
Eye Exam:	11/17/09	(8 weeks ago)	07/07/10	(2 months ago)	

Diabetes Performance Measures (As of last night)

- 1: Hgb A1c Done in last 6 months
- 2: Hgb A1c < 8.0%
- 3: BP < 130/80
- 4: LDL Cholesterol Done in last year
- 5: LDL Cholesterol < 100
- 6: Tobacco Non-user
- 7: Creatinine Done in last year
- 8: Micro-albumin Done in last year
- 9: Foot Exam Done in last year
- 10: Eye Exam Done in last year
- 11: Diabetic Education Done in last year
- 12: Flu Vaccine Done in last year
- 13: Pneumovax Done
- 14: Aspirin Use

Chronic Disease Algorithm

Diabetes Mellitus (DM)
Hypertension in DM

Source: Adapted from Mayo Clinic.

from outdated OR systems. Third, a few surgeons were driving up the complication rate and exposure to particulate matter, as they took excessive time to perform their procedures. Fourth, the lack of transparency and data sharing among physicians meant that outlier physicians had no idea they were outliers.

As a result, physicians, with management support, pursued the following solutions:

- All carts must remain in the OR throughout the procedure, with double checks to ensure that all required supplies were present before the surgery.
- Management purchased and installed high-grade ventilation systems with a high-efficiency particulate air filter in each OR.
- OR times are measured for surgeons with similar procedures and benchmarked both locally and nationally, with mutually agreed-on limits (two standard deviations above the mean).
- Surgeons are managed assertively through performance improvement initiatives and, if necessary, excluded from the program.

The outcome was a reduction in SSIs from 1.3 percent to 0.6 percent, which doesn't seem significant until you consider the financial impact of each SSI ($16,051 per infection × 280 fewer infections annually = savings of $4,494,280). The project was such a success that the organization extended it to many other surgical programs throughout its system, gaining savings in the tens of millions of dollars—not to mention more than a thousand fewer potentially fatal infections.

To summarize, disease management represents a multidisciplinary, team-based approach to standardizing both clinical and operational processes. In addition, interdisciplinary teams develop a best-practice approach and benchmark it against a traditional approach with metrics for both clinical and business processes. This transformation requires active participation by both physicians and management, who should fill in a matrix like the one in exhibit 11.7. This enables strategically important clinical processes to improve as the organization focuses on optimizing both quality and business outcomes collaboratively.

Post-acute Care

Post-acute care is an essential element of the population health infrastructure. It has the greatest impact on healthcare outcomes because a hospitalization only treats acute episodes of care and has little, if anything, to do with the thousands of day-to-day decisions that individuals make about their healthcare that affect their long-term morbidity and mortality. The decisions to take medications (or not), exercise (or not), observe a healthy lifestyle (or not), comply with evidence-based recommendations (or not), and eat healthy food (or not) are personal choices that have little to do with the influence of healthcare providers or organizations and everything to do with the personal perspectives and values of patients and their families. Therefore, what happens outside of a hospital or physician's office is of paramount importance if healthcare organizations want to have a meaningful impact on outcomes and costs.

At the heart of post-acute care is readmission prevention. The Centers for Medicare & Medicaid Services (2018) penalizes healthcare

Exhibit 11.7: Processes and Metrics Template

Processes	Metrics
Clinical processes	Key clinical metrics
Operational processes	Key operational metrics
Business processes	Key business metrics

organizations for unnecessary readmissions by 3 percent, and these standards were established for good reason:

- Of readmissions within 30 days after discharge, 75–85 percent are preventable.
- Of discharges, 51 percent do not have follow-up within 30 days (and they are 1,000 percent more likely to be readmitted).

Opinions within the healthcare field on the root causes of high readmission rates are diverse. Some point to failures in follow-up. Some care teams neglect to develop meaningful follow-up plans (e.g., they instruct patients to "see your regular physician" when the person may not have one). In fact, in approximately two-thirds of cases, no follow-up occurs. Moreover, organizations sometimes experience a delay in dictation of discharge summaries, or the summaries never reach the primary care or follow-up physician. Some problems may center on medications and discharge instructions—up to two-thirds of individuals are unable to understand the instructions provided, particularly with regard to their medications, and up to 70 percent are unable to afford (or choose not to pay for) expensive medications. Perhaps one of the major issues is that the healthcare system lacks patient and family incentives to participate fully in care. Some commentators, however, point to a lack of standardized discharge processes in hospitals, with significant variation in how they are handled throughout the nation. Regardless of the root causes, healthcare organizations that are serious about improving this failure-riddled process must redesign care for the twenty-first century in order to participate in at-risk or global budget agreements.

Yale New Haven Health System's structured transition care rounds and post-acute care program constitute an excellent example of readmission prevention and management of the post-acute process. The health system is made up of five hospitals (including its flagship, Yale New Haven Medical Center) and Northeast Medical Group, a large, physician-run foundation of primary care and medical specialists. Its staff no longer speaks in terms of "admissions" or "discharges," which imply the beginning and end of its responsibility, but rather says "transitions of care" from one venue to another. Its post-acute care programs consist of the following elements.

The health system has developed a standardized process that takes place with every patient every day of the year. Transition planning no longer takes place Monday through Friday from 9 a.m. to 5 p.m.; it is a daily, around-the-clock process. The post-acute process begins prior to every elective inpatient episode through both a risk assessment and proactive planning. Most elective inpatient episodes are predictable in their LOS, based on initial diagnosis and comorbidities, to within a fraction of a day, and thus post-acute planning takes place prior to hospitalization and can be adjusted as needed. The system also has adopted preoperative risk assessment for elective procedures of varying severity. This evaluation involves a pediatrician or an internist, supported by an anesthesiologist (or nurse anesthetist) and a care manager, to assess potential issues. Common clinical comorbidities discovered during this process include difficult airways, sleep apnea, diabetes, atrial fibrillation and other arrhythmias, and cardiac valve issues. This process reduces the cost per case, LOS, likelihood of readmission, ED visits, and risk- and severity-adjusted morbidity and mortality rates.

The transition planning process is a team activity led by a care coordinator (typically an APN with a deep knowledge and understanding of the internal and external system, including all relevant payer contracts). The team includes a physician, nurse practitioner, nurse, case manager, risk manager, and pharmacist. The pharmacist plays an essential role in medication reconciliation, determining whether the patient can afford the medications, drug interactions, potential allergies, follow-up counseling regarding medications, and assessment of patient and family understanding of medications. Yale's staff engages in structured discussions with patients and their family every afternoon throughout the planning process.

Documentation is completed in real time. This means that operative notes are completed as the procedure is finished, post-acute care unit notes are done on transfer to the floor, and discharge (or transition of care) notes are completed the day of transfer to an ambulatory facility or home. All relevant clinical and business information is up-to-date and shared with all relevant care providers and managers. Members of the staff make routine posttransition phone calls to ensure understanding of the plan, satisfaction with the service, and compliance with and understanding of all recommended treatments and medications.

Patients are stratified (red, yellow, green) according to risk factors, clinical and nonclinical determinants, and other socioeconomic factors so that additional resources and time can be devoted to working with those in greatest need and at greatest risk of relapse or return. Yale's metrics include rate of on-time transition, LOS reduction, readmission rate (adjusted by risk and severity), ED utilization rate, patient satisfaction, adjusted cost per case, and compliance with the Healthcare Effectiveness Data and Information Set and ambulatory metrics. It also monitors the functional recovery improvement index (actual vs. expected), pain control, bed days per 1,000 patients, averted admissions or ED visits, and overall adjusted cost of care—of each patient and in aggregate—over a rolling period.

The health system maintains collaborative risk-sharing agreements with key ambulatory facilities, including skilled nursing centers, retail pharmacies, urgent care centers, home health agencies, nursing homes, outpatient rehabilitation facilities, FQHCs, and ambulatory procedure centers. It also has contracts with large employers and relevant payers and health plans. These agreements ensure alignment. All clinical and business analytics are shared with all relevant providers and facilities to ensure transparency and integrity.

Yale also holds monthly meetings with aligned collaborators to discuss specific case reviews, comparative data and analytics, process improvement initiatives, and interfacility challenges. These meetings are essential to supporting partners, and they maintain both transparency and accountability.

Fee-for-service contracts will not incentivize the type of policies that Yale has adopted. For instance, St. Luke's was able to reduce unnecessary readmissions by 92 percent and reduce unnecessary ED visits by 75 percent—two improvements that would pose financial problems under fee-for-service. Thus, these programs must be done with other payment models (e.g., risk-based capitation, global budgets) so that they make good business and good clinical sense.

Retail Medicine

As access to routine care became more problematic over the 2010s, with average waits of several months in certain metropolitan areas, retail medicine through big-box retailers and pharmacies became a natural disruptive solution. It has the potential to plug this hole in the population health infrastructure. Patients have become consumers through the increasing use of high-deductible healthcare policies that increased out-of-pocket expenses and through the creation of health savings accounts. In addition, they have been squeezed out of the traditional market because of ever-increasing costs and cost shifting and are starved for low-cost options of acceptable quality.

Disruptive innovation takes place when an industry becomes squeezed and abandons the low end of its own market (i.e., low-margin services), allowing new entrants to work their way upstream. As hospitals and physicians were squeezed by low reimbursement and high costs in the late 1990s and early 2000s, they turned to high-margin work (e.g., elective, high-end procedures) instead of changing the business model. Thus, millions of Americans were left with little immediate access to routine care except through EDs or urgent care clinics, which are all relatively expensive and, in many cases, inconvenient and cost-ineffective.

By 2015, there were almost 3,000 retail clinics in the United States, with plans for almost 50,000 such facilities worldwide by 2020. These clinics are typically staffed by APNs under medical direction and focus primarily on urgent care and on treating 36 predefined, high-volume, low-risk conditions, carefully proscribed by clinic policies, with evidence-based, standardized approaches. Any potentially significant or serious condition is immediately referred, without charge, to a regular physician or an ED for definitive management and treatment. These clinics increasingly use low-cost diagnostics, and most have affiliation agreements with hospitals and physicians to ensure ready availability of consultations and higher levels of care if needed. They provide retail amenities, such as wellness checks, appointment reminders, and follow-up calls, and their costs are significantly lower than most urgent care centers, EDs, or even physicians' offices.

The benefit for the retailer is to combine multiple businesses (pharmacy, supermarket, department store, pharmacy benefits plan) under one roof, which dilutes fixed costs, lowers cost structure, and creates a more consumer-friendly environment in which to provide routine healthcare services for low-risk conditions. Walmart is currently adding telemedicine capabilities to its retail clinics to enable immediate medical consultation when needed through its Teladoc program. Walgreens treats many common diseases, such as diabetes and hypertension, through its retail outlets, and it plans to add many more through the use of evidence-based algorithms with physician oversight.

From a population health perspective, this means that healthy individuals now have a lower-cost option to receive treatment for minor, commonly occurring acute conditions such as ear infections, sore throats, rash without fever, minor lacerations, and sprained ankles. This alternative reduces cost, improves access and convenience, and relieves EDs and urgent care centers from nonemergencies that can be cared for in much lower-cost settings. Many retailers look to healthcare organizations to provide clinical consultation and expertise, covered lives, compatible electronic health records (EHRs) and HIEs, and strategic alignment. In addition, many organizations create retail facilities of their own as an essential element of comprehensive clinical integration services.

E-Health

One essential element of population health infrastructure is also a remarkable disruptive innovation: e-health. This expansion of telemedicine enables routine healthcare services to be accessible through an iPhone, personal computer, iPad, or other device. Many pundits feel that the primary access point to healthcare in the twenty-first century will be applications on smartphones. American Well, the largest e-health platform in the United States, reports that more than 100 million Americans accessed healthcare services via phones, computers, mobile devices, or retail kiosks in 2016. Many large employers now provide e-health applications to not only provide services but also monitor their health plans, pharmacy benefits management program, and employees' compliance with basic health recommendations (in exchange for a lower premium or deductible).

As of June 2016, e-health visits ran approximately $59 and are staffed by a physician or by an APN with medical direction. Services consist mainly of urgent care. Consumers can choose between a variety of clinicians, access their credentials and backgrounds, undergo a diagnostic exam using their phone or a retail kiosk, receive recommended treatment and prescription delivery via an affiliated pharmacy, and participate in follow-up care.

Although urgent care is the most common use of e-health, alternative applications for this new technology include on-demand inpatient consultations; ED case flow augmentation for low-risk, fast-track patients; home health care services; routine postdischarge and postoperative care; and behavioral health care. It also contributes physicians to the national pool, particularly for difficult-to-recruit specialists in geographic areas of scarcity.

Management of chronic conditions is another promising use. Many people with diabetes, hypertension, chronic obstructive lung disease or asthma, congestive heart failure, and similar chronic conditions can safely monitor their own diseases and be managed by practitioners. Using wireless technology and wearable devices, individuals can keep track of their health at home. The use of wireless technology enables practitioners to receive decision alerts that may result in an early, home-based intervention. E-health platforms can interface with physicians' offices, EHRs, HIEs, and healthcare organizations to communicate PHI freely and confidentially. This collaboration between care coordinators, primary care clinicians, and patients helps to manage long-term conditions in a more convenient and cost-effective way.

Many healthcare facilities (particularly in rural areas) lack a full complement of clinical specialists and subspecialists. E-health platforms enable any specialist (assuming a valid state medical license where the patient is located), from any venue, to evaluate and potentially treat a patient. The ultimate example of this is the e-ICU, which enables intensivists to care for patients throughout a geographic region, enabling the patient to remain in his community hospital and be cared for by qualified clinical personnel in local centers with the oversight of highly skilled specialists and subspecialists who work out of centralized tertiary and quaternary centers.

Families often seek care in EDs after hours because of lack of access, insurance, or financial means. E-health platforms provide a way to assess and manage stable patients with minor acute conditions, who often wait for hours to be seen after triage. Redirecting these patients often relieves the ED of backlog and the family of unnecessary waiting, and it provides a significantly lower-cost alternative for everyone concerned.

One of the key success factors for post-acute care is timely follow-up, and many private practices and clinics are not set up to handle routine transitions of care in a seamless manner. E-health platforms provide a way of managing routine, low-risk follow-ups for nonacute conditions without having to make appointments at a physician's office. E-health can be done at the patient's convenience. Routine examinations can be performed through a smartphone, giving practitioners a sense of whether this approach is sufficient or whether the patient needs to be referred for more traditional evaluation.

E-health may also affect behavioral health, a long-neglected component of the US healthcare system. It is often the root cause of many chronic diseases such as obesity, diabetes, alcoholism, opioid addiction, and smoking. E-health platforms provide convenient, low-cost colocation services (primary specialty care integrated with complementary care) that promote the effective treatment of chronic diseases.

With the persistent geographic maldistribution of physicians, APN, and physician assistants, e-health can provide an alternative source of qualified healthcare practitioners in rural and inner-city areas. The distribution of healthcare personnel will never be even, but e-health platforms provide a way of leveling the field so that everyone can access less costly, more convenient care, with any kind of medical or surgical specialist, at any time, from anywhere.

PUTTING IT ALL TOGETHER: MAKING THE TRANSITION FROM FEE-FOR-SERVICE TO RISK-BASED CONTRACTING

As mentioned earlier in this chapter, fee-for-service reimbursement is incompatible with a fully operative population health program. When a healthcare system successfully implements a population health program, costly care events decrease—because inpatient admissions, elective procedures, inpatient ancillary services, ED visits, and physicians' office visits all decrease. Such a paradigm shift in the model of clinical care requires a significantly different business model.

Many alternative payment models are, in effect, fee-for-service with a lower cost structure. These include the following:

- Pay for performance (top-decile performers subsidized by bottom-decile performers, based on performance metrics)
- Shared savings
- Bundled-payment programs for defined episodes of care (e.g., orthopedic, cardiac, and cancer service lines involving discrete procedures that meet quality metrics and reduce the cost of care)

These models promote lower costs, more standardized care, and adherence to quality metrics. However, they still fundamentally incentivize volume-based care, particularly with regard to high-margin elective procedures and high-cost therapies (e.g., chemotherapy).

What health systems truly need is some form of risk-based, capitated (per member per month), or global payment option that rewards the maintenance of health, prevention of disease, and provision of cost-effective interventions with positive outcomes. This transition will be difficult—it involves the transformation of a $3.2 trillion industry into a very different clinical and business model. Payers are beginning to make the adjustment through value-based at-risk contracts, large employers are creating significant incentives for employees to become more engaged in managing their own healthcare costs and outcomes, and many healthcare organizations are committed to making this change over a defined period.

David Pate, president and CEO of St. Luke's Health System, calls this transition the *yellow box*. His conception of it looks something like exhibit 11.8. The graph shows that fee-for-service will probably not disappear altogether. Rather, it will likely become an increasingly minor form of contracting compared with at-risk contracts that are based on defined healthcare outcomes and costs.

The transition requires a thoughtful strategic plan aligning transformation of the clinical care model with the business model so that a sustainable margin can be made throughout this time frame. But putting it all together requires a multistep process.

Step 1: Align All Key Facilities and Practitioners

The foundation for any transformational change in a healthcare system is complete alignment with facilities and practitioners who are willing to work with the organization to make the transition. Those who can't or won't make the transition cannot be aligned with this effort but can continue to contribute to the system in a

Exhibit 11.8: The Yellow Box

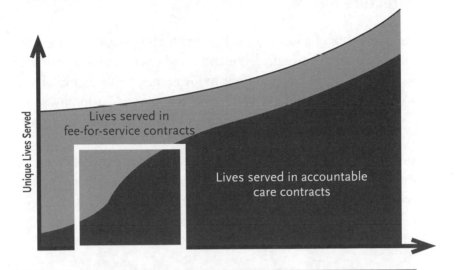

more individualized way, as long as they do not undermine the organization's effort or outcomes.

As mentioned earlier, at-risk contracts require clinical and business analytics to provide real-time, role-based information to both track and monitor individual and aggregate performance. These analytics are essential in any aligned relationship, whether between a healthcare system and an individual or a healthcare system and other aligned facilities.

Step 2: Build the Integrated Network Together

Each person or facility in a network brings a unique perspective and expertise to the table, and organizations that take advantage of the diverse talents within any integrated network will build more functional systems. Every system component should add both clinical and operational value to the system as a whole.

Step 3: Focus on Opportunities to Lower Cost Structure First

As covered in chapter 10, working with a physician–management collaboration to lower the labor and supply chain ratios is an obvious way for healthcare organizations to lower their cost structure. Doing so effectively can build a capital reserve that is necessary for investment in a population health infrastructure. Other significant opportunities include the transfer of care from high-cost venues (e.g., EDs, primary care clinics) to low-cost venues (e.g., retail medicine outlets, e-health visits) where appropriate. Again, these efforts are possible with traditional silos, but they work more effectively with aligned relationships that promote mutual clinical and business success.

Step 4: Focus on Palliative Care and Inpatient Disease Management

This step is listed first for the population health initiatives as it focuses on the top 1 percent of covered lives that make up 23 percent of costs. Improving both services will provide the most immediate and greatest cost reductions with the least amount of investment and effort. As Geisinger Health (Danville, Pennsylvania) has demonstrated, initiatives that focus on patients with the greatest risk, cost, and acuity provide the quickest return on investment. Healthy individuals with minor chronic conditions often take the longest to produce any return, if at all. Therefore, within either a capitated model or a traditional fee-for-service model, palliative care and inpatient disease management will improve margins significantly, regardless of the payment methodology.

Step 5: Build New Sources of Revenue

Any margin improvement program will ultimately fail if the sole focus is on lowering costs. Long-term margin can only be sustained with revenue growth, and healthcare has abundant opportunities to do so, such as e-health solutions, retail medicine, direct-to-employer contracting, and innovative reimbursement models designed to increase revenues and lower costs (e.g., bundled-payment models). Revenue growth is the engine that fuels every enterprise, and without it, waste-reduction programs (e.g., Lean, Six Sigma) will never realize their full potential. However, recall that effective population health programs for post-acute care may undermine inpatient volume and revenues. Healthcare must find new areas of growth to compensate for this loss and to fund transformation.

Step 6: Develop an Infrastructure for Ambulatory Population Health

Building a population health infrastructure should not be pursued seriously until an organization has an exit strategy for most fee-for-service contracts—effective post-acute care programs will cut deeply into pay-for-volume revenues. Careful coordination between clinical and contracting units must be maintained so that the transition can be appropriately synchronized. Many organizations attempt to balance avoidance of readmission penalties (3 percent of Medicare Part A funds) with maintenance of volumes, and now that pay-for-value contracts have emerged, this balance is ultimately unsustainable. Effective post-acute care, retail medicine, and e-health will significantly lower inpatient, ED, and physicians' office volumes. The shift must be planned so that the organization can be paid to avoid these cost centers in favor of optimizing health.

Step 7: Exit Fee-for-Service Last

As mentioned earlier in the chapter, no organization will eliminate fee-for-service contracts. However, they will not be the dominant payment model in the twenty-first century. Organizations that linger in fee-for-service arrangements will see their margins erode as most payers move to more profitable models. Thus, change should not be done for its own sake but for the betterment of clinical outcomes and business margins.

CONCLUSION

Population health will become the dominant care and business model of the twenty-first century because it represents the rationalization and more effective distribution of increasingly scarce resources. The model directs resources to those with the greatest needs (and costs), lowering the cost of the entire system while focusing on the optimization of outcomes. The traditional, one-size-fits-all model deprived the sickest minority of resources and gave the healthy majority too much, so rightsizing our industry will provide better performance at a far lower cost for all. Reimbursement methodologies that support preventive measures, lifelong health maintenance, and early interventions for life-threatening conditions and that eliminate wasteful or non-value-added services will support healthcare organizations in their move toward fulfilling their mission to optimize healthcare and not merely treat injury and disease.

REFERENCES

Centers for Medicare & Medicaid Services. 2018. "Readmissions Reduction Program (HRRP)." Modified March 20. www.cms .gov/medicare/medicare-fee-for-service-payment/acutein patientpps/readmissions-reduction-program.html.

Kindig, D., and G. Stoddart. 2003. "What Is Population Health?" *American Journal of Public Health* 93 (3): 380–83.

Morrison, R. S., J. D. Penrod, J. B. Cassel, M. Caust-Ellenborgen, A. Litke, L. Spragens, and D. E. Meier. 2008. "Cost Savings

Associated with US Hospital Palliative Care and Consultation Programs." *Archives of Internal Medicine* 168 (16): 1783–90.

Nash, D., J. Reifsnyder, R. Fabius, and V. Pracilio. 2010. *Population Health: Creating a Culture of Wellness.* Sudbury, MA: Jones & Bartlett Learning.

Ogden, C., M. D. Carroll, C. D. Fryar, and K. M. Flegal. 2015. "Prevalence of Obesity Among Adults and Youths: United States, 2011–2014." *NCHS Data Brief* 219 (November): 1–8.

World Health Organization. 2018. "WHO Definition of Palliative Care." Accessed April 19. www.who.int/cancer/palliative /definition/en/.

CHAPTER 12

Creating a High-Reliability Organization for the Twenty-First Century

Kathleen Bartholomew
John Nance
Jon Burroughs

ON THE 30-MINUTE *drive home from your board meeting, you find yourself mentally replaying the risk manager's quarterly report for your hospital—mostly because of the shocked look on the board members' faces when they heard her speak. The report discussed the hospital's progress on handwashing, falls, infections, and patient safety huddles. After the last avoidable patient death six months ago, the senior leadership team worked hard on initiatives to raise awareness of each employee's role in keeping patients safe. Yet it has happened again—a lapse in handwashing protocol has resulted in a death from a hospital-acquired infection. And this time to an 11-year-old child!*

"But what else could we have possibly done?" you ask yourself.

"A lot," comes the answer.

As you roll into your driveway, this is your final thought: If every organization is perfectly designed to get the results it consistently achieves, your hospital is perfectly designed to kill two patients per year!

If your healthcare organization already functioned as a high-reliability organization (HRO), patient harm or death from medical mistakes would be an extremely rare occurrence, if it ever happened at all. But many years after the pivotal Institute of Medicine (IOM) report *To Err Is Human*, healthcare is just now realizing that the improvements engendered by the HRO model are vital to the survival of healthcare institutions.

High reliability has a variety of meanings and includes sensitivity to operations and the system environment, respect for potential error, leaders who are willing to face facts, a reluctance to simplify interpretations, constant and vigorous awareness, the elimination of non-value-added autonomy, and an unwavering focus on continuous performance improvement (Wachter 2012). Healthcare HROs embody the philosophy, strategy, and tactics necessary to change from the old model of healthcare delivery (resulting in medical error as the third leading cause of death in the United States) to the new model of high reliability.

And here's the key: That transition is no longer optional. Why? Because the principles of high reliability work as well for healthcare as they do for other sectors, and that fact makes it an ethical mandate. If we know that a particular achievable standard of care can protect against terrible and wholly avoidable injuries and deaths, then those patients and their families—indeed, the nation—have a right to demand that a superlative standard of care be the minimum standard everywhere.

Could you look the family of that deceased 11-year-old in the eye and promise anything less?

Indeed, when a healthcare organization truly achieves high-reliability status through its willingness to make massive internal changes, the uniformity of care alone will eliminate the need to ask (when, for instance, your family is expecting a baby), "Do you know a good obstetrician?" Such questions are still necessary today because of the wildly variant methods, techniques, temperaments, and training—and unacceptably variant outcomes—of individual doctors and hospitals alike. But what would the medical world look like if you didn't need to ask for recommendations because you knew everyone practiced with uniform standards derived from careful evidence? It would look like an HRO.

Many in healthcare have grown weary of hearing about the safety achievements of commercial aviation, but the airline industry, and numerous other high-risk industries, are just as human in nature as healthcare, and therefore their ability to minimize catastrophes to near zero has much to teach the medical profession. When the toll of unnecessary deaths stands at 440,000 patients per year, how can anyone in healthcare reject such lessons as minimized variables and collegial communication (Golladay and Collins 2010)? If what we were doing for safety had been working, there could be a viable argument for ignoring high-reliability industries, but widespread success is decidedly not the reality.

Before any of us buy an airline ticket, we don't stop and ask a frequently flying friend, "Do you know a good pilot I can retain to fly my plane?" You trust both a specific airline and the airline system (inclusive of governmental regulations). You trust that all pilots are trained to the same benchmark and would not be in the cockpit if they did not meet those standards. You trust the airline to maintain its aircraft to the highest standards and to be honest and transparent with you when things go wrong. And, because of this demonstrated uniformity of excellence and demonstrated safety performance, you accept whatever pilots the airline assigns and whatever airplane it places at the gate.

Ask yourself a simple question. If your mother were brought to your hospital in dire need of the best care medical science can provide, would you be comfortable with any doctor, any nurse, or any service line treating her without your intervention? Your answer to that question frames the task ahead.

The fact that healthcare is more complex than the airline industry in no way relieves us of the responsibility to understand that lessons from aviation provide a road map for healthcare. The key elements of those lessons are the uniform, transparent, systemic dedication to zero harm as well as best practices, which are essentially absent in the traditional cottage industry model of medicine.

The difference between healthcare and aviation is healthcare's lack of a basic belief that adverse impacts on consumers can be driven to zero. For healthcare to be successful as an HRO, the energy and focus of the entire organization must fiercely follow that belief. The airline industry seismically altered its culture in the 1980s so that the focus transitioned from minimizing harm to eliminating it altogether, and the results have been dramatic and permanent. Correspondingly, every healthcare organization has a responsibility to change the convictions of its board, senior team, and all levels of its organization to align with this same focus and the same resultant goal of zero harm. Failing to do so, when we know the solution, is quite simply as unethical as it is potentially lethal.

Having thrown down the gauntlet, we can proceed to the heart of this chapter, which is the functional definition of, and pathway to becoming, an HRO in healthcare.

WHAT IS A HIGH-RELIABILITY ORGANIZATION?

By definition, an HRO is a human enterprise that carries an innate risk of creating substantial harm when its processes fail. Nuclear power generation, the airline industry, and high-rise and major industrial construction projects are all examples of fields with extraordinarily high public accountability and extraordinarily high potential for catastrophic failure. Yet these are industries that have reduced both the impact and the incidence of inherent catastrophic failure to near zero.

How have they accomplished such a dramatic improvement? By reengineering their internal structures as thoroughly as necessary in order to routinely prevent catastrophic failures and impacts once considered all but inevitable. Part of the restructuring is operational, but a profound and systemwide change in the mental perception of all personnel must also be present. In other words, it requires a major shift from a resigned allegiance to "the way we've always done it" to the uniform attitude that "there are better, proven methods we can adopt to keep our customers, employees, and communities safe from harm."

Reality Check

This chapter outlines the journey from here to there—from "some harm happens but we're trying our very best" to "we will accept nothing less than zero harm." That 11-year-old patient—and many others—would still be alive and unharmed if your hospital were, in fact, highly reliable.

It is not a pleasant experience for the board of an established hospital to be asked, "Are you a quality institution?"

"Well, of course!" is the instant answer. "Haven't you read the billboards, or seen our trophy case, or our award plaques?"

"Yes, but how do you *know*?"

As the question is pressed and the answers become less glib, boards often realize that despite some internal measures, great marketing, and an inherent pride, they really do *not* know whether they are running an excellent institution, a mediocre one, or a dangerous one—even when they know that a few patients are being deprived of their lives each year and many others injured by human error.

Leaders accept some harm and death because they have spent years immersed in a mental model in which bad things can and do happen despite all the good things done to prevent them. It is, in a phrase, normalized deviance on an institutional basis. This attitude is always a result of failing to introduce sustainable change to the most powerful force governing the course of any institution: culture. Senior leadership has a responsibility to create the conditions, for instance, in which all staff can and will speak up and say what they see, with the shared common goal of doing the best for the patient. This is called *patient-centric care*, and it is difficult to achieve, principally because the archaic cottage industry model of medical delivery is, instead, physician- and management-centric: Do as much as possible to support the physician, the executive, and their autonomy, and good things will trickle down to the patient.

The definition of *patient-centric*, by the way, is incredibly simple: Everything is subordinate to the best interests of the patient. Inducing, sustaining, and eventually inculcating these changes from the physician- and management-centric mental model to the patient-centric model is very difficult, even at the start. No human, no matter how wise, powerful, educated, or celebrated, can effectively see his own culture. It is akin to asking (if such communication were possible) a fish to describe water. Culture is all around; it permeates and frames everything we see, do, and perceive in the workplace—and yet asking someone for a quick and cogent description of that culture will initially draw a blank stare. Moreover, the power of cultural resistance to change—a group's own inertia—cannot be understated.

Studies show, for instance, that physicians will wash their hands less if no one is watching because they revert to the cultural norm. No member of a medical team is immune to this cultural resistance. In one hospital where bedside bar coding had been recently introduced, the night-shift nurses routinely printed off new coded armbands for each patient but wore them on their own arms to defeat a system that had dared challenge the way they had always done things. Culture completely invalidated the purpose of the process.

Thus, we soothe our consciences by imposing initiatives that the majority of the staff perceive as the flavor of the month, and we merely assume that the initiatives are going to be accepted and incorporated. But we don't follow through. We tolerate a nurse who is on her second 90-day improvement plan. We accept the behavior of our best surgeon when he gets upset in the operating room and throws things like a five-year-old. We fail to see the impact that cutting the education budget has on quality and safety outcomes. All of these examples have two things in common: They are the result of cultures in which patients were routinely harmed or killed, and they arise when leaders fail to prepare their institutions to embrace the seriousness and scope of the needed changes—in other words, to align values and vision.

You can count on *your* senior leadership team to understand these dynamic challenges, right? Not necessarily, and it is your task as the leader to inspect, not just expect, especially when change against the cultural grain is involved. To begin, does every member of your senior team really understand and share the values you are attempting to teach and maintain? The preliminary work for cultural change starts with senior executives who do not hesitate to openly share their concerns with each other, who have a high level of trust and transparency, and who openly engage in constructive conflict as a team. The foundation for high reliability starts with authentic leaders who consistently articulate vision and demonstrate values, building confidence and legitimacy through a continued process of self-awareness and reflection (Avolio and Walumbwa 2014).

However, more than 82 percent of people do not trust their boss to tell the truth, and a culture of silence is the norm. Most organizations today still function as a hierarchy with leaders who have a predominantly authoritarian leadership style. At the staff level, a nurse will not vocalize a major concern to a peer, manager, or physician primarily because of self-preservation (notice the pivotal shift in values—personal safety usurps everything, including patient safety). A study of more than 5,000 nurses revealed that they do not speak up as a result of the following motivations (Bartholomew 2015):

- Fear of making the situation worse
- Fear of being isolated from the group
- Fear of retaliation
- Lack of time
- Learned helplessness (why bother, as nothing will change?)

Self-silencing filters down from nurses to patients, and the result is a fear-based culture. A study of cancer patients at the University of Washington revealed that patients do not speak up, for the same reasons that nurses do not vocalize their concerns (Huff 2014). When leaders do not promote and support staff who share their "truth," patients hesitate as well, and a destructive silence prevails.

Ironically, innovation and change come from the complete opposite behavior—positive deviance. Unless we understand how humans operate in a group, we cannot create an HRO. The very basis of the HRO philosophy is that no human can be perfect all the time, so we need to create a system that is prepared for and expects human error.

WHAT DO WE KNOW ABOUT HARM?

Healthcare has a strong tendency to deliver disastrous consequences from process failures—and it therefore has an even greater public responsibility to be highly reliable. With 440,000 avoidable deaths per year in American hospitals alone (plus 4.4 million injuries), high reliability is a status neither achieved nor truly approached. Without question, this constitutes a national emergency that must be addressed by aggressive change (James 2013).

The Innumerable Varieties of Harm

Medication Errors

Medication errors are the most common means of harm, with more than 10,000 prescription medications and 300,000 over-the-counter remedies available. With a growing number of individuals treated for multiple chronic diseases, particularly as they age, more than 5 percent of all hospitalized patients experience some sort of adverse drug event at some point, of which 1 percent to 2 percent are fatal (Wachter 2012). Part of the issue is complexity, as experts have documented as many as 100 procedural steps between the creation of a prescription and the delivery and administration of that prescription. More than half of prescription errors occur in the ordering stage and the remainder in the administration stage.

Typical ordering and administration errors include the following:

- Ambiguity of orders (leading to wrong drug, wrong dose, wrong route of administration)
- Use of "do not use" abbreviations
- Mix-ups among sound-alike medications (e.g., Lamictal, an anticonvulsant, vs. Lamisil, an antifungal)
- Interruptions and distractions
- Nonstandardized dosing packages
- High-risk medications (top three: potassium; insulin; and heparin, a blood thinner)

Potential solutions are diverse. One possibility is computerized physician order entry (CPOE) with decision supports and barriers to medication errors. Computerization is also useful in health information exchanges (HIEs), which allow for medication reconciliation across the entire continuum of care. Answers can also be low-tech in the form of standardized, color-coded packaging. Rechecks and read-backs for high-risk medications and for all verbal orders to ensure accuracy and clarification are similarly straightforward. The liberal use of clinical pharmacists on rounds and for consultations as well as conservative prescribing (i.e., nothing prescribed that is unnecessary to treatment) also work.

Surgical Errors

Surgical errors make up 45 percent of all inpatient adverse events, and up to 17 percent of these may lead to a permanent disability (Gawande 2002). According to the Leapfrog Group (2018a), a consortium of large employers that focuses on healthcare issues, the majority of surgical errors arise from the performance of low-volume, high-risk operations and complex procedures.

The most common surgical errors include the following:

- Retained foreign bodies
- Surgical fires during an operation from cautery and lasers

- Wrong-site surgery stemming from refusal to perform universal protocol (e.g., Willie King in Tampa, Florida, underwent an unnecessary amputation of a lower extremity owing to the surgeon's refusal to check for the correct leg after an X-ray was mislabeled.)

Inexperienced practitioners and excessive complexity can lead to many of these errors.

In 2003, the Leapfrog Group published volume-based criteria to guide institutions when considering a complex procedure. They are listed in exhibit 12.1.

Many potential solutions for surgical errors center on the actions of the surgical staff. For instance, the World Health Organization's Safe Surgery Checklist has been shown to cause a 45 percent decrease in surgical morbidity and a 55 percent decrease in surgical

Exhibit 12.1: Evidence-Based Annual Volumes for High-Risk Surgeries

	Hospital	Surgeons
Coronary artery bypass	450	100
Percutaneous coronary interventions (stents for obstructed arteries)	400	75
Aortic valve replacement	120	22
Bariatric surgery	125	20
Abdominal aortic aneurysm	50	8
Esophagectomy	13	2
Pancreatic resection	11	2
High-risk deliveries	NICU with at least 50 neonates	N/A

Source: The Leapfrog Group (2018b).

mortality (Gawande 2009). Evidence-based, standardized setups and procedures will likely become standard, along with universal protocols with briefs (prior to procedures) and debriefs (following procedures). Crew resource management with established surgical teams for high-volume, high-risk procedures and access to simulators for infrequently performed, high-complexity procedures may help. Checkoffs with simulators will probably become a national standard, as it has already become in the aviation industry.

Other efforts focus on reducing staff error through making objects safer and more user-friendly. Bar-coded or radio frequency–labeled sponges and instruments may help detect retained foreign bodies. Strict prevention procedures, particularly with cautery and lasers, will reduce the risk of fire. Ultrasound-assisted invasive procedures (e.g., central line placement) will likely reduce perforations, hematomas, and bleeding.

Diagnostic Errors

Diagnostic errors represent 17 percent of all preventable errors and 5–10 percent of all inpatient errors, as demonstrated by autopsy. They represent the most common reason for paid malpractice claims, particularly among ambulatory patients. The most common missed diagnosis is heart attack, although delay in diagnosis and treatment of oncologic, neurologic, urologic, and surgical conditions are also common (Wachter 2010).

In the attempt to eliminate diagnostic mistakes, the physician's own approach may get in her way. The common practice of using a trial-and-error strategy (also known as *heuristics*), rather than an evidence-based approach to solving complex diagnostic problems, is responsible for many mistakes. Trial and error works fine for straightforward clinical diagnoses but not for complex ones, particularly when the patient suffers from multiple comorbidities and confounding variables.

There are myriad biases in healthcare. Anchoring bias (overreliance on first impressions) can be a trap; in specialty-specific biases, practitioners focus on their own field of expertise (e.g., cardiologists tend to find cardiology problems and prescribe heart-related solutions; they may not consider solutions for conditions that do not affect the heart). In bias against chronic patients who may be perceived to misuse healthcare services, doctors miss life-threatening conditions in patients whom they find personally difficult, resent, or have difficulty empathizing with. Atypical presentation bias occurs when individuals with common chronic conditions present with uncommon, life-threatening conditions.

The environment in which medical judgments are made is also a potential danger. Many organizations now maintain nondistraction zones where nobody is permitted to interrupt or distract an individual performing a critical function, such as mixing a high-risk medication or thinking through a complex, high-risk medical or surgical problem.

One of the challenges in healthcare is to convince a patient that seeing a highly skilled healthcare practitioner after a procedure is critical. Failure to present or follow up can lead to diagnostic error in the long term. Individuals who return repeatedly with similar diffuse complaints can be negatively labeled over time, and they may present unexpectedly with difficult-to-diagnose, life-threatening conditions.

Potential solutions to diagnostic errors are as diverse as their causes. The weakness of the heuristic approach can be lessened with decision support tools (e.g., IBM's Watson). Professionals clinging to an older model of autonomy may have difficulty acknowledging that the inherent complexity of their rapidly evolving profession may now require such tools. To the same point, anchoring bias can be addressed through rounding with multidisciplinary healthcare teams, particularly for difficult-to-diagnose conditions. The Mayo Clinic has pioneered this methodology.

Other improvements focus on changing the physician's process. Time-outs to reconsider less common and potentially dangerous conditions when the patient is not responding as expected may become common in the twenty-first century. Metathinking is also on the rise. In this technique, individuals (whether practitioners or leaders) can step outside of themselves briefly to look at a process objectively, determining whether it is reasonable or potentially prone to error.

Physicians must also cultivate awareness of potential situational biases. Awareness of these biases is the first step toward compensating for them and adapting around them when necessary.

One of the classic situations behind diagnostic error is the supposedly low-risk handoff ("Don't worry about Mr. Smith—he is being discharged tomorrow") that turns out to have a potentially mortal complication. Healthcare organizations can prevent this problem by developing the excellent habit of reevaluating all patients following a handoff, even those who appear low risk.

Human Error

Of course, the biggest risk factor in any human endeavor is, in fact, being human. Our fallibilities dog us at seemingly every turn. For example, fatigue of various types is a major cause of error. Tiredness and boredom are underestimated actors and represent the dangerous underside of burnout. When people no longer take pride in their work or empathize with patients, bad things inadvertently occur. For instance, alarm fatigue commonly leads to mishaps. When a unit has so many alarms or stimuli that the human mind habituates and ceases to focus, the situation can potentially turn fatal.

New technology can also contribute to complications. Poorly designed medical tools or devices can sometimes be difficult to use. A dilemma as simple as this can increase risk of errors, by raising the rate of misuse or injury. In addition, an unintended consequence of the electronic health record (EHR) is the absence of physicians, advanced-practice practitioners, and nurses at the bedside focusing on complex clinical problems they were trained to solve. Instead, they work in isolated areas where clinical conditions cannot be directly observed and communications cannot freely occur.

Much human error can be traced back to excessive variation. For example, almost 40 years ago, anesthesiologists standardized procedures, embraced universal equipment, and developed medication labeling designs, saving millions of lives. Outside of anesthesiology, however, variation in design and labeling of equipment, vials, tubing, and the like—made worse through the use of multiple vendors and manufacturers—is a familiar driver of non-value-added complexity and harm.

The medical field has developed many practical ways to combat human error. For instance, to reduce fatigue and boredom, one option is instituting team-based rotating duties. The Lahey Clinic in Burlington, Massachusetts, uses teams effectively to rotate clinicians through various clinical and administrative roles with the goal of keeping everyone fresh, knowledgeable, and supportively questioning each other's performance and perspectives. Many senior management teams also feel that rotations through operations, finance, and other sections encourage a deeper bench of expertise and the sharpening of critical skills. The aviation industry has been doing this for years with crew resource management, and it works.

To reduce the more specific problem of alarm fatigue, limit the use of alarms. The Joint Commission has originated a patient safety initiative to do just that.

Hospitals and health systems can take steps to make technology work for, not against, humans. To address the absence of medical professionals from patient rooms as a result of EHRs, clinically trained, certified coder scribes can work with physicians and clinicians. These professionals reduce per-unit costs, optimize physician and practitioner productivity, enhance the amount paid on every mistake-free (clean) claim, and, most important, enable clinicians to refocus on patient care. Hospitals should also automate as much medication reconciliation as possible to ensure accuracy. Consider robotic bar-coded medication systems. Many organizations realize that the chance of human error is too great in a process with 25–50 steps per script. Instead, a well-programmed automated process frees humans to manage the system rather than directly participate in every stage.

As in other sectors, standardization will ease many problems in the medical field. These efforts should be directed, in part, toward standardized equipment/medication labels and processes. This simplification will not only reduce potential errors but also decrease costs, optimize outcomes, and improve employee morale. Health systems can also minimize and standardize supply chain vendors. To reduce costs and optimize what is an inherently challenging management process, value analysis committees at many institutions enable physicians and executive leaders to collaborate on simplification of the supply chain. In Texas, for instance, Memorial Hermann's physician integration group eliminated almost $500 million in supply chain costs over a three-year period by standardizing all vendors and reducing their number while minimizing the potential for error.

Transition Errors

Transitions and handoffs have long been known to cause inadvertent medical error—most organizations still lack a standardized process. Unfortunately, handoff errors can result in medication errors, a lack of appropriate follow-up, missed lab or radiology results that may be significant, and shortcuts or workarounds that may place everyone at risk.

The medical field has at its disposal a number of tools to address this class of error. Hospitals can institute standardized processes for verbal interactions, such as SBAR (situation, background, assessment, and recommendation), that emphasize what is most important, find the risks most likely to occur, and recommend approaches to unexpected complications or relapses.

It is impossible for physicians, advanced-practice practitioners, and nurses to keep every essential piece of clinical data immediately available for every patient, so they need tools that are helpful in assisting practitioners to make guided decisions. Devices such as a low-tech whiteboard in patient rooms and high-tech smart cards with implantable microchips are useful. Important clinical information can be embedded in smart cards or placed on whiteboards to remind team members of key clinical, personal, and demographic information.

As for most elements of healthcare, an HIE can help reduce the potential for error. A workable HIE with clinical and business analytics enables practitioners, leaders, and stakeholders to have accurate and up-to-date information (with the patient's consent). This innovation enables more appropriate and timely care.

Another proven approach to transition-error reduction is the use of a universal discharge or transitions-of-care checklist that includes postdischarge (or, as it is now described, post-acute) calls. Most discharge planning is ad hoc, but organizations (e.g., Yale Medical Center) that have a completely standardized process have significantly reduced readmissions, increased compliance and follow-ups, and reduced morbidity and mortality. Postdischarge calls are an invaluable way to accomplish a number of important goals, such as the following:

- Confirming the patient's understanding regarding his care
- Ensuring compliance with medication reconciliation and follow-up appointments
- Clarifying discharge instructions while the patient is not under the influence of sedating medications
- Confirming the understanding and support of family members
- Receiving feedback regarding care, treatment, and service

Teamwork and Communication Errors

The phrase *teamwork errors* may be a misnomer because most healthcare is not yet provided in formal teams. In fact, although the United States has always had a very loosely team-based approach, with physicians doing physician work and nurses doing nursing work, most people do not consider patient care a coordinated, team-based activity. Rather, it is thought of as supportive of the physician–patient relationship across the continuum of care. This idea is simply a tradition, and organizations that have moved toward a more interdisciplinary approach see opportunities to improve efficiencies and outcomes. For instance, clinical pharmacists contribute medication reconciliation expertise and can explore cost-effective alternatives that support better compliance and reduce the cost of care.

After two jumbo jets on Tenerife Island (Spain) collided on a runway in part as a result of pilot error, killing 583 passengers, the aviation industry discovered that reducing the differences in authority and status of individuals who work together decreases errors by fostering improved communication. Unfortunately, the medical field has far to go to accomplish a similar improvement, and many physicians still feel uncomfortable addressing questions from team members about treatment decisions. For physicians and executives, the deep-seated paradigm of professional autonomy is difficult to give up because it is a deeply ingrained and unconscious behavior. Yet the conflict of autonomy versus team leadership is the battle line between the status quo and high reliability.

Healthcare-Associated Conditions

Healthcare-associated infections occur in approximately 5–10 percent of all admissions, resulting in approximately 100,000 preventable deaths annually (Yokoe et al. 2014). With the growing Medicare payment withholds for central line–associated bloodstream infections, hospital-acquired urinary tract infections, and Clostridium difficile infections, hospitals take on a great deal of financial (in addition to clinical) risk in not properly addressing these issues. The Institute for Healthcare Improvement has created widely promulgated standardized-practice procedure bundles for the prevention and mitigation of these conditions; however, the traditional culture of autonomy still prevails and inhibits the widespread adoption of important, evidence-based improvements.

In addition to these clinical bundles, other infections, such as methicillin-resistant Staphylococcus aureus, are emerging as important patient safety issues as a result of the misuse of antibiotics. The incidence of blood clots has also risen thanks to the lack of proper preventive measures after certain types of major surgery (e.g. pelvis, joint). Experts anticipate that standards in these areas will rapidly evolve to protect the public from both problems. Other increasing patient safety issues include pressure ulcers (responsible for more than 50,000 deaths annually), falls (affecting 50 percent of nursing home patients, 20 percent of which result in serious injury), and delirium (a root cause of falls) (Wachter 2012).

WHAT WOULD A HOSPITAL LOOK LIKE IF IT FUNCTIONED AS AN HRO?

To bring about the bold vision of hospital-as-HRO, it may help to visualize the details of an ideal institution.

Leadership

High reliability starts at the top. In a true HRO, the organization knows the leader as an authentic person; employees can articulate her vision and personal values and why she cares. Budgetary policy is supportive—resources are appropriate to the patient, not the budget. In an HRO, when managers are asked, "Do you have what you need to do your job?", the answer is yes. Charge nurses are acknowledged as experts who understand the criticality of each patient's needs as well as the experience level of every nurse and are trusted stewards of the organization's resources, as well as the patient's safety. In an HRO, frontline nurses staff according to values using the typical staffing grid as a guideline rather than a strict mandate.

Patients

In a high-reliability hospital, patients have full and open access to their EHRs, and they are considered the inviolate owners of all of their health information. Moreover, any harm done to them is transparent and personal. If a patient is harmed or dies, a family member is asked to present at a board meeting and to the hospital staff to illuminate the consequences of error and personalize its impact.

Staff

In an HRO, all staff are skilled communicators who are trained and practiced in confrontation- and conflict-management skills, and they do not hesitate to speak up, as they understand that they are critical members of the team. Staff routinely ask for peer feedback and have each other's backs at all times to foster trust and ensure reliability. No disruptive behavior is tolerated from anyone of any rank or seniority in the hospital. If it occurs, staff stop the behavior or the procedure immediately and address the issue directly with the person and then up the established chain of command if necessary.

Teams

A high-reliability hospital uses teams of multiple configurations. First, the physician, nurse, and patient together establish a daily goal. No patient has surgery unless the case has been brought before a team of physicians, and there are no preference cards (instrument requests for each physician and practitioner in the operating room) because the surgeons have decided collectively what best practices are for each surgery and have standardized all setups and procedures.

A team-based culture extends beyond patients and medical staff, however. All employees have been educated in clinical resource management or Team Strategies and Tools to Enhance Performance and Patient Safety (a similar model) and have mastered communication competencies. These approaches create standardized practices, communication protocols, and techniques that reduce unnecessary variation and optimize outcomes in high-risk, error-prone situations.

Potential Structures

The changes required to bring about high reliability in hospitals are both sweeping and granular. Structural solutions designed to improve reliability are discussed in the following section, including changes to leadership, teamwork, training, and staff engagement.

Leadership

HROs avoid top-down leadership and work to sustain plentiful contact between staff and the senior team. For instance, some institute mandatory weekly rounding by all leaders and managers and periodic rounding (or shadowing) by board members for an entire 8- or 12-hour shift. This innovation is preceded by training for leaders on meaningful rounding to acquire real-time information and build trusting relationships. Leaders can further flatten the hierarchy by following frontline staff, inviting them to follow executives, sharing meals, asking for feedback, and performing 360-degree surveys. All of these strategies inspire a shared responsibility. Examine your institutional culture. Do the same rules apply to everyone? Only when vision, values, and behaviors match can true cultural change begin.

Teamwork

Superior teamwork plays a major role in making a health system highly reliable. Physician–nurse engagement is a piece of the puzzle. As a rule of thumb, a minimum of 6 to 8 physicians and nurses should meet monthly in every department. The guiding principle of these gatherings should be that a lack of time together means a lack of improvement. Most organizations can seize many other opportunities for deeper engagement of the medical team as well. For example, provide education to the group on the history and culture of doctor–nurse relationships. Develop a dyad model of leadership (physicians and nurse leaders forming working partnerships). Convening a nurse–physician council or even a nurse–physician summit also helps. Such summits can level the playing field by opening with doctors and nurses who share their most recent medical errors. Participants can describe the current physician–nurse norms and work on establishing new norms together. These events demonstrate an

HRO's investment in fostering, nurturing, and maintaining collegial relationships, which makes for smoother institutional functioning.

Staff members must trust their organization before they cooperate fully with its vision of high reliability. Hospitals should never abandon a team member in the case of an adverse occurrence. Support each other through full and open discussion of truth. Sanction or remove those who abandon their team or team leader by misrepresentation, who refuse to share all available information, or who attempt to assign blame and shame after an adverse occurrence.

HROs build departmental and interdepartmental safety huddles into the team schedule to answer the following questions:

- Where will our next patient safety disaster or near disaster come from?
- What steps should we take to immediately address and improve person-to-person communication and establish relationships across traditional silos?

These huddles make harm visible to teams. Every employee should be able to tell the story of how the last adverse event occurred and the improvement put in place to prevent further harm.

Training

High reliability is built on a foundation of training and continuous feedback and correction. Provide ongoing, repetitive education and recurrent team training conducted by different sources, both internal and external to your organization. Invite folks from other industries and share success stories publicly. Use videotaped simulation that can be customized to approximate real working situations and environments for team training, and as soon as possible begin training facilitators who can train others. Employees benefit from online educational tools and resources, but hospitals must follow up with measurements of communication competency and annual team evaluations.

High-quality hospitals and health systems make a continuous effort to support education on communications and relationships. Culture change arises from training focusing on language and behavior. Increase your budget for ongoing staff and leadership development, but make sure to carry out educational initiatives in a cost-effective way. For example, results of any such initiative must be visible, and gains must be shared to maintain the momentum. Any substantial culture change that arises from educational efforts is bound to create potential relationship challenges; provide unstinting support for those facing such conflicts.

Staff Engagement

In the hospital community, high reliability requires participation by all. Elicit deep thinking from the front lines in all departments on how to solve problems and address challenges by setting up advisory groups with informal membership. Leaders should embrace continuous engagement and ongoing discussion; they can shepherd midlevel managers and directors into the role of facilitator after coaching education.

Because good engagement requires alignment, successful institutions harmonize medical staff bylaws with the corporate bylaws and include identical behavioral standards in annual performance evaluations.

WHY HAS HEALTHCARE FALLEN SO ABYSMALLY SHORT?

Mounting an effective attack on the US healthcare system's massive shortcomings requires a clear understanding and appreciation of the mechanisms of both systemic and personal failure, which, in truth, are common to every other human institution with an equal potential for disaster. We must understand the basic engine of medical mistakes, misadventures, and sentinel disasters, and that starts by understanding the disastrous role of the traditional medical belief in professional human infallibility.

In a nutshell, human beings, no matter how well trained in any profession, are incapable of guaranteeing continuous perfection—not because of any deficiency in our training or professionalism but because we have inborn shortcomings that deny us the ability to always perceive things as they really are or should be. Communication, perception, and assumption errors may be suppressed but can never be fully eradicated from the performance of even the best and the brightest professional human in any discipline. Yet when tradition misguides an entire profession to disregard that reality, we create a terrible inevitability of harm.

It has been said that "any human institution built on the expectation of continuous perfect human performance has hard-wired failure into its very structure" (Abrahams 1997). The essence of that reality is that a system that cannot completely expunge human error—and yet that is built on the assumption of a complete absence of human error—virtually guarantees that the mistakes that eventually occur will be surprises for which the system is unprepared. These dangerous surprises are allowed to metastasize to their most disastrous conclusion.

Even a cursory examination of closed-claim insurance files from medical disasters invariably underscores this point: Wrong-site surgeries, retained objects, missed diagnoses, incorrect medication application, and a host of other deadly mistakes all have well-known and highly predictable causes, and there are corresponding effective methods of catching, preventing, or neutralizing them before they affect a patient's well-being. However, when a hospital or medical team inadvertently shepherds a causal chain of mistakes to an injurious outcome, the vast majority of the time a principal causal factor was either lack of knowledge of a safer way to proceed or a refusal to use recommended preventive measures. Both root causes stem from the traditional belief that good doctors, nurses, and medical teams are not allowed to make mistakes, and therefore will not.

The medical profession perpetuates such disasters by refusing to recognize the desperate lack of a robust "focused factory" of standardized, best-practice approaches that can aid in producing predictably good outcomes and minimizing the opportunity for errors. The medical field has journals staffed by hardworking and diligent editors, but a collection of publications cannot alone provide the baseline information available worldwide to inform physicians and healthcare institutions alike about the best practice in any given treatment protocol, response, or surgical technique. That must be done by a team of committed individuals continually working toward improving their processes while minimizing potential error through a series of rapid-cycle evaluations of high-risk situations.

The scandal of nosocomial infection illustrates the lack of systemic understanding of these truths. Of 440,000 patients lost every year to medical error in US hospitals, almost half die from a hospital-acquired infection. The lethality of failure to follow strict infectious prevention procedures is no surprise. In fact, the IOM's (Kohn, Corrigan, and Donaldson 2000) estimated death rate in 1999 from nosocomial infections ranged from 24,000 to 48,000 (figures we now know were very low). Yet a recent study found that physician handwashing rates—directly connected to nosocomial rates—are still terrible and fall sharply when there is no system for observation or for reinforcing the rules. Boards of directors are constantly amazed and chastened when their often-prideful citation of improvement in handwashing protocols is put in perspective: A handwashing rate of 82 percent, for instance, means that only 18 percent of your patients are in danger of dying from a nosocomial infection transmitted by a doctor. Clearly, one major problem is a failure to understand the clear and present dangers and to accept the fact that the way we have always done things will no longer suffice—ethically, legally, and morally.

REFERENCES

Abrahams, J., dir. 1997. ". . . *First Do No Harm*." New York: American Broadcasting Company.

Avolio, B. J., and F. O. Walumbwa. 2014. "Authentic Leadership Theory, Research, and Practice: Steps Taken and Steps That Remain." In *Authentic Leadership Theory, Research, and Practice*, edited by D. V. Day, 331–65. New York: Oxford University Press.

Bartholomew, K. 2015. *Ending Nurse-to-Nurse Hostility: Why Nurses Eat Their Young and Each Other*. Marblehead, MA: HCPro.

Gawande, A. 2009. *The Checklist Manifesto*. New York: Henry Holt and Company.

———. 2002. *Complications: A Surgeon's Notes on an Imperfect Science*. New York: Metropolitan Books.

Golladay, K., and A. B. Collins. 2010. *Adverse Events in Hospitals: National Incidence Among Medicare Beneficiaries*. Department of Health and Human Services Office of the Inspector General. Published November. https://oig.hhs.gov/oei/reports/oei-06-09-00090.pdf.

Huff, C. 2014. "Speaking Up for Patient Safety." *ACP Hospitalist*. Published March. https://acphospitalist.org/archives/2014/03/patientsafety.htm.

James, J. 2013. "A New, Evidence-Based Estimate of Patient Harms Associated with Hospital Care." *Journal of Patient Safety* 9 (3): 122–28.

Kohn, L. T., J. M. Corrigan, and M. S. Donaldson. 2000. *To Err Is Human: Building a Safer Health System*. Washington, DC: National Academies Press.

Leapfrog Group. 2018a. "High-Risk Surgeries." Accessed January 25. www.leapfroggroup.org/ratings-reports/high-risk-surgeries.

———. 2018b. "Surgeon Volume and Surgical Appropriateness." Accessed January 25. www.leapfroggroup.org/surgeon-volume.

Wachter, R. M. 2012. *Understanding Patient Safety*. New York: McGraw Hill Medical.

———. 2010. "Why Diagnostic Errors Don't Get Any Respect—and What Can Be Done About Them." *Health Affairs* 29 (9): 1605–10.

Yokoe, D. S., L. A. Mermel, D. J. Anderson, K. M. Arias, H. Burstin, D. P. Calfee, S. E. Coffin, E. R. Dubberke, V. Fraser, D. N. Gerding, F. A. Griffin, P. Gross, K. S. Kaye, M. Klompas, E. Lo, J. Marschall, L. Nicolle, D. A. Pegues, T. M. Perl, K. Podgorny, S. Saint, C. D. Salgado, R. A. Weinstein, R. Wise, and D. Classen. 2014. "A Compendium of Strategies to Prevent Healthcare-Associated Infections in Acute Care Hospitals." *Infection Control and Hospital Epidemiology* 35 (8): 967–77.

CHAPTER 13

Building a Culture of Service Excellence for the Twenty-First Century

Jake Poore

IMAGINE THIS LETTER just landed on your desk:

> *Dear CEO,*
>
> *I want to take a moment to thank you and your team for saving my son's life—but I want you to know that I will never come back to your hospital again. You see, a few weeks ago, I received a call that all mothers dread. It was your dispatcher telling me my son was hit by a car on his way to school and that he'd been brought to your emergency department. He's recovering now, thanks to the skilled doctors and surgeons on your team. But in those first few moments after I heard the words from the dispatcher, my heart sank. I dropped everything and raced to your hospital.*
>
> *I wasn't sure where to park, so I double-parked near the ED entrance, kept my car running, and hopped out to ask the*
>
> *continued*

395

continued from previous page

security guard if I was in the right place. But before I could utter a word, he said, "You can't park there—please move your car." I tried again, but he said, "No parking zone, ma'am. You'll need to move your car to the main lot."

After I parked my car, I hurried through the hospital doors, where I frantically asked the security guard where I could find my son. He slowly turned a clipboard toward me and said, "Name and ID, please."

I scribbled my name and he pointed me toward the triage window. I don't know what the word "triage" means, but I rushed over and peered through the little hole in the darkened glass only to see two employees casually chatting about their weekend. "Excuse me," I said. "I'm looking for my son. Please, has he been admitted here?" Seemingly agitated by the interruption, one of the employees said after looking at the admissions list, "He's been moved up to the med/surg unit on the third floor." She turned back to her coworker, and they resumed their conversation.

I made a few wrong turns before locating the elevators. When I stepped out on the third floor, I asked the unit nurse about my son. "Oh, he's been sent to radiology," she told me.

I raced down to radiology only to have the nurse tell me, "Sorry, ma'am, he's in surgery now."

AND THAT IS WHEN I LOST IT.

I was so frustrated and angry. How could everyone be so immune to what I was feeling, what I was experiencing? I felt like an intruder in this so-called place of healing.

Fast-forward to today, and my son is home recovering. The doctors and nurses treated my son's injuries expertly, and for that I'm grateful. But the rest of your staff? Well, it's obvious you're not investing in them, because if you were, my situation would have been quite different.

continued

continued from previous page

I'm writing this letter to challenge you to get your people together—get your team together—because I assure you, my story isn't unique. Another child will be hit by a car tomorrow, next week, or later this afternoon, and another mother will arrive at the hospital with the same fear in her heart. She'll be confused. She'll be anxious. And she'll be scared.

The question is, will you and your team—your entire team, including the security guards, the parking attendants, the receptionists, and everyone else—be prepared for her?

Sincerely,
A Grateful but Disappointed Mom

One of the questions on the Hospital Consumer Assessment of Healthcare Providers and Systems (HCAHPS) asks, "Would you recommend this healthcare system to your family and friends?" How do you suppose this mother answered that survey question? What criteria will she use to determine her answer? If her response is based solely on clinical excellence and outcomes, the answer to this question may be yes. But clinical excellence alone does not reflect the totality of patients' expectations.

When you have consistent levels of clinical excellence mixed with inconsistent levels of service quality across multiple team members or departments, your patients' survey responses will likely mirror that inconsistency—or worse. Think back to the mother's letter and consider the actions and attitudes of everyone she encountered before she actually met the people caring for her son: a parking lot security guard, a front desk security guard, triage nurses, a unit nurse, and a radiology technician. When you consider these factors, her answer to the "intent to refer" question is likely to be a definitive no.

When we talk about building a culture of service excellence that consistently delivers exceptional patient experiences across the continuum of care, let's begin by defining what we mean by the *patient experience*. One of the most widely accepted, comprehensive definitions of *patient experience* comes from the Beryl Institute (2018): "The patient experience is the sum of all interactions, shaped by an organization's culture, that influence patient perceptions across the continuum of care."

Clearly, patient experience is far more nuanced than merely expressing satisfaction or dissatisfaction with clinical outcomes alone. Everything the patient sees, hears, smells, and feels throughout the hundreds of touch points in his journey affects and influences—both positively and negatively—his total experience of care. In our example, every person who interacted with this mother had a role in coloring her experience, though she wasn't the actual patient. Everyone in healthcare needs to realize that although the patient is our purpose, he is not our only customer.

This isn't the first time this kind of situation happened at our fictional hospital, and it won't be the last. Shouldn't the institution have a plan? When another child is hit by a car and brought to the emergency department, what should the ambulance driver ask? What should the security guard and valet parking attendant know? What should the front desk receptionist, the triage check-in team, and the unit floor nurse say? How can you set them up for success for the next patient interaction?

When it comes to healthcare in the twenty-first century, clinical excellence alone is no longer enough. While individual talents may vary, doctors, nurses, and other clinicians generally have the training, tools, and technological infrastructure required to deliver quality clinical care. By and large, when a patient sees a healthcare provider, clinical excellence is assumed. So how can healthcare systems compete? With the exception of the few healthcare systems and providers that compete on the basis of technological advantage, the great differentiator for healthcare systems in the twenty-first century lies in how well they deliver service excellence.

Are patients willing to forgive providers for minor medical mistakes (a blurry image on a mammogram, for instance), but what if the provider was rude to her? The patient will not only look for another provider but will gladly tell everyone she knows about how poorly she was treated. To the patient, what separates a good experience from a bad one is in the service she received. Without the knowledge to effectively evaluate clinical expertise, patients rely on what they know: they are experts on how well they were treated. How well (or poorly) were their clinical *and* nonclinical needs met? How was their total experience? In contemporary healthcare, clinical excellence is assumed, but service excellence is expected.

This increased emphasis on service is happening for many reasons, not the least of which is that patient and consumer expectations have risen as a direct result of our robust service-based economy. In addition, out-of-pocket costs have increased, and more detailed information on healthcare standards is available on the internet. Patients expect to have their medical concerns handled expertly by highly skilled clinicians. But, at the same time, they also have high expectations for the compassion, care, and human kindness with which they are treated by both medical and nonmedical team members.

It's important to remember that most patients aren't comparing you to the healthcare system down the street or even in the next town; they're comparing you to the coffee place that remembers their name and unique coffee order (even when they haven't visited that coffee shop in a week). They're comparing you to the hairstylist who remembers to ask about their daughter's graduation. They're comparing you to Ritz-Carlton, Southwest Airlines, Zappos, and yes, even Disney—where customer service excellence is the key differentiator and competitive advantage.

Patient satisfaction surveys reflect not only clinical outcomes but service outcomes as well. This fact means there are financial implications tied to high scores on questions that focus on clinical excellence as well as service outcomes. Healthcare systems that fail to elevate the service side of healthcare (no matter how solid their clinical expertise) risk not only the loss of unhappy patients but also a reduction in reimbursements. This statement may be bold, even frightening, but the financial imperative for the healthcare sector to up its game and build a culture of service excellence is undeniable.

While it may seem unfair to place healthcare in competition with the nearest Ritz-Carlton, the reality is that the opportunities for differentiation are greatest on the service excellence side of the equation, as long as you continue to provide clinical excellence that consistently meets expectations. It's a daunting challenge, but I believe today's healthcare organizations will be able to meet this challenge and emerge stronger as a result.

Patients are not medically trained experts, but they are experts in what they do know from their life experience: They want you to call them by their preferred name. They want you to speak to them in a language they understand (no medical jargon or confusing medical terms). It should go without saying that patients want to be treated with kindness and respect.

The disconnect happens when one department really hits it out of the park and wows the patient with personalized, individualized care—but then, the patient is transferred to another department where the service falls short. "What just happened?" the patient thinks. "I was having a good experience and now these folks are treating me like I'm on an assembly line!" Patients do not experience healthcare vertically, in one department or silo; patients (and their families) experience care horizontally, across all lines of your business. While you and your team may be highly trained in delivering excellent clinical outcomes, your patients' perceptions are shaped by both the clinical and the nonclinical or service excellence aspects of care that they experience throughout the continuum of care.

By definition, every touch point along the patient experience journey is important: the housekeeper who cleans his room; the dietitian who delivers his food; the nurses and doctors who directly administer care; the volunteer who delivers flowers; the billing team that handles and processes bills, insurance, and payments; and so on. The question becomes, How do we create and hardwire a culture of service excellence across an entire healthcare system?

HOW TO SYSTEMATIZE A CULTURE OF SERVICE EXCELLENCE

The keys to creating and systematizing a culture of service excellence are threefold:

1. Involve all employee groups (and a few patients) as stakeholders and architects in the design of the organization's new cultural blueprints, including an organizational true north and a set of operational priorities.
2. Define what your healthcare system stands for and what you will no longer stand for by keeping the good things and getting rid of what I call *graffiti*, with the goal of having everyone on the care team aligned toward one shared vision and able to say, "This is how we do things here."
3. Hardwire your new culture by documenting "the way we do things here," rewarding it when you see it, and correcting it when you don't.

STEP ONE: INVOLVE ALL EMPLOYEE GROUPS

To deliver consistently exceptional patient experiences, you must create a culture that supports and delivers systemwide service excellence from the boardroom to the waiting room to the exam room to the break room. The first step is for leaders to gather a group of thoughtful, responsible, multidisciplinary team members together so they can identify and clearly articulate two things: their organizational true north and a set of operational priorities about which everyone can say, "that applies to me."

One of my first consulting clients, Sheltering Arms Rehabilitation Center (Virginia), underwent the cultural transformation process.

The leaders quickly realized that what they were doing was more than just a prescriptive quick fix. They were undertaking a serious commitment that would provide benefits far beyond just improving the patient experience.

"You can't just change your scores in a meaningful way without making some fundamental changes in your organization," said Jim Sok, then president and CEO of Sheltering Arms. "This process is for anybody that's considering trying to build a stronger culture within their organization to not only help get better patient satisfaction scores, but also to build stronger employee loyalty and to build stronger patient–employee relationships within the organization."

A cultural transformation is more than just providing scripts for people to follow or telling your team to "be nicer." You can't impose a culture and expect it to take hold. The cultural transformation process cannot be an edict, a new initiative, or another program of the month from the boardroom or the C-suite that is expected to trickle down to every employee with full implementation and buy-in. These things may work in the short term, but after a while they fail. Why? Because employees are smart. They can spot the next flavor of the month a mile away.

Instead, the culture needs to grow organically—from the ground up, with full participation from every employee group in the organization. That's the real secret to building a successful cultural transformation. When employees are involved in building and creating their organization's cultural blueprints, they have authorship. Authorship leads to ownership, and ownership leads to mutual accountability, which means they will police it and monitor it even when the leaders aren't around. This participation is the key to building a culture of service excellence, and this is the reason why other prescriptive "do this, say that" programs or checklists don't work for any sustained period.

After your staff agrees on "how we do things here" during this grassroots process, they will then define the elements of the organizational culture with a service promise that aligns everyone to a true north. This isn't the mission or vision statements that you hang on your wall or post on your website. Your true north is a short, internal statement that unites and aligns the entire organization toward delivering the same goal. It is a clear, end-in-mind statement of what everyone promises to do to deliver the organization's mission and vision every day—or, as my team and I like to say, it's your mission and vision in work clothes.

Your true north must be short, memorable, and relevant to all. It is something that is customer driven and that every employee can equally contribute to making a reality. Every job and every role is vital to its overall success. Dignity Health Medical Foundation's true north is, "We unite healing and human kindness." For the Walt Disney World Resort, that statement is called the Disney Service Theme, and the first three words are what all cast members (employees) remember: "We create happiness by providing the finest in entertainment for people of all ages, everywhere."

I was fortunate to enjoy an 18-year career at Disney, and during that time, the most important lesson I learned is that you must first have employee alignment in order to create the "magic" consistently. If you don't, you unknowingly create a culture of silos, fiefdoms, and islands, where everyone does their own thing.

Because Disney is guest driven, they consistently ask visiting guests why they intend to return year after year. Guests respond with the following:

1. The place is clean.
2. The employees are friendly.
3. They had fun.

Clean. Friendly. Fun. Always those three. Always in that order.

So how do you get 65,000 cast members to pick up trash? You can't just say, "Do this or you're out of here." You tell them that picking up trash and keeping the place clean is the number-one key driver to guest loyalty; if we do this, then they will come back. At Disney, no one really wants to pick up trash, but everyone wants to create happiness!

Chapter 13: Building a Culture of Service Excellence 403

Operational Priorities

Your operational priorities are a set of agreed-on standards that are prioritized in order of importance to empower employees to make nonemergent decisions on the spot. Along with the true north statement, the operational priorities must also be in place to provide a practical blueprint for how every interaction should occur as well as to be a decision-making filter for everyone to use when conflicts arise in the course of delivering service excellence to patients and to each other (internal customers). Together, the true north statement and the operational priorities become your healthcare organization's new cultural blueprints that will serve as the foundation for systematizing a culture of service excellence.

Disney's true north begins with the words "we create happiness." Disney's operational priorities are safety, courtesy, show, and efficiency. (The next time you're at a Disney theme park, I challenge you to find one cast member who can't recite these operational priorities quickly and in order. They can do it!)

But Disney's priorities are not your priorities. You and your staff have to decide on what yours might be. Is safety also first in your organization? As busy as things can get at Walt Disney World, courtesy is still prioritized above efficiency. (Disney does feel that efficiency is important—with millions of guests a year and long lines for rides, it certainly is. But it's not more important than courtesy. What about in your organization?)

As leaders, our job is to make the implicit explicit and to make the invisible visible. If the culture is not explicit, if employees cannot say with shared knowledge of a common goal that "this is the way we do things here," then the old adage of "culture eating strategy for lunch" will win. Consider grand rounds. Grand rounds are a teaching tool, akin to Monday morning quarterbacking, where physicians and healthcare leaders identify the things they would have, should have, or could have done differently. The purpose is to thoroughly examine and discuss specific medical cases. But when these rounds are completed, what reinforcements are in place at the organization to ensure the next set of employees will know how to handle the situation if it occurs again? Where is the if-then statement?

Healthcare professionals are expected to deliver care with peace of mind for patients. But how can they do that when many don't feel as though they have employment with peace of mind? Working in a "gotcha" culture, or a culture where it seems as though no one really has your back, can be toxic—not only to the employees living it but also to the patients they serve.

However, when everyone is working in a culture with a common set of operational priorities, and everyone is looking through the same lens, employees are empowered and reassured that the organization has their backs. Monday morning quarterbacking takes on a new life. Now, using the operational priorities, every employee can analyze the situation for the best possible outcome and share that outcome or solution with all employees in her department and throughout the organization to ensure consistency. Ultimately, this becomes more than just a random act of kindness or a service recovery to fix a problem. It's been systematized so that everyone in the institution can say, "This is now the way we do things here."

Connecting People to Purpose

Everyone has a role on the care team. The challenge is that sometimes employees operate as if they are wearing blinders, and they are consciously or unconsciously encouraged to do just that. They become so focused on their specific job tasks that they remain blind to their role on the care team. It's your job, as a leader, to rip the blinders off and make sure everyone on the care team knows the important role they play in the healing process. This is the real secret behind creating a culture of service excellence: connecting people to purpose.

One of the most effective ways to widen people's perspectives and connect them to purpose is to show them that they're more than just their job title. Have you ever heard people describe their job saying, "I'm just a . . ."? For instance, they'll say, "I'm just a groundskeeper," "I'm just a transporter," "I'm just a reception-ist," or "I'm just a technician." Like blinders, these labels prevent employees from seeing the bigger picture and understanding where they fit in the continuum of care that makes up the patient experi-ence. This lack can cause employees to become singularly focused on specific job tasks with no connection to their greater role in the healing process.

Stories from the Field: Glorified Dishwashers and Tray Passers

Several years ago, I was invited to shadow the sterile processing unit at a hospital out west. The entire team was skilled and profes-sional, but they had blinders on. They only saw themselves as (in their words) "glorified dishwashers." They believed they were just the people who cleaned the surgical instruments.

I asked them to consider what would happen if the tools and instruments weren't properly cleaned, sterilized, and prepared for surgery. Increased risk of infection, complications during and after surgery, and poor clinical outcomes, they responded. They realized the vital role they played in the healing process and saw the bigger picture. They understood that their role in the patient experience was more than just their individual job description or title. They weren't glorified dishwashers—they were responsible for providing clean and sterile instruments that heal.

Consider another example. I remember working with one food and beverage team who considered themselves to be just tray passers. Day in and day out, they filled patients' orders for food and drink and delivered them multiple times a day and overnight to patients' rooms.

Just as I had done with the sterile processing unit, I asked this team to consider what would happen if the food they prepared and delivered was incorrect or contrary to dietary restrictions, or if the silverware or plates were dirty. Patients could become sick. Patients could have an allergic or other medical reaction. Patients could be infected with germs from dirty plates and silverware, they responded. It became clear that their role on the care team was more than just passing trays from the kitchen to the delivery cart to the patient. My job was to move them from the task orientation defined in their job titles and descriptions and connect them to purpose. They weren't just tray passers; they had to see themselves as part of the care team. They provided food and drink that heal.

Tangible Versus Intangible Assets

The central purpose of a healthcare system can be found in the clinical expertise of its doctors and nurses. They represent the tangible assets: Patients get examined, receive medicines or other treatment, and so on. The intangible assets are the kindness and compassion demonstrated by doctors and nurses and by the people you don't necessarily expect to be on the care team. This includes housekeepers, security guards, gift shop employees, valet parkers, volunteers, billing clerks, environmental services workers, and more. All of these people are your aces in the hole, so to speak, when it comes to living a culture of service excellence.

Connecting people to purpose is the key to successful cultural transformations because it engages the human side of healthcare— the human side of the patient experience. By tearing down the vertical silos defined by job tasks and removing the blinders, everyone on the care team knows her role in the total patient experience and in the healing process across the continuum of care.

The magic ingredient that makes other organizations stand head and shoulders above others is their ability to connect people to purpose. It's why Southwest Airlines is called the Love Airline (even their stock symbol is LUV). It's why Ritz-Carlton employees believe and say, "We are ladies and gentlemen, serving ladies and gentlemen." It's why at Disney, every cast member is working toward his one stated goal of creating happiness.

At 21 years old, my first job at Disney was to sell balloons on Main Street. It isn't hard to sell balloons, right? Yet I went through three days of intensive training. I learned how to sell balloons in on-the-job training, but during those three days I also learned that I was one of hundreds of touch points in the visitor's experience at Disney. I could be the first. I could be the last. I could be somewhere in the middle. If my job was to sell balloons, but my *purpose* was to create happiness, what did that mean? Like the tray passers and the sterile processing unit, it's about connecting people to their purpose.

I remember early one morning before any guests had arrived at Disney, my leader told me to look down the street toward the castle. He said, "Jake, what do you see?" I was a little confused.

"Well, I see the castle, sir," I replied.

"Yes," he said. "But do you see any trash on the ground?"

I didn't see any! Because every cast member is aligned toward the same common goal, or what I call their *operational true north*: We create happiness by providing the finest in entertainment for people of all ages, everywhere. The park employs custodial cast members who sweep the streets and keep them clean. That day, however, I learned an important lesson: My task was to sell balloons, but my purpose, or role, in creating happiness and satisfying that key driver of cleanliness was to pick up trash when I saw it (and not just wait for the custodial cast member to do it).

Your team likely has a pretty good grasp of the clinical or business (for nonclinical staff) side of the equation. They're competent at their individual job tasks, which is probably why you hired them in the first place. The next step is to engage the human side of healthcare. By doing this, you connect the head (clinical expertise and knowledge) with the heart (human kindness and service excellence). When the head and the heart are engaged and committed, the hands will follow.

Uniting Clinical and Service Excellence

Think of the patient experience as the double helix of a DNA strand: The clinical excellence strand is no longer enough to sustain healthcare systems over the long term. It is merely one half of the double helix.

The challenge is to unite healing (clinical excellence) with human kindness (service excellence) so that it becomes part of your organizational DNA. We do this by filling the gaps between healing and human kindness, by building a culture of service excellence. When done correctly and consistently, this new culture of clinical and service excellence will be the key differentiator that will set your organization apart from other healthcare systems.

Moving from Episodic Care to a Complete Care Experience

The move from volume to value, from episodic care to a complete care experience, is well under way. The logical focus is on the caregiver at the bedside or in the exam room, but much of the patient experience has been influenced before patients even see a clinician. Prior to seeing a doctor or a nurse, patients likely will have seen or interacted with many people: the parking attendant, a security guard, the volunteer at the main entrance, the housekeeper cleaning the lobby restrooms, the gift shop attendant, the front desk registration, the accounts payable worker, and so on.

Imagine the entire patient experience as a kind of relay race with a wooden baton as the patient experience that's handed off from touch point to touch point. The goal, of course, is to have a smooth transition, or what I call a *warm handover*. When the patient experience falters, however, instead of being passed along intact, the baton gets whittled down. What's worse is that we often don't even realize it's happening.

Can't find a parking spot? Whittled. Confusing signs? Whittled. Volunteer distracted by a personal phone call? Whittled. Can't find the office or exam room? Whittled. Dirty plates and silverware in the cafeteria? Whittled. In every interaction and at every touch point of the patient experience, we're either whittling away or we're passing the baton intact to another member of the care team. Often, the baton is whittled—and the patient's experience is colored—*before* they even see the doctor.

More than ever before, your bottom line depends on good communication, excellent clinical and service outcomes, and exceptional patient experiences with good handoffs from one area to another. Healthcare systems face many challenges today, including rising costs and drastic changes in payment processes and reimbursements. Each of these challenges directly affects a healthcare system's bottom line. Most healthcare organizations are making some effort or initiative toward specifically improving patient experiences, but when it comes to building an organization-wide culture of service excellence to improve the patient experience for good, the question isn't why. It's how.

STEP TWO: DEFINE WHAT YOUR HEALTHCARE SYSTEM STANDS FOR

Transforming Your Organization to a Culture of Service Excellence

You can't create a road map of where you want to go as an organization unless you know your starting point. During this critical first step in the cultural transformation process, the goal is not to make big plans or roll out another unsuccessful initiative or program of the month. The goal is to understand where you are as an organization right now. There are lots of ways to assess an organization, but your challenge is to do it from the patients' perspective.

One simple tool my team uses as part of its assessment process is to make use of the easily available digital video technology all around us. Just grab a camera or your smartphone and snap a photo identifying every single step along the patient experience journey. But be sure to do it from the patients' perspective! (I often receive strange looks when I lie down on a hospital gurney in a suit and tie and take photos of the ceiling tiles above. But think about it: Isn't that what the patient sees when he's scared and being wheeled down the hall before a procedure? How would you feel about hospital-acquired infections if you looked up and saw dirty ceiling tiles before surgery?) This process will provide a clear picture (literally) of what your hospital or healthcare system looks like through the patient's eyes.

Where do patients park their cars? Snap photos of the parking lot signage, parking spaces, valet parking attendant (if applicable), access to the healthcare system, landscaping, trash cans, and ramps. Where do patients enter your building? Snap photos of the doorway, entrance signs, greeter (if there is one), floor, carpet, lights, and directional signs. Keep going until you've captured the entire experience from beginning to end. Are there light bulbs out? Scuffs on the floor? Holes in the wall? Chipped paint? Misspelled signs? Clutter in the hallways? Trash on the floor?

Now notice your employees. Are name tags worn by everyone or just a handful of employees? Are the name tags visible and easy to read, or are they turned around so no one can see them? Are the employees smiling and making appropriate eye contact with patients, families, and each other? Or are they checking their phones or chatting about last night's happy hour in common areas within earshot of patients?

Now notice your own examination room. Are the instruments organized or strewn about on a table? Is the equipment clean? Is the décor up-to-date? Are patients' personal files stored electronically, or are they scattered about the nursing station desk?

Keep walking. Does your care team have a place to go on their break, or do they share a restroom with patients and visitors? Are they forced to smoke outside your building so that everyone entering or exiting will see them? Is your waiting area filled with old magazines, dated artwork, and dead plants?

They say you can never really know a person until you've walked a mile in her shoes. Indeed, to be able to see and experience things from another person's point of view is a great gift. It can change our perspective, foster empathy, and create better understanding. In healthcare, as in most other fields as well, we tend to get caught up in the daily grind without always noticing what's right in front of us. So how can we really know what patients (or visitors, employees, vendors, family members) are seeing, feeling, and experiencing at our healthcare systems?

Organizational chaos and inconsistency reign when everyone sees things through their own lens—their own silo—with blinders on. After looking at the patient experience through the patients' eyes, an organization must come together and collectively decide what they currently stand for and what they will or will not stand for anymore.

Identifying and Eliminating Verbal and Physical Graffiti

A key component in creating a culture of service excellence and defining who you are as an organization is weeding out any ambiguity. You must have an explicit culture in which everyone can say, "This is what we stand for, and this is what we will no longer stand for." Anything that distracts or detracts from the ideal patient experience is what I call *graffiti*. Graffiti can be either verbal or physical and can include things such as the following:

Physical Graffiti
- Trash in patient areas
- Sounds of power-washing the floors in the middle of the night

- Employees walking past trash
- Poor directional signage
- Employee name badges flipped over (or no badges at all)
- Heavy perfume, cologne, or cigarette smell on a doctor's or nurse's clothing

Verbal Graffiti
- "It's not my job."
- "Sorry, I'm not allowed to have overtime."
- "I don't know."
- "Next!"
- "I'm off the clock."

There are many examples of verbal and physical graffiti. The point is to recognize it and then eliminate it, continuously—it has a tendency to creep back.

Building a Culture of Always

The hardest organizations to change are the ones that are already pretty good. The need for change is not a major source of pain. Maintaining the good status is also not a driving force. It's hard to identify what great *is*, because you're already very good.

We're all guilty of this, aren't we? Too often, we become comfortable with good or good enough instead of striving for more— reaching for that last inch that drives great experiences. As the popular phrase in business goes, "Good is the enemy of great."

A Quick Exercise

I often ask my audiences to do a little exercise with me. You can do it too, right now. Ready? Without getting out of your seat, reach one hand as high above your head as you can. The height of your hand represents the pinnacle of service excellence, right? Perhaps.

Now, raise your hand just an inch higher.

Most of us can always reach just a little higher. My question is, Why didn't you reach that high the first time?

I do that exercise often with audience members, and when I ask them why they didn't reach that high the first time I hear things such as, "Well, we had to stretch first." Or, "We didn't know that was the height we could reach until you pushed us."

That extra inch is what we're talking about. It's the hardest inch of all.

Having some people reach to the new height isn't going to create consistency in the continuum of care. But getting everyone to reach high at the same time? That's alignment. That's consistency. And that's what patients expect.

Good to Great and Sometimes Versus Always

In the business world, good is the enemy of great. In healthcare, I believe that sometimes is the enemy of always. Great companies not only create experiences that reach higher heights (or go the extra mile), they also seem to get everyone in the organization to deliver it—consistently—creating a culture of always.

What makes Disney or Ritz-Carlton so consistently excellent? Is it a handful of really great employees? No. Do they get there by hiring good people? No. "Good" is hiring good people and letting them be free to do good work, as they see it. But great? Great is making those patterns systemic. The result of great is having customers who ask, "What do you put in the water here that makes everyone here so great?"

So how do you get to great? How do you get to a culture of always? Organizations achieve these states by building a culture with a set of shared operational priorities and common behaviors that everyone knows, understands, and follows—"the way we do things here."

Consider the following:

- Some doctors shake hands with patients; some don't.
- Some sit and listen to the patient's story before diagnosing; some interrupt within 18 seconds to "move things along."
- Some nurses introduce themselves; some don't.
- Some offer to close the patient's door to keep out noise; some don't.
- Some food service people offer to help elderly patients open plasticware and milk cartons; some don't.

Besides doctors and nurses, did you know the average patient interacts with more than a hundred care team members along her healthcare journey, clinical and nonclinical employees alike? This broadness of experience is why it's so critical to include everyone when your goal is to improve patient experiences. Every interaction a patient has with medical and nonmedical staff helps to shape the patient's perceptions of their experience. Here's the bad news: On patient satisfaction surveys, we get zero credit, which means zero reimbursement dollars, for answers of "Sometimes." Remember, federal financial reimbursements are tied to patient satisfaction surveys. These surveys only give credit for "Always" answers. For healthcare administrators, improving the patient experience isn't just something that's nice to do; it's an imperative.

STEP THREE: HARDWIRE YOUR NEW CULTURE

The next step in building a culture of service excellence is to hardwire your desired cultural blueprints into the DNA of the organization. You must operationalize them so that everyone on the care team is aligned toward one common goal and can say, "This is how we do things around here."

Part of the process of hardwiring your new culture across the healthcare system includes having robust service recovery and employee recognition programs in place, as well as a department playbook to document how departments do things. Together, these three powerful tools can help to reinforce and strengthen your organization's culture of service excellence.

Service Recovery

When mistakes happen, and they will, organizations need a process to make things right at the moment they occur (as long as it is not a serious situation where safety and liability are issues). But finding the solution to a problem or giving out a free coffee coupon to a disgruntled patient or visitor is only a temporary solution.

The best service recovery efforts work to resolve the situation as efficiently and as effectively as possible, but they also document the process so that everyone on the care team can learn from the experience. It's a two-pronged approach: Address the situation at the front line, before it escalates, and report it so everyone can learn how to prevent or mitigate similar situations in the future. A good service recovery program allows employees to handle many issues on their own or with the assistance of a leader. Often, people don't want anything (e.g., a refund, something for free). Most times, people just want to be heard. They want to voice their frustration, and they want someone to listen to them. Customers also would like members of the leadership team to fix any significant perceived problems and issues so that they do not happen to others and would ideally like evidence that this has taken place. Regardless of the situation and the reason behind it, service recovery is an effective tool for providing exceptional customer service.

On-the-Spot Recognition: Catching Your Employees in the Act

Ask any of your employees to finish this phrase: "The only time I see my boss or hear from my manager is when I do something _____." They would probably finish the sentence with "when I do something wrong." Imagine if this dynamic were reversed. Imagine if employees didn't feel as though they had to walk on eggshells around their leaders, fearful of making even the slightest mistake. Imagine if they were recognized, in the moment, for doing things the right way. Encouragement and positive accolades may seem trite, but they can be a powerful motivator. Many companies and organizations hold an end-of-year event where they recognize employees for years of service, for work on a project, or for their overall contributions to the team. These events are nice, but are they really the best way to recognize employees? Is once a year enough, or does it seem contrived and a little forced?

I challenge leaders to switch things up a bit. Instead of looking for things your employees are doing wrong, why not catch them doing things right? Recognize employees for following through and raising the bar on the way we do things here. Be sure to copy their leader and human resources so it can be placed in their file. This way, you let the accolades build. When it's time for the employee's review, there will be visible proof of how that employee is living your new organizational culture. When you publicize what's being recognized (while honoring employees' privacy), others will say, "Hey, I can do that, too." It raises the bar across the organization.

Always Plays

Borrowing from the world of sports, a department playbook is a resource for every employee. It contains specific descriptions of service excellence (i.e., the way we do things here), which are designed, defined, and agreed to by the staff and are documented as plays. With "sometimes" the enemy of "always," we further designate these as always plays.

One client created an always play to address a confusing office layout at one of its clinics. When searching for the exit, patients were constantly turning the wrong way and sometimes entering another patient's room. To solve this problem, the employees came up with the idea that the provider who ends the visit with the patient (a doctor or a nurse) would walk the patient to the front reception desk—always. Not only did this help alleviate the problem of lost or wandering patients, but it also gave the doctor or nurse a little bit more time with the patient to address any last-minute concerns as they walked to the front desk. This "always" play is recorded in their department playbook, and everyone holds each other accountable for walking patients to the front desk. It's a simple process improvement tool that empowers employees to address customer service issues and create solutions to make things better.

New Employee Orientation

A vital piece of cultural transformation is new employee orientation. This process involves preemployment screening, interviewing, hiring, and training. When it's done right, new employees will become ambassadors of your culture. They will know what you stand for as an organization and what you don't stand for. They'll have an arsenal of tools available to prepare them to be ready not only on day 1 but also on day 2, day 3, and so on.

CONCLUSION

Building a culture of service excellence requires a shift in thought. Too often, we seek and embrace what we believe to be the right prescriptive program or initiative that will turn things around and make employees deliver better service. But imposing a culture won't work. Why? Because when a culture is imposed on employees, it may work for a little while, but over time it will fade away. Employees will go back to doing things the way they've always been done. Patient satisfaction scores will drop. Letters such as the one from the mother at the beginning of this chapter will appear more and more frequently on the CEO's desk—or worse, in the local newspaper, on social media, or on a ratings website. If you get a letter, consider yourself lucky. Eight out of ten people don't complain (to you). They just leave and tell everyone else.

There is no magic elixir or recipe for raising HCAHPS scores; improving the patient experience; or delivering exceptional service to patients, employees, and families. If you're really committed to building a culture of service excellence across your healthcare systems, you must be willing to commit time and resources to undergo a cultural transformation. Because delivering service excellence can't be just something you do or say. It has to become *who you are* as a healing organization.

REFERENCE

Beryl Institute. 2018. "Defining Patient Experience." Accessed April 25. www.theberylinstitute.org/?page=definingpatientexp.

CHAPTER 14

Legal Challenges for Clinically Integrated Networks

Brian Betner
Michael Greer

[Clinical integration is] an active and ongoing program to evaluate and modify practice patterns by the network's physician participants and create a high degree of interdependence and cooperation among the physicians to control costs and ensure quality.

—Pamela Jones Harbour, Federal Trade Commission Commissioner, 2009

THE CONCEPT OF clinical integration, or at least the phrase, is ubiquitous in healthcare today. In some respects, clinical integration has become a strategy (marketing or otherwise) for organizations in pursuit of the Holy Grail in healthcare—high-quality, cost-effective care delivered in an efficient, coordinated, and patient-centered way. Everyone in the healthcare sector has heard the phrase *clinical integration* and can generally articulate what the concept means to them, but clinical integration in its current legal state has only been around since the mid-1990s and did not take off as a model until the past decade. In fact, clinical integration did not even start as a model of care. Instead, it started as an antitrust concept but has gradually evolved into an accepted legal model as providers focus on continuity of care, quality of care, and value-based reimbursement.

THE PRICE-FIXING PROBLEM

To better understand the genesis of clinical integration, it is helpful to understand the underlying antitrust concern it is intended to address. Under the antitrust laws, it is unlawful for competing providers to get together and jointly negotiate pricing with commercial payers. The Supreme Court has determined this type of conduct is considered price fixing and is per se unlawful under the antitrust laws. Readers should know that in the antitrust context, *per se* has a very specific connotation. If the government is pursuing a case under a per se theory, all the government has to do is prove that an agreement exists between two competing providers. Importantly, it does *not* have to show the agreement between the two competing providers has caused any type of competitive harm. The purpose of the antitrust laws is to prevent harm to competition, so you would think the government must prove harm to competition (i.e., higher prices or lower quality). But the courts have decided there are certain types of activities that are so egregious and problematic that those activities will be considered per se unlawful without the need to go through a complex and expensive trial. For example, any type of "naked" price-fixing agreement among competing providers (i.e., an agreement to act as a cartel), "naked" market allocation agreements, or bid-rigging agreements are considered per se unlawful.

On the other hand, there are certain activities that competing providers undertake that actually promote competition, so the courts have decided in these instances that the *rule of reason* will be applied.

When the rule of reason is applied, there is a complex and expensive investigation of the procompetitive benefits and the anticompetitive effects to determine whether, on balance, the activity is good or bad. Because these types of investigations are so complex and expensive, if the government deems the rule-of-reason standard should be applied to an activity, the government will simply drop the case. This pattern means, ultimately, that the most important question is whether the government will apply the per se standard or rule-of-reason standard to a specific activity.

CLINICAL INTEGRATION IS BORN

Given this background, it is probably not surprising that a provider cannot simply meet with its competitor in a dark and smoky bar and agree to charge payers 500 percent of Medicare. This type of activity is clearly a naked price fix and would lead to payers, and ultimately patients, paying too much for healthcare services, so the government would pursue a per se case. As the healthcare sector evolved in the 1990s, however, a strange thing happened. The field saw hospitals and physicians form various types of provider networks, such as physician–hospital organizations, preferred provider organizations, and independent practice associations.

These provider networks certainly were not simply competing providers fixing prices in a smoky bar. But these provider networks also jointly negotiated prices with payers on behalf of competing providers, which the government found problematic. In 1994, the Department of Justice, with the Federal Trade Commission, issued updated guidance in which it described two methods for provider networks to avoid naked price-fixing concerns. The first method was to use a messenger model approach, through which the provider network would simply "messenger" offers between payers and providers. The second method was to financially integrate the provider network. Statement 8 of the 1994 Healthcare Statements specifically addressed ways to satisfy the financial integration requirement, including using capitation, percentage of premium, substantial withholds, and other risk-sharing methodologies. Essentially, the government wanted to see providers sharing downside risk in order to align incentives into offering more efficient care. If the provider network was financially integrated, then the government would use the rule-of-reason standard and walk away.

Not surprisingly, there was pushback from providers, who thought a sole focus on financial integration would limit their ability to create new and innovative care models for enhancing quality of care. In response to the criticism, the Department of Justice and the Federal Trade Commission updated their guidance in 1996. The 1996 Healthcare Statements introduced the concept of clinical integration as another method for providers to avoid naked price-fixing concerns. The new Statement 8 of the 1996 Healthcare Statements said that absent financial integration, provider networks could still involve sufficient integration to demonstrate that the provider network was likely to produce significant efficiencies. This integration could be shown if the provider network implemented "an active and ongoing program to evaluate and modify practice patterns by the network's physician participants and create a high degree of interdependence and cooperation among the physicians to control costs and ensure quality." The law noted that such a clinical integration program should do three things: (1) include mechanisms to monitor and control utilization to control costs and ensure quality of care; (2) selectively choose network providers to further these efficiency objectives; and (3) require the significant investment, both monetary and human, to accomplish the necessary infrastructure and capability. As with financial integration, if the government deemed the provider was sufficiently clinically integrated, it would use the rule-of-reason standard and walk away.

As we can see, with the 1996 Healthcare Statements, the concept of clinical integration was born. But there were still a lot of questions. What exactly did a clinical integration program require? What kind of mechanisms were needed? How much investment of time and money was necessary? Over the ensuing years, the government has issued a number of advisory opinions offering guidance, and it has become clear that the 1996 Healthcare Statements' description was misleading in the sense that the government requires a much more complicated program than initially suggested. However, one common theme is clear: There is no cookie-cutter model and no black-and-white answer. The solution is based on the specific facts and circumstances of each provider network. Ultimately, the provider network must produce significant efficiencies that benefit consumers and that cannot be generated individually by the participating providers.

CLINICALLY INTEGRATED NETWORKS: ANTITRUST FRAMEWORK

Although there is no recipe that will effectively apply to all situations, through the various advisory opinions, enforcement actions, and other guidance, we can glean what is necessary for a provider network to be deemed clinically integrated. The key is collaboration and interdependence among participating providers that result in significant quality, utilization, and cost-improvement efficiencies in the delivery of healthcare services.

Step 1: Indicators of Sufficient Clinical Integration

This first step in the antitrust framework is the most time consuming and the hardest to implement. It involves the formation and operation of the clinically integrated network and includes numerous operational substeps, discussed in the following sections.

Substantial Contributions of Financial and Sweat Equity
Providers have to be fully involved from the beginning, both in terms of making financial contributions to the clinical integration program, such as an annual fee or information technology hardware

and software costs, and putting in time on committees and other operational functions of the clinical integration program.

Careful Choice of Providers

Members of the network must select those likely to comply. The goal of any clinical integration program is to generate efficiencies and increase quality by changing practice patterns. Not all providers are interested in this outcome, so while the clinical integration program certainly needs to have sufficient participation to provide coverage, it also needs to be selective to make sure participating providers are aware of the stringent requirements and will comply in an ongoing basis with those requirements.

System for Exchange of Relevant Medical Information

All members of the clinical integration program should be able to pass on information with ease, preferably via electronic health records (EHRs) or electronic health information exchanges. This sharing allows providers to coordinate care more easily and permits the clinical integration program to monitor provider adherence to protocols and measure performance against benchmarks.

In-Network Referrals

A hallmark of coordinated care and interdependence is that providers keep referrals within the clinically integrated network to the maximum extent possible.

Clinical Protocols or Practice Guidelines

Arguably, the most important aspect of a clinical integration program is the creation of clinical protocols designed to improve quality and utilization, allowing the healthcare organization to "build a better mousetrap." It is critical that the participating providers spend the time and effort to create these clinical protocols, work to implement them, analyze their effectiveness, and repeat the process. These protocols should be formally adopted by the clinical integration program and applied to all network patients.

Development of Goals or Benchmarks

The clinically integrated program, working with participating providers, should establish goals in the areas of quality, efficiency, and cost that support improvement over its current performance.

Measurement of Providers' Compliance

Protocols and benchmarks are meaningless unless the clinical integration program can measure providers' performance and compliance with the guidelines. A clinical integration program should be able to collect, store, and analyze data through data warehouses, scorecards, and dashboards.

Review and Assessment of Individual and Aggregate Performance

Along with measuring providers' performance, the clinical integration program must review and analyze both individual and aggregate performance in relation to the protocols and benchmarks.

Identification of Providers Who Fail to Apply the Guidelines

The clinical integration program should monitor and enforce its performance standards via formal programs, and providers must participate in ongoing quality assurance monitoring activities, including audits.

Performance Improvement and Corrective Action Programs

Individual participating providers should have consequences for not meeting the goals or benchmarks. The first step should be a performance improvement program. Preferably, this type of plan would be formulated by other participating providers.

Development and Implementation of a Sanctions Process

Integrated entities must create a process to sanction participating providers who habitually fail to meet network goals or refuse to follow the clinical integration program's policies, including possible expulsion from the clinical integration program and, potentially, financial sanctions or rewards based on performance. After a performance improvement plan is established, the next step should be a consideration of corrective action, which may include sanctions or possible expulsion from the clinical integration program.

Step 2: Ancillarity of the Joint Negotiation for Pricing

Once the clinical integration program is deemed sufficiently clinically integrated by the standards of regulatory precedent, the second step in the antitrust framework is to determine whether joint price negotiations are ancillary or "reasonably necessary" for the clinical integration program to achieve its proposed efficiency and cost benefits. Said another way, what about the clinical integration program makes it necessary to allow independent competing providers to negotiate prices jointly? Admittedly an amorphous standard, this step is often overlooked when conducting an antitrust analysis of a clinically integrated network.

There is no bright-line standard and there may be several acceptable rationales, but the government has only endorsed one "ancillarity" justification: Broadly speaking, for the clinical integration program to generate maximum efficiencies, participation by all providers, in all contracts, is important. In turn, the only way for this to happen is for the clinical integration program to negotiate contracts for all of its providers. It is important for all providers to participate in all contracts for a number of reasons, but this condition can often be a point of contention for participating providers who want the ability to opt out of certain contracts entered into by the clinical integration program.

Step 3: Rule-of-Reason Market Analysis

Establishing sufficient integration and ancillarity means that the clinically integrated network's joint negotiations are not a per se unlawful price-fixing agreement; however, it does not mean they are per se legal or that the antitrust analysis is complete. Instead, the antitrust analysis then requires balancing the clinically integrated network's market power, if any, and offsetting efficiencies under the rule of reason. Under traditional rule-of-reason analysis, the question ultimately boils down to whether payers have sufficient alternatives if the clinically integrated network attempts to exercise market power by raising prices, and secondarily, whether the clinically integrated network can prevent or impede the formation or operation of other networks.

The first, and most important, element of the rule-of-reason analysis is whether the clinically integrated network has market power and thus is likely to have anticompetitive effects. This power is primarily determined by evaluating the network's market share in *each* of the service lines included in the network. As a starting point, the 1996 Healthcare Statements—specifically Statement 8 regarding physician network joint ventures, which would include clinically integrated networks—provide an antitrust safety zone for nonexclusive networks whose participating physicians constitute 30 percent or less of the physicians in each physician specialty; for exclusive networks, the safety zone is 20 percent. Clinically integrated networks that fall within the safety zones will not be challenged, absent extraordinary circumstances.

Clinically integrated networks that exceed these market share thresholds, however, will not necessarily raise antitrust concerns; instead, the government will consider other factors, including the proportion of providers in any service or specialty. The government also considers the incentives given to the providers, the presence of competing networks or non-network physicians, the potential for "spillover" effects from the network's activities (e.g., participating physicians obtaining competitively sensitive information through the network and using it to coordinate prices or insurance contract negotiation or participation outside of the network), and, similarly, the existence of collateral agreements (e.g., agreements or provisions that refuse to deal with competitors outside of the network or deny them necessary access to key facilities).

As the earlier discussion suggests, whether the clinically integrated network is exclusive is complex and very important to the antitrust analysis. The government will evaluate not only whether the network is expressly exclusive but also whether it is de facto exclusive—or stated differently, nonexclusive in fact and not just in name. Market indicators of nonexclusivity (in addition to express contractual provisions) include the existence of viable competing networks with adequate provider participation, participation by network physicians in other networks or contracting directly with payers (or evidence of their willingness and incentive to do so), earning substantial revenue from those networks or payer contracts, absence of evidence of departure from other networks or payer contracts, and absence of any indication of coordination among participating providers regarding prices or other terms in contracts with competing networks or payers.

GOING BEYOND ANTITRUST

Clinical integration is a concept born from the perils of the antitrust enforcement, but there are a number of other legal considerations that create a greater challenge for the development and effectiveness of clinically integrated networks. It is important to keep in mind that the current healthcare landscape is largely built on a regulatory framework that is in some cases older than 30 years—many years prior to more recent efforts focused on innovation, population health, and value-based reimbursement. Despite meaningful efforts at innovation in healthcare delivery through reimbursement policy, much of the current healthcare regulatory framework does not expressly or adequately contemplate the concept of clinical integration and similar innovative arrangements.

By definition, clinical integration involves the alignment of providers who are not part of the same organization or legal entity and who will deliver and coordinate care. This new arrangement may stress traditional concepts of scope of practice and autonomy and will generate referrals for healthcare services within the network. Couple these necessary competencies with the demands of value-based reimbursement that emphasizes and creates accountability around quality, cost savings, standardization, and clinical efficiency, and you create a number of potential legal entanglements and challenges. Development and implementation of clinically integrated networks require not only a thorough understanding of the legal framework and considerations associated with these activities but also a keen perspective on healthcare operations and provider relationship dynamics. Well-designed and innovative clinically integrated networks should consider the regulatory and operational issues discussed in this section.

Fraud and Abuse Considerations

Many observers consider compliance with federal and state fraud and abuse laws to be the most significant challenge or burden to formation and effective operation of a clinically integrated network. These laws are often viewed by the sector as barriers to the various forms of provider alignment that clinical integration is striving to achieve. Existing fraud and abuse laws and their application tend to focus on fee-for-service reimbursement structures and compensation for services rendered or other tangible exchanges and do not clearly contemplate incentives for health, wellness, and cost containment. Following is a rundown of the principal federal fraud and abuse legal barriers.

Stark Law
The federal physician self-referral law, commonly referred to as the *Stark law*, provides that if a physician (or immediate family member of a physician) has a financial relationship with an entity, then the physician may not make a referral to the entity for the furnishing of designated health services (DHS) for which payment may be made under Medicare or Medicaid; the entity may not present or

cause to be presented a claim under Medicare or Medicaid or bill any third party for DHS furnished pursuant to such a prohibited referral. It is important to keep in mind that the Stark law is a strict liability law, which means that proof of intent to violate the law is not required. So, for all practical purposes, a financial relationship either complies with the law or it does not.

The term *referral* is broadly defined under the Stark law to include any request by a physician for an item or service. A *financial relationship* includes an ownership or investment interest in, or a compensation arrangement with, an entity. Ownership or investment interests may be through equity, debt, or other means. The term *compensation arrangement* is defined very broadly to include most transfers of remuneration between a hospital or other DHS entity and a physician (e.g., space lease, medical director agreement). All financial relationships to which the Stark law applies are either direct or indirect. The Stark law provides a specific definition of *direct* and *indirect* financial relationships. An indirect compensation arrangement exists in three situations. First, there is an unbroken chain of any number of persons or entities that have financial relationships between the referring physician and the DHS entity. Second, the referring physician receives aggregate compensation from the person or entity with whom the referring physician has a direct financial relationship that varies with, or takes into account, the volume or value of referrals generated by the referring physician for the DHS entity. Third, the DHS entity has knowledge of the fact that the aggregate compensation varies with, or takes into account, the volume or value of referrals.

In some circumstances, a physician can "stand in the shoes" of her physician organization, resulting in a "direct" arrangement by operation of law, even when, in fact, there is not a direct relationship. This situation occurs when (1) the only intervening entity between the physician and the hospital or other entity furnishing DHS is his physician entity or (2) the physician has an ownership or investment interest in the physician organization. A common example is a medical director agreement between a hospital and a physician group.

If a hospital has a medical director agreement pursuant to which a group furnishes a physician to provide medical director services, then the Stark law may ignore the existence of the group and treat the arrangement as creating a direct financial relationship between the physician and the hospital (even though, in fact, it is not direct). A *physician organization* is defined as a physician, a physician practice, or a group practice (as defined by 42 CFR 411.352). Among other things, a *group practice* is a single legal entity comprising at least two physicians, through which the physicians provide substantially all the patient care services furnished by the physicians, and the services are billed under the group's billing number.

The Stark law defines the term *designated health services* to include the following items or services: clinical laboratory; physical therapy, occupational therapy, and speech and language pathology; radiology and certain other imaging; radiation therapy and supplies; durable medical equipment and supplies; parenteral and enteral nutrients, equipment, and supplies; prosthetics, orthotics, and prosthetic devices and supplies; home health; outpatient prescription drugs; and inpatient and outpatient hospital services.

The Stark law prohibits providers from submitting claims for payment to Medicare or Medicaid, or any other third-party payer, including the patient, for services furnished pursuant to a prohibited referral. The Stark law also provides certain statutory and regulatory exceptions to the prohibitions set forth in the law. Every financial relationship between a referring physician and a DHS entity must meet a Stark law exception to comply with the Stark law. Sanctions for not complying are significant. In addition to a prohibition on billing and payment, violations can also result in civil money penalties up to $15,000 per claim multiplied by the amount of improper payments, up to $100,000 for "circumvention" schemes, and possible exclusion from participation in federal healthcare programs. These penalties do not include potential liability emanating from alleged False Claims Act violations, which can be both civil and criminal.[1]

In order to comply with the Stark law, the requirements of an exception must be met. It is important to evaluate all financial relationships existing prior to and during the formation of a network. Because fair market value compensation is a critical consideration when evaluating compliance with the Stark law, total or so-called aggregate compensation flowing from an entity to a physician for multiple arrangements often comes into play. Clinically integrated network entities are rarely the actual parties performing and submitting claims for reimbursement, but financial relationships among referring physicians and entities that submit claims to Medicare or Medicaid for DHS will inevitably implicate the Stark law. Depending on the clinically integrated network's structure and the nature of its physician relationships, available Stark law exceptions include bona fide employment, personal services, fair market value, indirect compensation, EHR items and services, and risk-sharing arrangements.

A particular challenge when assessing compliance with the most appropriate Stark law exception is determining whether performance-oriented incentive compensation is consistent with fair market value. Today, there is no generally accepted methodology for calculating fair market value for common clinical integration performance incentives, such as shared-savings payments, pathway compliance, or clinical outcomes.

Antikickback Statute

Unlike many other industries that customarily reward business development, the exchange of remuneration (basically, anything of value) intended to influence referrals reimbursable by a federal healthcare program is illegal. Given that clinically integrated networks are essentially joint ventures among competitors and referral sources, it is important to evaluate all potential referral sources, flow of funds, support activities, and delivery of services to avoid even the appearance of improper remuneration that could violate the federal antikickback statute (AKS). The AKS is a criminal law that prohibits any person from knowingly and willfully soliciting, receiving, offering, or paying remuneration—directly or indirectly, overtly or covertly, in cash or in kind—in return for purchasing, leasing, ordering, or arranging for or recommending purchasing, leasing, or ordering any good, facility, service, or item for which payment may be made in whole or in part under a federal healthcare program. The AKS is broadly written and was interpreted by the courts in the 1985 *United States v. Greber* case to have been violated "if one purpose of the payment was to induce future referrals."

Under the Affordable Care Act passed by Congress in 2010, a person need not have actual knowledge of the AKS or have a specific intent to commit a violation of the AKS. The AKS contains safe harbors, which, if met, protect the parties to the transaction from AKS liability. However, the failure to comply with all portions of the safe harbor does not result in automatic violation of the AKS. Similar to the Stark law, safe harbors relevant to clinical integration activities include employees, personal services and management contracts, EHR items and services, and risk-sharing arrangements with managed care organizations.

In the absence of safe harbor protection, a clinically integrated network arrangement will be evaluated based on a "facts and circumstances" test that considers all elements of its structure and operations and the intention of the parties to determine AKS compliance. Many design elements and factors can be incorporated into network development and support the legitimate purpose of a clinical integration effort, including network efficiencies, documented need for services, shared governance, clinical guidelines development, and availability of in-community specialty and subspecialty services. Even when structured conservatively, many successful network arrangements will inevitably affect other competitors in the same market or service area, and these competitors can be expected to file complaints.

Civil Monetary Penalties Law

The Civil Monetary Penalties (CMP) law, among other violations, prohibits a hospital from knowingly making a payment, directly or indirectly, to a physician as an inducement to reduce or limit services provided to Medicare or Medicaid beneficiaries who are under the direct care of the physician. Until the CMP law was modified in 2015, the use of gainsharing incentives to modify physician practice patterns was widely considered an illegal or risky practice.[2] *Gainsharing* is an incentive program that involves the sharing of financial gains from various cost-saving measures, most commonly involving an arrangement between hospitals and a physician or group of physicians. This loosening of the CMP law, however, does not necessarily reduce all risk associated with incentive arrangements designed to control costs and increase efficiencies. The CMP law is potentially abrogated by any arrangement that involves cost-saving activities, such as device standardization, vendor selection, and so on.

A number of favorable advisory opinions have been issued by the Office of Inspector General of the Department of Health and Human Services that provide a road map of sorts for organizations interested in pursuing gainsharing arrangements. These advisory opinions outline a number of favorable characteristics, including the following:

- The arrangement is appropriately monitored to ensure patient care is not adversely affected.
- The organization has the flexibility to use most cost-effective, clinically appropriate items and supplies.
- Cost-savings-related financial incentive is reasonably limited in duration and amount.
- Compensation is conditioned on various safeguards to avoid stinting, cherry-picking, and increasing referrals.

Liability under the Stark law, the AKS, and the CMP law is not academic, as fraud and abuse enforcement activities are nearing an all-time high. A number of innovative, population health–oriented programs sponsored by the Centers for Medicare & Medicaid Services have been paired with broad waivers to these laws.[3] The waivers are issued specifically to address the inflexibility of the collective federal fraud and abuse laws in accommodating financial incentives focused on improving quality outcomes, cost savings, and clinical efficiencies.[4]

Healthcare leaders must understand that fraud- and abuse-related liability often derives from the planning phases and not solely from the implementation of arrangements that involve unlawful benefits to and among referral sources. To the extent that there is an investigation into the structure of and relationships within a clinically integrated network, all participants should expect their email, internal presentations, and various drafts of documents to be reviewed to determine the intent of the parties. The federal government has made it abundantly clear that fraud and abuse enforcement focuses on the involvement of individuals when assessing corporate wrongdoing. For this reason, the full range of internal activities related to network development (e.g., readiness assessment, risk assessment, network development) may be subject to review and scrutiny.

Tax-Exempt Organizations

Clinically integrated networks, as previously discussed, are essentially joint ventures among independent providers. These joint ventures will inevitably include participation by tax-exempt organizations, which are commonly hospitals. Any joint venture involving nonprofit and for-profit parties should be carefully structured to enable the tax-exempt participant to further its charitable purposes and to avoid placing any participating tax-exempt organization at risk for violating Internal Revenue Service (IRS) rules regarding private benefit and inurement. Importantly, clinically integrated networks that do not participate in the Medicare Shared Savings Program are unlikely to be eligible for exempt status. In the 2016 private ruling 2016115022, the IRS denied tax-exempt status to a commercial-only accountable care organization (ACO) on the grounds that a substantial portion of its activities were focused on negotiating agreements with third-party payers. According to the IRS, this commercial payer focus is considered a "substantial nonexempt purpose." The private inurement and benefit rules are implicated when any part of the net earnings of an exempt organization inure to the benefit of any private shareholder or individual.

The fundamental purpose of these prohibitions is to ensure that charitable assets are preserved for public benefit and not diverted to private use. This preservation is largely achieved by ensuring that financial arrangements among tax-exempt organizations and network "insiders" and "outsiders," such as board members and contractors, are designed to be consistent with fair market value. Violations of the private benefit and private inurement rules can lead to revocation of tax-exempt status.

Health Insurance Portability and Accountability Act, Privacy, and Security

Patient information and associated quality data are at the heart of all clinically integrated networks. A network must have a health information technology infrastructure capable of supporting the broad range of activities associated with EHR access and sharing, performance measurement, and data analysis of patient information. Central to this infrastructure is an EHR system that serves as a shared medical record platform for network participants. Clinical integration itself does not create privacy and security issues otherwise uncommon to routine healthcare operations, but the combination of multiple provider types as well as the complexity of data sharing and analysis typically involved in network activities create their own challenges. These challenges must be assessed against a host of federal and state privacy and security laws.

Most notable of these laws is the Health Insurance Portability and Accountability Act (HIPAA) and its corresponding privacy and security rules.[5] The HIPAA Privacy Rule regulates the use and disclosure of protected health information (PHI), and the Security Rule addresses required safeguards and protections involving electronic PHI. HIPAA applies to covered entities and their business associates. As a general rule, HIPAA prohibits the use and disclosure of PHI except as specifically permitted under the Privacy Rule or a patient authorization. Most clinically integrated network activities will fall into a Privacy Rule exception for what is referred to as treatment, payment, and healthcare operations. Because clinically integrated network participants are invariably either covered entities or business associates of the participating covered entities, network activities must be structured to comply with all applicable HIPAA requirements and best practices.

Beyond HIPAA, many states have established confidentiality and consent laws that regulate or impose restrictions and requirements on patient-related information. These laws, in many cases, may be more rigorous than HIPAA and take into consideration the provider type and the nature of the information (e.g., mental health, substance abuse).

In recognizing these challenges, clinically integrated networks should carefully evaluate their structure and the ways in which patient information will be used and disclosed among network participants by developing administrative, physical, and technical safeguards that provide for the following:

- Appointment of a designated privacy and security representative or officer
- Creation of an organized healthcare arrangement for the network participants to enable confidential sharing of protected materials related to PHI and peer review
- Development of a notice of privacy practices that clarifies the relationships among network participants and their use and disclosure of patient information
- Addressing release of information requests by third parties and individuals
- Security breach investigations and risk assessments
- Access rights and controls for participants; audits and monitoring of network participants' use of and access to patient information
- Management of access and transfers of patient information contained in a shared EHR

State Law Considerations

The reimbursement of healthcare (and ensuing fraud and abuse enforcement) tends to be regulated at or focused on the national or federal level, but the delivery of healthcare remains largely concentrated at the state level. Clinically integrated network formation and operation involve many state-level issues. Unlike more predictable federal perspectives, state regulation of healthcare takes into consideration a wider range of cultural priorities and perspectives.

State and Medicaid Laws: Kickbacks, Physician Referrals, and Fee-Splitting

As a result of their role in administering state Medicaid programs, many states have a substantial regulatory framework focused on similar fraud and abuse matters. These laws generally tend to mirror federal laws, but they focus on claims, referrals, and relationships involving Medicaid funds and are enforced by the state's attorney general or Medicaid fraud-control units.

Licensure

State licensing laws, both for individual professions and facilities, are largely based on traditional concepts of provider autonomy or even outdated treatment timelines associated with pre-acute, acute, and post-acute care patterns. In many instances, a state's licensing framework will not have been updated to accommodate many of the competencies that clinically integrated networks require or seek to develop. These competencies include expanded scopes of practice for nonphysician providers, hospitals' expanded role and emphasis on pre-acute and post-acute care, quality review by provider types other than hospitals, providers' use of cutting-edge technologies to treat patients, and many others. In many cases, providers can seek an advisory opinion or variance from the appropriate state licensing agency. In most cases, however, the agency will not be prepared to opine on activities that fall outside of its acknowledged regulatory guidance. Other than requiring provider licensing, some states see the increasing role of provider networks and have legislated specific registration or similar requirements for provider organizations that form to function as a clinically integrated network.

Corporate Practice of Medicine

The corporate practice of medicine is a legal doctrine that generally prohibits corporations, entities, or individuals (i.e., nonphysicians) from practicing medicine or employing a physician to provide professional medical services. This doctrine proscribes physicians from entering into employee relationships, partnerships, or other arrangements with nonphysicians where the physician's practice of medicine may in any way be controlled or directed by a nonphysician. Physicians can generally enter into independent contractor arrangements with nonphysicians. Many states, however, have created exceptions that permit a range of corporate employers, including hospitals and health maintenance organizations. Because clinical integration necessarily involves some aspect of centralized and standardized delivery of care, it is important to consider in the development stage whether any state law on the corporate practice of medicine touches on network activities to minimize malpractice risk to the network and potential nullification of participation agreements.

State Peer Review Laws

Peer review confidentiality is largely a matter of state law.[6] Most state peer review laws and related judicial scrutiny follow an elemental or formulaic process that strictly stipulates whether statutory protections will be afforded. This formulaic process typically involves a predictable, plain-meaning analysis of whether the statutory requirements were met. These approaches tend to not be well understood or easily incorporated into network activities in which care that is delivered and evaluated outside of more traditional care environments, such as hospitals, is taken into account. With some exceptions, state peer review laws will involve several common concepts regarding who can initiate the peer review process, what activities and information are subject to the process and privilege, the timing of the process beginning and end, with whom privileged information can be shared, and when privileged information is waived or when confidentiality does not apply.

To be sure, clinically integrated networks are not specifically addressed by most state peer review laws because these laws were adopted prior to the relatively recent reform driven by various market forces and the Affordable Care Act. For this reason, careful attention should be given to structuring networks and their care assessment activities in a manner that will at best meet the letter of state law and, if possible, the spirit. Peer review privilege challenges are routine, but few state courts have fully assessed the role of nonproviders and nonlicensed organizations, such as clinically integrated networks and ACOs, in the peer review process.

Insurance and Any Willing Provider Laws

Clinically integrated networks that assume risk in their contracting activities may also be subject to state insurance laws. Whether the risk is of the nature and type that triggers insurance jurisdiction will almost certainly depend on the nature of the risk (e.g., risk of contingent, uncertain loss vs. clinical performance), how the participating providers are compensated for their clinical services (e.g., capitation or withholding vs. upside shared savings), and the nature of the contracted relationships (e.g., whether the network and providers are downstream or upstream from an insurer). A network that is subject to state insurance laws, whether by design or otherwise, may be required to register or become licensed as a health insurer or managed care organization with the appropriate state agency. This registration or licensure requirement will typically involve a host of conditions related to financial strength or solvency, network adequacy, consumer communications and grievance procedures, and state auditing or reporting requirements. In addition, several states have *any willing provider* laws that require health insurance carriers to allow providers to participate in networks if certain conditions are met. While the scope of these laws is generally limited in nature, as the laws exclude self-funded employer arrangements and Employee Retirement Income Security Act plans, consideration should be given to whether narrow-network development would be frustrated by state laws that could limit the ability to exclude certain providers.

REFERENCE

Harbour, P. J. 2009. "Clinical Integration: The Changing Policy Climate and What It Means for Care Coordination." Federal Trade Commission. Published April 27. www.ftc.gov/sites/default /files/documents/public_statements/clinical-integration -changing-policy-climate-and-what-it-means-care-coordination /090427ahaclinicalintegration.pdf.

NOTES

1. The False Claims Act makes it illegal to submit claims for payment to Medicare or Medicaid that are known or should be known to be false or fraudulent. False Claims Act enforcement often stems from a whistleblower provision that allows individuals to collect a percentage of recoveries.
2. The Medicare Access and CHIP Reauthorization Act (MACRA) of 2015 limited the CMP law by adding the words "medically necessary," the effect being that only inducements made to reduce or limit medically necessary services to Medicare or Medicaid beneficiaries would be prohibited.
3. No fewer than ten federal programs incorporate fraud and abuse waivers, including the Pioneer ACO Model, the Medicare Shared Savings Program, the Bundled Payments for Care Initiative, the Comprehensive Care for

Joint Replacement Model, and the Next Generation ACO Model.

4. MACRA also includes a directive that the secretary of the Department of Health and Human Services conduct a study and report to Congress with options for amending certain fraud and abuse laws to permit gainsharing or similar arrangements between physicians and hospitals that improve care while reducing waste and increasing efficiency. This report was issued on May 19, 2016.

5. Also of importance are federal and state confidentiality laws pertinent to drug and alcohol abuse treatment. A federal law titled Confidentiality of Substance Use Disorder Patient Records strictly regulates the disclosure and use of alcohol and drug patient records maintained in connection with any federally assisted alcohol and drug abuse program.

6. The Patient Safety and Quality Improvement Act of 2005 provides federal privilege and confidentiality protections for patient safety information generated pursuant to a prescribed evaluation system process involving patient safety organizations (PSOs; see also www.hhs.gov/ hipaa/for-professionals/patient-safety/statute-and-rule). Some clinically integrated networks, particularly those with activities that cross state lines, should explore whether a PSO is appropriate for their structure and care delivery platform.

CHAPTER 15

Intermountain Healthcare: An Evolving Integrated Delivery System

Jon Burroughs

INTERMOUNTAIN HEALTHCARE (SALT Lake City, Utah) is an example of a healthcare system that decided early in its history to develop an integrated clinical delivery system going far beyond what a stand-alone hospital delivery system could do. It was established as a secular not-for-profit entity in 1975, when the Church of Jesus Christ of Latter-day Saints (LDS) donated its 15 community-based hospitals in the hopes of developing them into a world-class healthcare system. Over the next 40 years, Intermountain grew to a $6.9 billion system with 22 hospitals; 180 clinics; 3,500 total affiliated physicians; a medical group with more than 1,600 employed physicians and advanced-practice practitioners; and SelectHealth, a not-for-profit health plan subsidiary that covers more than 850,000 people. One of the things that sets Intermountain Healthcare apart is its integration of technology with advanced clinical and business analytics. These analytics are supported by the largest healthcare-based enterprise data warehouse (EDW) in the world, which integrates evidence-based clinical decision-making with the business of providing cost-effective care. This chapter takes an in-depth look at this unique organization and its component operational building blocks as an example of how healthcare systems throughout the country can move toward a more integrated delivery model and successfully compete in an increasingly pay-for-value world.

EARLY AND CURRENT VISION

Intermountain Healthcare's "secret sauce" is its strong corporate support for visionaries who were not content with how healthcare was delivered (and consumed) in the United States. The original mission was to grow by becoming better, not bigger. The organization recognized early that clinical integration was the key, so initial efforts focused on integrating the disparate hospital organizations through unified quality assurance, standardized policies and procedures, and an integrated and unified management process.

By 1985, the organization's internal preferred provider organization (PPO) and health maintenance organization (HMO) were breaking even. It shifted its attention to unifying and integrating the organized medical staffs with standardized bylaws, policies and procedures (e.g., credentialing, privileging, peer review), and quality metrics. At that time, the hospitals began integrating through the merger of various governing boards into regional boards overseeing facilities in defined geographic regions.

In 1994, the Intermountain Physician Task Force led to the creation of the Intermountain Physician Group, which encouraged local and regional physicians to begin to work together toward common clinical and quality goals. This cooperation enabled the creation of clinical programs that work together to standardize evidence-based practices.

There are currently 10 clinical programs supported by 13 clinical services (e.g., lab, imaging), each of which has its own specialized clinical and operational projects and goals. This basis has led to Intermountain's current mission to help people live the healthiest lives possible, to continue to refine its clinical integration, and to focus on population health.

The entire system is overseen by a corporate board made up of approximately 24 members, including the system CEO; the CEO of the medical group; and a large number of physicians who develop and approve systemwide goals and strategy for quality and service, finance, and operations. There are 31 additional boards; 16 are associated with hospitals and hospital regions, with the remainder pertaining to the medical group; community care foundation; and SelectHealth, the subsidiary health plan. The Intermountain Community Care Foundation provides grants to more than 35 community clinics that serve as safety net organizations, and the Intermountain Healthcare Foundation draws revenue from its capital campaigns and community-wide fund-raising to serve the organization's mission throughout Utah, Idaho, and beyond. To ensure a strong clinical perspective and focus, approximately one-third of the 470 trustees throughout the system are members of the healthcare professions.

One of Intermountain's early leaders, Homer Warner, MD, served as a cardiologist and is considered by many to be the father of medical informatics. He collaborated with colleagues at LDS Hospital and the University of Utah on building one of the first electronic medical records in the 1960s, and he envisioned the future digitization of healthcare. He saw technology as a means to integrate clinical decision-making in a seamless way and not merely as an end in itself. He predicted the growing use of telehealth to connect caregivers with patients throughout the region and the globe.

Dr. Warner also foresaw the evolving roles of healthcare practitioners in the next century and was heard by many to state that "a physician should never do what an advance practice practitioner can do who should never do what a nurse can do who should never do what a technologist can do who should never do what a clerical person can do." This attitude set the stage for a more team-based approach to healthcare, which was virtually unknown at that time, with the assignment of specific roles based on training and expertise.

Early leaders saw the value of a vertically integrated insurance product to eliminate the nonvalue overhead cost of external insurance providers and align insurance-based incentives to drive evidence-based clinical outcomes. SelectHealth was established in 1982, and from its inception, it focused on health promotion and a strong connection with the marketplace.

Brent James, MD, Intermountain's former chief quality officer, was one of its early visionaries. He believed strongly in reducing non-value-added clinical variation by integrating evidence-based practices into the clinicians' routine work to the greatest extent possible. Since the early 1980s, when he and pulmonologist Dr. Alan Morris worked with physicians to dramatically reduce the mortality rate of acute respiratory distress syndrome (ARDS), physicians have continued to work with Intermountain clinicians to create standardized approaches to more than 70 clinical conditions. These approaches are based on review of the literature, with continuous follow-up adjustments as initial results are generated, in an effort to optimize quality and reduce costs. Since the early ARDS success, these initiatives have, to name a few improvements, cut adverse drug events in half, cut mortality rate for pneumonia by more than 40 percent, reduced admissions to the neonatal intensive care unit, dropped elective inductions of pregnancy prior to 39 weeks' gestation from 30 percent to 2 percent, and cut the mortality rate for coronary artery bypass graft surgery in half. Although these quality initiatives have saved thousands of lives over the years, they have cost Intermountain Healthcare millions of dollars as a result of the perverse incentives of fee-for-service reimbursement!

To operationalize its quality methodology, Intermountain created its Advanced Training Program (ATP), a 20-day course for clinical executives and quality improvement leaders that provides instruction in basic and advanced quality methods. The ATP highlights the Intermountain integrated-quality approach with examples of past successes and opportunities to participate in ongoing projects. Many graduates have gone on to pioneer programs of their own throughout the country, and beyond, that demonstrate similarly impressive results. The ATP includes the following major topics:

- Guideline and protocol development and implementation
- Outcome measurement
- Health services research methods
- Health policy and economics
- Cost-based accounting
- Medical informatics
- Severity-of-illness measurement and application
- Total quality management and continuous quality improvement theory and methods for healthcare
- Teams and teamwork

Every ATP participant is required to complete a quality improvement project and is assisted by a quality analyst throughout the duration of the program, an integral part of the learning that enables graduates to continue their projects outside of the classroom and make a difference in their various clinical settings. Intermountain also conducts an annual ATP Alumni Conference for graduates of the program to discuss their current projects and to share best-practice innovations they have discovered to improve clinical outcomes so that ongoing learning can be disseminated throughout the organization.

REORGANIZED STRUCTURE

In October 2017, Intermountain Healthcare announced a new internal structure to serve patients and communities better. In place of its current geographically defined administrative regions, the organization is creating a new systemwide structure with two main groups: the Community Care Group and the Specialty Care Group.

The Community Care Group focuses on keeping people well through prevention and excellent primary care—for example, ensuring people get the health screenings and immunizations they should have, helping them manage chronic diseases such as diabetes, and providing them with outpatient treatments for relatively minor medical needs. The Specialty Care Group is focused on specialist and hospital inpatient care, delivering the right care in the right way at the right time.

Intermountain's new internal structure is based on how patients use health and healthcare services and reflects new communication tools and processes that allow for faster and more direct contact among patients, caregivers, and organization leaders. The new alignment creates more value for those the organization serves, including the underserved, to whom charity care is provided in times of need.

This change is part of the ongoing innovation at Intermountain, and it is being undertaken from a position of strength. Intermountain has made many similar bold moves over the years: creating an insurance company (SelectHealth), forming a medical group with about 1,500 employed physicians, and developing world-class clinical programs—all working together to help people live the healthiest lives possible. Innovations such as these have contributed to Intermountain becoming a recognized leader and one of the world's most respected healthcare institutions.

Intermountain expects that its new internal structure will result in more consistently excellent patient experiences, whether at hospitals, clinics, other venues, or online. The changes will help the organization continue to provide the highest-quality care at the lowest sustainable cost.

PHYSICIAN ENGAGEMENT AND ALIGNMENT

Any healthcare executive will tell you that *engagement* (defined as a sense of ownership and often confused with morale) and *alignment* (defined as overlapping self-interests among clinical, operational, and organizational goals and values) are necessary to any high-performing organization, and Intermountain Healthcare is no exception. From its advent, physicians have been considered to be strategic partners working alongside the executive team and management in all significant clinical and business endeavors. The organization does not focus on the traditional pluralistic model, asking whether a physician is employed or self-employed, but rather expects every physician to be aligned in partnership with Intermountain whether they choose to be employed or not. It has a centralized credentials verification organization (CVO) for the system, and each affiliate physician is required to be credentialed through at least one of its facilities. The CVO performs delegated credentialing on behalf of SelectHealth and other health plans and payers that partner with the organization. Every physician agrees to certain nonnegotiables to be part of the organization. These requirements are memorialized through the professional provider participation agreement with SelectHealth. Some of the most important of the 18 commitments the agreement contains are discussed in the following sections: accept responsibility for performance, share performance data, provide equal access for all patients, and disclose all conflicts of interest.

Accept Responsibility for Performance

Intermountain-affiliated physicians must accept responsibility for their performance on quality, patient engagement, and cost measures. This acceptance includes both a commitment to excellence and a willingness to participate in financial rewards (or penalties) based on performance.

Moreover, physicians must comply with evidence-based clinical standards and business best practices as defined by Intermountain. The provider must contribute to a culture of continuous shared learning and improvement by participating in the development and adoption of these standards and practices and by identifying ways they can be improved.

Share Performance Data

Most high-performing organizations recognize that data and analytics transparency drive improved performance as a result of the Hawthorne effect (the powerful impact that knowing one's performance is observed has on actual performance). Thus, all physicians, clinicians, and managers must agree to unblinded reporting of all relevant clinical, operational, and financial data and analytics throughout the organization. Again, this requirement reflects the understanding that the industry as a whole is moving toward the same level of transparency through publicly reported data (e.g., Healthgrades, ProPublica, Leapfrog safety scores, Hospital Compare, Physician Compare), and thus the organization must do so as well.

Provide Equal Access for All Patients

Intermountain-affiliated physicians must provide equal access, including reasonable access for uninsured patients. They should demonstrate an interest in population health management as well as the ability to manage the health of a patient population. They must participate in relevant local value-improvement projects as applicable.

Value Analysis

Most larger healthcare organizations currently have a value analysis committee made up of physician and executive leaders to make systemwide decisions about adopting new technologies and clinical paradigms and choosing vendor relationships. Waste in the supply chain, as well as the inappropriate use of new technologies and paradigms, can be a significant driver of non-value-added costs and can undermine optimal clinical outcomes. Thus, Intermountain considers its value analysis process to be foundational in linking physicians and executives to make decisions that have a significant impact on quality and cost.

Disclose All Conflicts of Interest

Many physicians and executives have legacy relationships with healthcare suppliers and vendors that can have a significant impact on clinical decision-making. Thus, the organization takes the integrity of clinical and operational decision-making very seriously and requires all clinicians and managers to disclose all potential conflicts of interest (similar to federal sunshine laws). Once they do, deliberative clinical and operational bodies can determine whether they are significant from an organizational perspective. Everyone is expected to comply with the recommendations and requirements of these bodies if they wish to work in the system.

INTERMOUNTAIN MEDICAL GROUP

Founded in 1994, the Intermountain Medical Group is the large multidisciplinary organizational arm in the system through which physicians may seek employment. No requirement exists for employment in any given specialty, as all physicians must sign an agreement with SelectHealth and Intermountain that includes key nonnegotiables, including those listed earlier; thus, all physicians are considered aligned with the fundamental goals, objectives, and values of the organization. There are more than 1,400 physicians in the physician group, which makes up less than half of all affiliated physicians throughout the system. Care for everyone is payer blind, so that they experience no variation or inadvertent adverse impact on clinical decision-making. In fact, Intermountain Healthcare has a financial assistance policy that provides means-tested support for hospitalized patients whose income falls within 500 percent of the federal poverty level. It maintains a similar policy for those treated in the clinic setting, provided that they fall within 300 percent of the federal poverty level. A significant number of medical directors are given 20 percent allotted time for administrative duties and meetings as a part of their compensation models, and they have negotiated key performance indicators (KPIs) that are a part of their at-risk percentage. The culture of physician leadership is strong. Physicians take great pride in their strong national brand as well their efforts to raise the bar to sustain that brand. In addition, with the growing at-risk features of every compensation model, physicians who cannot (or will not) meet organizational expectations, as determined by both physicians and management, do not stay in the system very long. The organization understands that the at-risk component of all clinical contracts will increase to mirror the national trend, and it continually works toward that goal.

To support physicians and their ability to produce optimal outcomes, the organization launched a comprehensive physician well-being program in 2002 to promote physician and practitioner health, consistent with The Joint Commission standards. Ongoing survey scores that track morale, cohesiveness, collegiality, adaptability, expression of opinion, and ability to get things done are high, and everyone feels that this program is an investment that reaps immediate rewards.

CLINICAL PROCESS IMPROVEMENT INITIATIVES

One of the key differentiators of Intermountain Healthcare is its widespread adoption and active use of process improvement techniques, which deliver continuous quality improvement for both of its clinical and business outcomes. Its Institute for Healthcare Delivery Research prioritizes systemwide quality, safety, and service needs and goals through the creation of strategic, operating, and quality plans. These plans are generated by total quality management research and educational plans to facilitate governance and operating board discussions of quality priorities. The institute also initiates programs throughout the system to disseminate quality improvement techniques and to advance key quality improvement projects.

To coordinate this effort, the organization created governing and operating councils to oversee and coordinate specific geographic regions, ensuring that clinical and business information and intelligence are spread effectively throughout the system (though this is currently being restricted to provide more efficiencies and value to patients). Such governing and operating bodies include the following:

- *Guidance Council.* At the corporate level, it disseminates systemwide quality, operational, and financial goals and objectives and holds regional operating councils accountable.
- *Regional operating councils.* In each defined geographic region, the councils ensure that regional quality, operational, and financial goals and objectives are being met.
- *Value analysis committees.* These communities create an interdisciplinary process to determine the introduction, dissemination, or continued use of clinical, technological, operational, or business paradigms; make major vendor decisions; and evaluate the cost-effectiveness and safety of major initiatives.

Every geographic region and clinical unit performs an annual inventory of the more than 1,440 clinical conditions treated throughout the population health continuum. These conditions are prioritized based on volume, cost, and variability in order to identify the items of top importance. In 2016, clinicians and managers found that 62 hospital-based and 42 ambulatory conditions were responsible for 95 percent of total resources and outcomes. This discovery determined which conditions should be prioritized as a process improvement focus. One of the benefits of having such a sophisticated health information management (HIM) infrastructure is that these process improvement teams have ongoing access to more than 58 data registries. These registries provide predictive analytics and point-of-contact data capture that enable the analysis of specific conditions and processes.

The 104 clinical conditions that constitute Intermountain's top priorities have been sorted by the organization into the following ten clinical programs:

- Cardiovascular care
- Neurological sciences
- Musculoskeletal services
- Surgical specialties
- Women's and newborn services
- Intensive medicine
- Intensive pediatrics
- Intensive behavioral health care
- Oncology
- Primary care

All of these clinical programs have access to telehealth services such as telepharmacy, tele-intensive care unit (ICU), and e-health for lower-acuity care. These services are fully integrated into the electronic data and analytics infrastructure to provide real-time information regarding the outcomes and costs of services.

Within these 10 clinical programs are 60 clinical development teams. They assume ownership of one or more care processes and are made up of a team of specialists qualified to recommend evidence-based approaches to high-risk, high-variability, high-volume processes. The key is to blend algorithms into the workflow to ensure a seamless and less complex process, supporting the recommended clinical procedures. This is supported by clinical decision support software through Intermountain's electronic health record (EHR) vendor, Cerner, along with IBM pattern-matching software. This software has decision alerts and Bayesian sorting that create a hierarchy of decision support elements in a prioritized way, ensuring that the highest-impact clinical decisions come first. As a result of the variation found in the ambulatory setting, where there tends to be less oversight and greater autonomy, there are now more than 14 development teams in primary care reporting directly to the Guidance Council to reduce non-value-added variation, improve quality, and reduce costs. All clinical teams are led by physicians and comprise advanced-practice practitioners, care management nurses, social workers, psychologists, and executive facilitators who work together to create and operationalize pathways that are, in turn, tracked electronically.

Throughout the organization, all pathways are modified monthly (based on major events such as new information, new products and services, or unexpected adverse outcomes that reflect a less-than-optimal clinical process). Each protocol or pathway is disseminated throughout the system so that there are no duplicative, redundant, or contradictory clinical processes anywhere in the system. All clinical processes are monitored and tracked from an operational and financial perspective to ensure sustainability and improvement.

Projects are classified according to whether they have a potential immediate impact on organizational performance (type 1) or whether they are important from a research and academic perspective (type 2). Many published articles originate from these projects, and all clinicians and managers receive credit for this work. Projects are also categorized by whether they pertain to clinical support services, service quality and engagement, administration (e.g., information technology, operations), and aligned financial incentives (shared accountability).

A prime example of such a recent improvement initiative and its clinical and financial impact is Intermountain Healthcare's work with patients with severe sepsis and septic shock. As most clinicians and clinical managers know, this single diagnostic entity is responsible for approximately 10 percent of all ICU admissions and 30 percent of all ICU deaths, and it carries a mortality rate nationally of approximately 20 percent, with a national annualized hospital cost of almost $30 billion. To address such a pervasive issue, the clinical team assigned to the project performed the following steps:

- Confirmed that the treatment of sepsis was a high-priority, high-volume, high-cost, and high-risk process
- Built a cross-functional (i.e., interdisciplinary) team to own and manage the process throughout the organization
- Drew a conceptual model with a map of the process from clinical, operational, and financial perspectives
- Developed a series of statements of aim to articulate specific and measurable clinical, operational, and financial objectives for the project
- Built a data dashboard system (including a data definitions and specification manual) to collect, interpret, and report progress data throughout the system
- Aligned incentives (at-risk contracts and incentivized quality metrics) to drive continuous performance improvement

The clinical team's statement of aim for this project became, "To institutionalize a system for screening patients for potential sepsis who present in the emergency department." The initial goal was to appropriately screen 75 percent of all patients who were eventually diagnosed with sepsis, and the stretch goal was 90 percent. The implementation team members consisted of five physicians, a nurse, a phlebotomist, an administrator, and a research assistant.

To analyze every step from clinical, operational, and financial perspectives, the team drew up workflow and swim lane process maps for this screening process. A workflow process map looks at every step in a process, whereas a swim lane process map illustrates which steps are controlled by which roles (e.g., physician, nurse, phlebotomist, registrar).

A sepsis screening tool was designed to help identify patients who may have sepsis, and an 11-step sepsis bundle was developed to create a clinical and operational algorithm that all relevant clinicians and support services agreed to follow and that became mandatory throughout the system. The bundle included two steps: (1)

the resuscitation phase and (2) the maintenance phase. Once the pathway was introduced and implemented, clinical, operational, and financial metrics were followed to determine the impact of this new process on clinical and business outcomes.

The bundle and the measurement and reporting system led to an early observation that variation in antibiotic use was an issue. Therefore, specialized efforts were made to ensure that antibiotics could be standardized throughout the system by prepackaging them with standardized order sets and decision alerts to ensure compliance. The 21 emergency departments (EDs) throughout the Intermountain system did additional work to identify improvement opportunities in their own environments, tested those ideas, and shared them with the rest of the system when appropriate.

Over a six-year period, the mortality rate for sepsis and septic shock dropped by more than 50 percent—from 21.2 percent to 9 percent—with an average of 100 more lives saved annually. The bundle also resulted in shorter lengths of stay and a total cost savings of 15–20 percent per case.

Thanks to ingrained professional habits and processes, this project was not easy—optimal adherence took several years to achieve. Even so, compliance drove mortality and costs down, while key learnings from this project spilled over to other critical care and high-cost, high-risk clinical entities, such as ARDS and pulmonary failure.

Intermountain Healthcare participated in the creation of the High-Value Healthcare Collaborative in conjunction with the Harvard Medical School, which brought together 13 delivery systems to share data on joint quality improvement projects. Intermountain's contribution included the sepsis project in addition to projects such as hip and knee replacement, diabetes, congestive heart failure, spinal surgery, and the optimization of operating room times and lengths of stay as well as other strategic quality initiatives. Through this collaborative process, a data mart brings together all of the clinical data throughout the enterprise to focus on specific challenges.

MENTAL HEALTH INTEGRATION

Mental health care is considered essential for every clinical area and is a required component of Intermountain Healthcare's population health approach. Former surgeon general David Satcher, MD, defined mental health as "a state of successful performance of mental and physical functioning resulting in productive activities, fulfilling relationships with others, and the ability to adapt to change and cope with adversity" (Satcher 2000). All clinical areas focus on moving interventions further upstream to address the root causes of disease. For instance, in cardiovascular disease, the most important risk factors are smoking and obesity. Both of these often result from people self-medicating for depression, anxiety, bipolar disorder, or posttraumatic stress disorder. Failure to address the root causes of smoking and obesity only leads to an endless cycle of recurrence and return to old habits, which defeats the organization's investment.

The Intermountain Healthcare Mental Health Integration (MHI) program is blended into all primary care practices and specialty care. It enacts a team-based approach to behavioral health that draws on the resources and best practice recommendations of the National Alliance on Mental Illness, the nation's largest grassroots advocacy organization for mental health.

The team includes a variety of members. First, of course, are patients and their families, who are empowered to lead most of the behavioral health initiatives. The primary care provider who initiates the mental health process on behalf of her patient is also included, as is the mental health integration coordinator, who facilitates the process, supports operational logistics, enters data into the EHR, and coordinates the team. A care manager, a health advocate, and a care guide provide support through coordination between the healthcare team, the patient, and his family; track and measure clinical progress; and report findings to the team. Each team also includes a mental health specialist, who is a licensed mental health practitioner such as a psychiatrist, psychiatric social worker, psychologist, or psychiatric nurse practitioner. This specialist provides clinical and technical support for the team and works with the primary care provider and staff to clarify the clinical diagnosis, create a differential diagnosis, and develop a holistic care plan and treatment options that match the patient's and family's identified health concerns.

The team works together to create specific and measurable clinical goals and objectives that are tracked against operational and business outcomes, such as variable cost and total cost per case, to ensure that interventions are effective and sustainable. For instance, MHI teams discovered that addressing depression effectively reduces unnecessary ED visits and crisis interventions by more than 50 percent.

The MHI teams go through a multistage process when they initiate care at the recommendation of a primary care practitioner:

- *Level 1 (potential care).* The initial operational team members review the complexity of a defined patient population; potential barriers to implementation; information workflow design necessary to track and measure progress; format for an MHI scorecard or dashboard to follow progress over time; and cost variables, including ED and physician visits, crisis interventions, and so on. Then they identify resources (including personnel) required.
- *Level 2 (adoption).* The team is assembled and the clinical and operational workflow process is designed by team members and then tracked through an MHI scorecard or dashboard. Clinical and business goals are established (e.g., reduce symptomatology, decrease ED visits and readmissions).
- *Level 3 (routinization).* Deployment is monitored, discussed, and modified over time, with clinical and operational workflow used and routinized, while metrics are modified and stretch goals are developed once initial goals are obtained.

The hard work of the MHI teams has lead to a number of key learnings, summarized in exhibit 15.1.

Once baseline mental and physical health information is completed, the primary care practitioner performs a baseline evaluation and physical examination to determine potential physical and somatic components of the issues raised. Initial assessments are divided into mild, moderate, and high categories of complexity. Those with mild complexity receive routine care with their primary care practitioners, who use the MHI guidelines and the care manager

Exhibit 15.1: Intermountain Healthcare Mental Health Integration Program: Key Learnings

Timeliness of interventions: The longer the gap between crisis and initial intervention, the more significant the crisis becomes, increasing the cost and complexity of later interventions.

Suicide screenings: All participants receive screening for suicidal thoughts to ensure that risks are not missed, particularly among individuals with more subtle or complex presentations.

Consistent and ongoing measurement: Results and patterns in people's lives often emerge that are unexpected and significant, which need to be addressed in a timely way by the MHI team.

Specific focus on children and adolescents: Younger patients are often overlooked, and they require their own unique approach to behavioral management. Children are challenging because they often cannot verbalize feelings and concerns; adolescents are challenging because they seek privacy and often require a more customized and nuanced approach.

Mental health assessments: All people undergo a standardized process to evaluate the complexity of their health concerns and the appropriateness of their participation in the program and to ensure that team resources can focus on areas that will provide the optimal health benefit.

or health advocate on an as-needed basis. Patients with moderate complexity work with a primary care practitioner, care manager or health advocate, and a mental health specialist (e.g., psychiatrist, psychiatric nurse practitioner) and use the MHI team to clarify the diagnosis, focus on treatment options, and monitor their condition over time. People with high complexity work with a primary care practitioner and a care manager or health advocate, and they maintain direct and regular contact with a mental health specialist. This specialist works directly with patients' families to assess and stabilize the patients' immediate environment. These individuals may also require specialized inpatient and outpatient assessments and treatment.

MHI packets contain assessment tools and materials to help MHI teams and their patients and families to understand the complexity of their health concerns and find the right level of team-based care. For adults, the packets contain materials such as a baseline evaluation cover letter, an initial history and consultation, a family rating scale, a patient health questionnaire, anxiety and stress disorder ratings, a mood disorder questionnaire, and an adult attention deficit hyperactivity disorder (ADHD) symptom checklist. The packets for children and adolescents contain items such as a baseline evaluation cover letter, an initial history and consultation, parental screen and family rating scale, Vanderbilt ADHD parent and teacher ratings, a patient health questionnaire, anxiety and stress disorder ratings, development disorder symptom ratings, a parent–young mania rating scale, home and school impairment scales, and a cover letter for schools.

The results of all of these assessments and tools are tracked over time, in conjunction with both clinical and operational results, to ensure that the interventions are both efficient and cost-effective. Intermountain Healthcare feels that the MHI has given it the greatest return on investment in its efforts to optimize healthcare outcomes for people with more complex, difficult-to-manage conditions.

HEALTH INFORMATION MANAGEMENT INFRASTRUCTURE TO SUPPORT CLINICAL INTEGRATION

None of the clinical initiatives discussed thus far would be possible without Intermountain Healthcare's sophisticated HIM infrastructure. The following section describes the practical application of this essential infrastructure as it translates infinite data sets into actionable, role-based clinical and business information that supports clinical integration at all levels of the organization.

Data come from a variety of sources, including the following:

- Clinical information from the evaluation of patients both inside and outside the system
- Claims data from billing and coding documentation, based on patient encounters
- Information from diagnostic and therapeutic tools, such as pacemakers, electrocardiograms, electroencephalography, pacemaker defibrillators, and implantable devices
- Financial information, such as cost of care, diagnosis-related group (DRG), length of stay, and case-mix index
- Patient satisfaction information, such as Hospital Consumer Assessment of Healthcare Providers and Systems scores and Press Ganey scores
- Unstructured data, the most significant of which are the nonclinical determinants of care such as demographic information, DNA, RNA, genomics, zip code, education, lifestyle, socioeconomic information (income), and so on

The data are fed into Intermountain Healthcare's EDW, which is the largest repository of healthcare data in the world. Through a process called *extraction, transfer, and loading*, along with data integration and modeling, difficult-to-interpret data are turned into information that can be organized into role-based dashboards or scorecards.

Overarching decisions about this data conversion are made by a data governance committee comprising physicians, healthcare administrators, and HIM experts who develop policies regarding various aspects of data, including management, life cycle, security, privacy, integrity, credibility, and access. Decisions are made about which individuals (including patients) in which roles receive which information. Thus, the dashboards and scorecards are distributed to operational and clinical units (including a patient portal) so that managers and clinicians can access information in real time that will optimize quality and minimize costs.

Further refinement of this information is performed by an adaptive data warehouse that takes interrelated information about a specific clinical condition or operational process and analyzes the information to seek meaningful patterns across the continuum of care. For instance, this process may be used to report any of the following:

- Clinical outcomes or time-driven, activity-based costs for a clinical condition across the continuum of care; this may involve combining analytics from multiple collaborating organizations that may or may not be a part of Intermountain Healthcare
- Statewide or regionwide healthcare outcomes and costs for a specific clinical condition (e.g., diabetes) or a group of interrelated diseases (e.g., infectious diseases)
- Contribution margin and net income calculations for the healthcare system for a given DRG, health plan, or payer contract
- Identification of specific variables related to readmission rate, ED utilization, or morbidity and mortality indexes
- Customized health maintenance profiles, with decision-support tools for individual patients, through patient portals

- Predictive analytics based on the collation of beneficiary registries to determine which people are at the greatest risk

Role-based analytics for each member of the organization support distributive accountability that enables individuals responsible for a clinical or operational unit to take responsibility for driving key performance outcomes. Private employers and health plans increasingly use the same analytics to incentivize beneficiary engagement through decreased premiums, deductibles, and copays in much the same way.

Outcomes from clinical and business intelligence enable the organization to make strategic decisions regarding the relative success (or not) of the following:

- Clinical programs and algorithms
- Operational improvement initiatives
- Cost-reducing measures
- Business plans and pilot programs
- Payer contracts
- Contractual incentives
- Collaborative business and clinical relationships
- Outsourcing contracts
- Decisions to lease or buy
- Merger and acquisition decisions

Disease management (as the sepsis bundle discussed earlier) is a more complex process, as most patients present with multiple comorbidities and behavioral issues juxtaposed with the primary clinical diagnosis. In addition, most people are covered by commercial or public payers that are interested in specific metrics pertaining to the management of the beneficiary's total healthcare outcomes and costs. Thus, the HIM infrastructure is applied according to the following steps:

1. Contracting analytics are compiled based on all KPIs generated by the payer and the healthcare system.

These analytics include clinical, claims, financial, and nonclinical determinant data that affect clinical and margin outcomes.

2. Population health data are separated into clinical and business intelligence on an individual (beneficiary) basis to adjust the information by risk and severity on a per member per month basis.

3. Risk- and severity-adjusted individual analytics are given a final score based on risk- and severity-adjusted categories (e.g., Medicare's hierarchical condition categories), and specific components of care are attributed to specific payers, health plans, and healthcare providers and organizations for assignment to care management teams.

4. Appropriate healthcare pathways or algorithms are assigned to each person based on a comprehensive list of his diseases and comorbidities.

5. Care pathways or algorithms determine which care modules or teams are assigned management of the patient. For instance, this step determines which patients receive behavioral health support, as discussed previously, and at what level those resources are delegated.

6. Patients are assigned a specific geographic region within Intermountain Healthcare based on the patient's demographics, specific resources that are required, and whether that geographic region has the scope of services necessary to support the requisite care.

7. Dashboards and scorecards are developed for each patient to track specific clinical, financial, utilization, compliance, and service metrics, and a variation analysis is performed to compare outcomes with standards benchmarked nationally.

8. Care pathways, clinical modules or programs, operational processes, and payer contracts are modified on an ongoing basis based on clinical and business intelligence findings.

Intermountain Healthcare uses predictive analytics in its primary care practices based on the creation of criteria for participation and risk- and severity-adjustment ratings. Patient-level data are collected, including demographics, biometrics, behaviors, medications, allergies, and contraindications to medications. This information is collated with payer- or health plan–related data that include, for example, morbidity and mortality indexes, cost index, and overall risk based on the patient's risk-stratification score.

From these data, a risk- and severity-adjusted score is developed to prioritize appointments, delegate resources, and assign practitioners based on the level of care needed. This degree of granularity throughout a large, complex system is difficult, if not impossible, to achieve without a robust HIM infrastructure—which is why the electronic tools described earlier are necessary to drive top-decile clinical and operational performance and qualify a healthcare system for premium payment.

EVIDENCE-BASED MANAGEMENT: AUTOMATING THE SYSTEMWIDE SUPPLY CHAIN

Every healthcare organization's supply chain has posed has many long-standing challenges, including high logistics costs, high cost of professional preference items, lack of collaboration between management and physicians, and lack of good real-time analytics. Supply chain costs vary from 13 to 27 percent of total operating revenues throughout the country, and Intermountain realized that mastering this operational variation was one of the keys to providing cost-effective healthcare services. The initiative started in 2005 with a comprehensive assessment by McKinsey that led to significant organizational changes intended to improve supply costs. A chief procurement officer position was created on the supply chain management team, with consolidation of its warehouses reporting to a systemwide supply chain and operations organization. This new configuration combined the following operational components into a seamless system:

- Choosing and developing strategic relationships with suppliers and vendors
- Developing process improvement techniques to reduce costs, improve service, and reduce inventories
- Sourcing materials, components, technologies, and services
- Managing logistics, warehouses, parts, and distribution inventories
- Managing internal operations and providing an interface between customers, suppliers, and distributors
- Managing quality through the use of Lean and Six Sigma techniques
- Continuing to streamline the supply chain process to optimize service, quality, and cost structure

Several years later, the system went through Lean and Six Sigma processes to eliminate waste and to streamline and standardize operations to enable digital tracking. Requisitioning transitioned to the web (the precursor to cloud-based monitoring), and the supply chain was simplified by reducing the number of vendors and physician-specific requests while making the remaining relationships more strategic and mutually beneficial. The initial savings were enormous, and each sourcing manager overseeing an area of specialization drove $1.5 million annually in savings, with a return on investment of approximately 10:1.

Recently, the supply chain is taking steps toward integrating into Intermountain's EHR so that supply chain choices and costs can be tracked in real time, with feedback to ordering physicians to further standardize preference items and vendors. A procurement steering committee made up of clinicians, supply chain managers, and executives provides governance and oversight of the supply chain process.

Because the value analysis process is conducted for affiliate physicians and managers throughout the system, capital and supply chain costs can be accurately budgeted, tracked, and managed through analytics and decision support tools. Thus, producers of supplies may interface directly with the supplier network that inventories and distributes supplies. In turn, the network may collaborate with the supply chain optimization process, which is connected with the clinical care network and finally to patients, making a seamless transition to and from the patient through the supply chain system.

Intermountain Healthcare's supply chain system currently constitutes a $2 billion annual cost, and its recent improvement efforts have resulted in not only savings of more than $700 million over the past ten years but also, more important, a complete incorporation of this essential operational support service and the organization's clinical integration efforts.

TELEHEALTH THROUGHOUT THE SYSTEM

Telehealth is an essential component of Intermountain's system, linking it to providers, facilities, business partners, payers, and consumers to ensure aligned and coordinated services. It is considered complementary to existing urgent care, consultations, emergency, cardiology care, stroke, and critical care services, and it helps business partners support employee health plans and population health. It presents the opportunity to provide value-added services where they previously could not exist. The following sections include some of the many ways in which telehealth is used.

Behavioral Health

Utah and Idaho are both rural states with many people hundreds of miles from behavioral health services. Behavioral health specialists can provide round-the-clock crisis intervention and psychiatric consultative services for both adults and children via smartphone, tablet, or personal computer. Such interventions result in either ongoing care or emergency transfers when necessary. Three-way consultations are possible that enable primary care physicians to participate and provide input based on their knowledge of the patient's family and of socioeconomic issues that may be important and relevant.

Stroke

Telehealth, which provides a direct connection with EDs and neurologists throughout the system, is essential to enabling potential stroke patients to receive thrombolytic therapy in a timely way. Many would not receive lifesaving treatment for acute ischemic stroke without the ability to consult with experts who are certified to determine whether thrombolytics are necessary and appropriate within the vital three- to four-hour period from onset of ischemic symptoms.

Cancer Care

The Centers for Disease Control and Prevention (CDC 2018a, 2018b) estimates 7,500 patients in Idaho and 11,000 patients in Utah will receive a cancer diagnosis every year. Many patients with cancer require ongoing chemotherapy and radiation treatments that necessitate logistically challenging travel and substantial expenditure of resources. Telehealth enables those living in rural or remote areas to directly connect to oncologists and other cancer-related specialists, enabling treatment at their local facilities through consultative services and evidence-based algorithms. Telehealth supports a more cost-effective approach to lengthy treatment that is often expensive, complex, and challenging.

Diabetes

Diabetes is now a chronic disease affecting more than 30 million Americans, and it requires an enormous amount of education, monitoring, and empowerment of patients to be successfully managed (CDC 2017). Telehealth enables diabetes educators to provide ongoing help to patients who are developing a deeper understanding of the managerial nuances of the disease and the many medications sometimes necessary to stabilize it. In addition, endocrinologists and other diabetes specialists can consult regarding the inevitable relapses and setbacks, which helps to minimize both risk and disruption in their patients' lives.

Language Services

Utah is home to a diverse population that includes native Spanish speakers and people who speak various Asian languages. Many of these individuals require translation services, particularly when a sudden illness or emergency strikes that requires adequate patient understanding and informed consent. Through telehealth platforms, translators are available around the clock, throughout the system, to support patients' and families' comprehension. Services of this type have been demonstrated to enhance compliance with evidence-based recommendations, which not only improves clinical outcomes but also lowers the overall cost of care.

Pediatrics

Given the paucity of pediatric subspecialists in rural areas, the treatment of children with chronic conditions can be problematic. Telehealth permits access to subspecialists at Primary Children's Hospital, particularly for chronic, complex, difficult-to-manage issues such as developmental disorders, chronic metabolic diseases, and postoperative care for major craniofacial surgeries. Specialists work directly with pediatricians, family physicians, and other primary care providers to ensure that patients and their families have ongoing access to specialized services to support a better outcome and optimized service.

Obstetric and Neonatal Care

Telehealth has proven essential for the care of pregnant women and their children in rural areas.

Genetic Counseling

Many women discover genetic abnormalities in themselves or their unborn children during pregnancy and require genetic counseling after diagnostic testing. This care can be difficult to access for those in remote areas; telehealth enables seamless communication between mothers, their primary practitioners, and regional specialists to develop diagnostic and therapeutic plans.

Lactation Support

For many women, lactating can be challenging, and telehealth brings lactation specialists into hospitals when one isn't available locally. Lactation may improve the health of infants and young children, and this service promotes the health of the child and the relationship between mother and child.

Newborn Critical Care

Many babies born prematurely require sophisticated specialized care for months, or even years, following their initial stabilization and treatment. This care is often multidisciplinary and requires numerous specialists participating and consulting in a team-based approach. Thus, telehealth provides an important link between tertiary and quaternary centers to ensure that babies continue to receive optimal care throughout the complete course of their recovery and development, even if they live miles from major pediatric centers.

Wound Care

Most wounds heal spontaneously; however, some complex wounds require ongoing specialty care and treatment that is challenging from remote and rural areas (e.g., hyperbaric therapy, ongoing debridement). Telehealth provides a platform for specialty consultation for both patients and their primary care providers, supporting ongoing management and care through evidence-based algorithms and protocols.

Simulation and Training to Improve Care

One of the more innovative applications of telehealth is its use in simulation to train clinicians, staff, and personnel to handle unexpected emergencies. The Intermountain Healthcare Simulation Learning Center is a sophisticated, 10,000-square-foot training facility located at LDS Hospital in Salt Lake City, with ten on-site and remote teaching laboratories scattered throughout Utah and southern Idaho. Telehealth is incorporated into simulation exercises through the display of vital signs, heart and fetal monitor tracings, and other clinical indicators so that clinicians can practice handling emergencies that may be life-threatening and require a correct immediate response.

The center provides a variety of simulation courses and exercises, ranging from basic to advanced and from general to specific. For example, it teaches a number of courses on basic workplace skills. Employees can learn how to use iCentra in an effort to help all clinicians and staff navigate the EHR and fully integrate the evidence-based algorithms, pathways, and clinical alerts embedded in the system. Workplace Violence is a three-hour de-escalation course for physicians, nurses, staff members, and managers, who will inevitably encounter workplace conflict that may rapidly escalate if not properly handled.

The center provides profession-specific training as well. Nurse residency embeds simulation as a routine part of its one-year program to support the smooth transition of nurses from nursing school to the clinical environment, reinforcing leadership skills and professional confidence. Nursing unit orientation incorporates simulation for every nursing unit to support rapid-cycle learning acquisition of the unique skills required on each clinical unit as a natural part of the orientation process. Operating Room Entry Orientation is a ten-week course that complements the training that operating room nurses learn in nursing school. It helps them learn the practical skills necessary to transition into busy operating environments following training.

Physicians benefit from the center's learning opportunities as well. Basic Aseptic Technique is a course that teaches surgical trainees proper approaches to working with surgical patients. Physician task training enables physicians to practice specific procedures and skills on mannequins, including central and arterial line placement, interosseous needle placement, lumbar puncture, managing difficult airways with advanced equipment, and chest tube or needle decompression of pneumothoraxes.

Leadership skills are taught as well. For example, crisis resource management techniques reinforce leadership approaches to disaster situations when clinical resources may be overwhelmed. A course titled Root Cause Analysis helps participants learn to prebrief, debrief, and analyze complex clinical situations, laying the foundation for leading and facilitating root cause analyses. This process is ideal for follow-up on unanticipated sentinel events throughout the system.

Connect Care: E-Health Visits for High-Volume, Low-Risk Care

Intermountain Healthcare also uses telehealth to provide visits for high-volume, low-risk conditions. Many other organizations, including Stanford University Hospital (California) and Sentara Healthcare (Virginia) provide a significant percentage of primary care visits through e-health platforms, and Intermountain felt that it was important to provide this lower-cost, easier-to-access alternative. A physician or advanced-practice clinician can be accessed within two minutes; conduct an examination via smartphone, tablet, personal computer, or employer-based kiosk; and provide a diagnosis and course of treatment in 10 to 15 minutes, all at a cost of approximately $59 per visit. The primary purpose of this modality is currently urgent care; however, Intermountain is working to use similar technology for specialty consultations, postoperative visits, home visits, and behavioral health management.

Intermountain feels that telehealth is the healthcare delivery model of the future. The organization is gearing up to enable evidence-based care throughout the system—and beyond—at a fraction of the cost.

SELECTHEALTH

SelectHealth, the insurance arm of Intermountain Healthcare, was established to reduce costs and to align incentives that lead to clearly defined healthcare outcomes. Population health was used to frame the approach so that incentives could be aligned around providing high-value care and engaging patients and families in making decisions about their health and care.

Most of SelectHealth's payer models involve some form of patient engagement through at-risk arrangements to incentivize healthy behaviors, good healthcare choices, and nonclinical determinants that have a significant impact on outcomes. For instance, the prepaid capitated Medicaid contract requires a small $5 copay for each visit to the ED to encourage other alternatives. SelectHealth also provides healthcare tools to support prevention, reminders for appointments or screening evaluations, and other steps in the complex healthcare process to support compliance. It helps people set up health savings accounts to enable each beneficiary to accumulate over time the financial resources necessary to cover deductible costs. SelectHealth also has a long-term strategic alliance with St. Luke's Health System (Idaho) to work together to achieve better health, better care, and lower costs for individuals and the communities served by the affiliation.

One of things that distinguishes SelectHealth is its provision of behavioral and mental health services in the majority of its health plans. Intermountain Healthcare has found that up to 50 percent of patients with a chronic disease have an undiagnosed or untreated behavioral issue (e.g., depression, anxiety, bipolar disorder, substance abuse), and more than 50 percent have unaddressed socioeconomic issues (e.g., low-quality housing, poor nutrition, exposure to pollutants or violence). One of the tenets of population health research is that acute clinical interventions and care account for less than 20 percent of the factors contributing to healthcare outcomes (see exhibit 15.2).

Thus, both SelectHealth and Intermountain require a behavioral health component in their disease management programs, and SelectHealth requires it in most of its health plans. Without addressing the underlying root cause of a healthcare issue, outcomes and costs are not significantly affected. For instance, the greatest risk factor for heart disease is smoking, and the primary reason for smoking is the self-medication of some form of mood or affective disorder such as depression, anxiety, or bipolar disorder.

In 2016, SelectHealth introduced a new health plan called SelectHealth Share, which was specifically designed to offer health plans to employers and employees with predictable and sustainable

Exhibit 15.2: Determinants of Health Outcomes

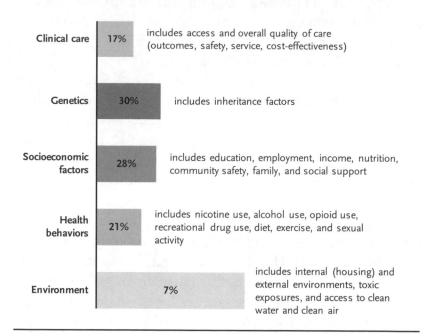

Clinical care — 17% — includes access and overall quality of care (outcomes, safety, service, cost-effectiveness)

Genetics — 30% — includes inheritance factors

Socioeconomic factors — 28% — includes education, employment, income, nutrition, community safety, family, and social support

Health behaviors — 21% — includes nicotine use, alcohol use, opioid use, recreational drug use, diet, exercise, and sexual activity

Environment — 7% — includes internal (housing) and external environments, toxic exposures, and access to clean water and clean air

insurance premiums over a three-year period. They are able to do that by partnering with Intermountain Healthcare's supply chain, population health, and quality improvement initiatives, designed to save more than $2 billion over a five-year period. A few examples of initiatives used to achieve these cost savings include the following:

- Standardizing and simplifying the supply chain through the elimination of non-value-added vendor relationships and supplies (e.g., one vendor per major product)
- Standardizing clinical pathways for high-cost, high-risk conditions such as sepsis, ARDS, neonatal care, and so on
- Creating interdisciplinary disease management programs for such issues as bowel surgery or surgical-site infections to standardize both clinical and operational processes

SelectHealth feels that its collaborations with leading health systems support the systems' ability to pass on clinical and operational cost savings. Its insurance products and services enable it to provide innovative health plans and improved healthcare outcomes at more affordable and sustainable costs.

CONCLUSION

In its formative years, Intermountain Healthcare envisioned clinical integration with a seamless connection between its clinical and business operations. This connection would be supported by an HIE with clinical and business analytics. Whereas most healthcare systems will evolve in other ways, Intermountain serves as an instructive example of how a clinically integrated delivery system committed to a population health approach can operate successfully, by focusing on improving healthcare outcomes while minimizing cost structure and waste. Complete engagement and alignment of physicians and operational leaders is key, as well as an organizational commitment to the values of customer service and excellence.

Clinical integration is a journey, and although nobody can conclusively predict what the future healthcare delivery model will be, the necessity of improving healthcare outcomes continuously, while reducing costs, requires a far more integrated and aligned healthcare delivery model than exists today. All healthcare organizations will be compelled to move in this direction if they are to survive.

REFERENCES

Centers for Disease Control and Prevention (CDC). 2018a. "Idaho vs. United States Comparisons." US Department of Health and Human Services. Accessed May 17. https://nccd.cdc.gov/statecancerfacts/Table.aspx?Group=5f&TableType=INCI&SelectedState=Idaho.

———. 2018b. "Utah." Accessed May 17. US Department of Health and Human Services. https://nccd.cdc.gov/statecancerfacts/state.aspx?state=Utah.

———. 2017. "New CDC Report: More Than 100 Million Americans Have Diabetes or Prediabetes." US Department of Health and Human Services. Published July 18. www.cdc.gov/media/releases/2017/p0718-diabetes-report.html.

Satcher, D. 2000. "Mental Health: A Report of the Surgeon General." *International Journal of Psychosocial Rehabilitation* 31 (1): 5–13.

Conclusion

Jon Burroughs

As the healthcare industry moves increasingly toward value-based payment (with an emphasis on health and well-being to prevent and mitigate illness, injury, and mental health disability), hospitals, physician practices, and other traditional business models will naturally evolve toward clinically integrated systems. These new systems will provide comprehensive healthcare services across the continuum of care and will rely decreasingly on external entities (e.g., payers, providers, health information management [HIM] support) to accomplish these goals. Other industries have already gone through the transformation of digitization, standardization, commoditization, and globalization; now it is up to healthcare, the most complex industry of all, to complete this necessary change.

Each chapter, written by various contributing authors, covered one operational facet of this new enterprise, and the recurrent themes discussed here are consistent throughout the book.

1. **Traditional stand-alone operational units must consolidate into systems that can provide comprehensive healthcare services across the continuum in a cost-effective way.**

    Traditional healthcare business models were built in the twentieth century to support the physician–patient relationship and the utilization of hospitals for significant mental or physical illness and injury. The emphasis was on

481

episodic care of acute conditions. With the exception of early childhood pediatrics and concierge practices for an affluent clientele, little emphasis was placed on prevention or on mitigating strategies—the traditional fee-for-service reimbursement model was based on acuity and severity of illness or injury, not on high-volume, low-acuity work.

To focus on health and the prevention of illness and injury in the twenty-first century, new, more comprehensive, more inclusive operational and business structures must be built that link the traditional physician practice and hospital to schools, long-term care facilities, home health providers, public health agencies, and other entities that affect the health and well-being of individuals. Systems must offer comprehensive services throughout the continuum, and they must be paid according to successful prevention and mitigation, instead of rewarding care for the most acute and complex illnesses and injuries through payment incentives.

Integrated networks must function as seamless entities, underpinned by a HIM infrastructure that will enable cloud-based information to be immediately accessible, reporting on real-time clinical and operational outcomes. Contracts with public and private payers, employers, and individuals will increasingly be made for payment on a per member per month or global budget basis. Significant incentives will drive improved outcomes at a fraction of the expense.

2. **Physicians, executives, and healthcare leaders must work together in partnership toward shared clinical and business strategic goals and objectives.**

In the traditional healthcare system, physicians, nurses, executives, and ambulatory healthcare leaders worked separately in their own professional silos, guarded by their professional associations, to protect their turf from incursions. Today, we must work in partnership to succeed or fail together. To generate improved outcomes, clinical and operational or financial expertise must be melded into seamless processes that enable a higher level of performance. The growing HIM infrastructure will reduce the need for physicians, nurses, and management; however, these professionals must be able to manage complex operational entities that require broad-based clinical and business or operational skills. The twenty-first-century healthcare enterprise will be distinguished by aligned arrangements, whereby healthcare leaders who are capable of managing significant organizational structures will be rewarded based on measured and mutually agreed-on outcomes. Therefore, traditional clinical and business roles will be melded into clinical executive roles that require both clinical and business acumen. Clinical executives will work in triads (physician, nurse, and operational executive) in an increasingly matrix-based structure made up of multiple partners, customers, and stakeholders, who will create shared accountability.

3. **A population health infrastructure (e.g., palliative care, disease management, post-acute care, retail medicine, e-health) is an essential foundation for managing the healthcare of people and populations across the continuum.**

In the twentieth century, regardless of whether an individual was sick or healthy, the physician's office and hospital were the major business models available to care for any healthcare issue. Population health is the twenty-first-century redistribution and rationalization of resources to optimally benefit subpopulations of covered lives who require significantly different levels of healthcare services. Those with life-threatening illnesses will receive palliative care services, those with chronic diseases will receive comprehensive disease management, those with minor acute problems will receive retail medicine, and the healthy majority will have a personalized healthcare plan and access to e-health. Thus, the vital few—the sickest people most in need of costly services—will receive the lion's share of the resources, while the healthy majority will be empowered to self-manage their healthcare with software and e-health support.

This system makes sense because it provides a return on investment for those with the greatest needs, the greatest risks, and the greatest costs while not spending significantly on those with the least need. In addition, population health focuses on nonclinical determinants (e.g., genetics, socioeconomic status, healthcare decisions, environmental factors) that have a profound impact on healthcare outcomes but had few dedicated resources in the past.

4. **A twenty-first-century HIM infrastructure is necessary to monitor clinical and business services across the continuum, producing real-time dashboards and decision support tools.**

HIM is a required foundation for any clinically integrated network. It provides all staff with role-based information in real time that can be used to manage and optimize clinical and business outcomes. Retrospective data are rapidly being replaced with concurrent and proactive analytics so that immediate interventions can be performed that will positively affect the quality and cost of care.

Thus, all organizations will require an enterprise data warehouse to convert disparate data into the actionable information that is essential for each clinician and manager who works to optimize care and cost. In addition, organizations must be linked through cloud-based services, which can share information globally by any authorized individual, to care for any person, anywhere on the globe, any time of day.

Predictive analytics will enable organizations and individuals to prioritize more effectively and to manage higher-risk patients who may need proactive strategies before their healthcare issues become both significant and expensive.

5. **Suppliers must realign their business models to focus on clinical and business outcomes that lower costs and support optimal clinical outcomes, not merely generate a return for stockholders and investors.**

Converting to a more capitated environment has been a lengthy process in the United States. One of the root causes of the delay is the vested interests of everyone (particularly suppliers) in generating profit margin through a volume-based business model. Thus, the business model for suppliers, physicians, and executives must be realigned to enable incentives and margins that are based on mutually agreed-on healthcare and business outcomes.

Unfortunately, as a result of the necessity of long-term investments, realignment takes time and requires systemic changes—in both the business entities themselves and the legal, regulatory, and accreditation framework that inadvertently inhibits or even blocks advancement. In addition, suppliers will need to invest in wireless technologies, analytics, and software that will support the growth and development of the new ambulatory care economy, which will be based on health and the prevention of illness, not the expansion of interventional acute care services.

6. **Disruptive innovation will continue to flourish, with significant investment and potential rewards for entrepreneurs who are willing to build the new healthcare infrastructure.**

New entrants will continue to challenge traditional ideas of how healthcare services may be profitably offered. E-health reduces the cost structure by almost 95 percent, and retail medicine can handle a significant amount of work traditionally managed in an emergency department or ambulatory office.

Therefore, healthcare organizations must be open to reinventing how care is imagined and delivered to ensure optimum outcomes at a minimum cost. In addition, consumers will increasingly migrate to innovative models that meet their busy lives, seeking out affordable options that provide necessary services that are sufficient for their needs.

Healthcare executives and physicians have sometimes been characterized as risk averse, and this tendency will not serve high-performing organizations that wish to innovate to succeed by writing new rules that support more cost-effective care. Thus, there is a renewed entrepreneurial spirit that requires innovative thinking and leadership to create business models that will support organizational success at a time of pent-up demand for affordable services.

7. **A new matrix management culture will evolve that relies on complete transparency, shared information, and trust to create aligned contracts that lead to optimal clinical and business outcomes.**

Traditional line authority has been replaced with matrix management structures that support collaboration, partnership, and a more complex and robust chain of accountability. Leaders will work interdependently while being empowered to achieve greater levels of self-management through the accessibility of actionable information with decision support alerts. Thus, the cultural shift in management will require a different personality, capable of adaptability, agility, and responsiveness to multiple customers and stakeholders in a more dynamic and empowered environment.

8. **Enterprises, clinicians, payers, and consumers must become aligned through at-risk arrangements in order to optimize clinical and business outcomes.**

   As matrixes continue to grow and develop, increased accountability requires aligned contractual relationships that place a significant percentage of total compensation at risk for mutually agreed-on outcomes, both within and between systems. Patients and consumers, who have been traditionally viewed as dependent on physicians and healthcare systems, must now become at-risk partners to optimize their own cost-effective outcomes. Although incentives are already present in the private sector, they will be created in the public sector to ensure compliance and will have a substantial impact. Payers and employers will increasingly partner with practitioners, healthcare systems, and beneficiaries through transparent, dynamic, at-risk arrangements to control outcomes more effectively and to ensure that both the clinical model and the business model are sound and self-sustaining.

Many mourn the loss of the cottage industry healthcare model, in which a single physician carried the weight of a community on her shoulders supported by a stand-alone community hospital. Physicians saw something noble, and even romantic, regarding this individualistic, dedicated ethos characterized by devotion, idealism, and self-sacrifice.

We are in a different time now. The complexity of technology, systems research, and societal expectations now requires a different clinical and business model that is customized, available on demand, and responsive to patients who no longer emulate stereotypes and social expectations. Our country is now ready to embrace the optimization of health as the foundation for a healthcare industry that has lagged behind systems in other industrialized nations, even as it excelled in its capacity to heal the sick and injured.

Building the twenty-first-century enterprise won't be easy, but it is necessary to fulfill the promise of higher-quality lives achieved using a more sustainable business model that is based on service and partnership in a very different world from the one that came before.

Index

Note: Italicized page locators refer to figures or tables in exhibits.

489

About the Editor

JON BURROUGHS, MD, MBA, FACHE, FAAPL, is president and CEO of The Burroughs Healthcare Consulting Network, Inc., and works with some of the nation's top healthcare consulting firms to provide best-practice solutions and training to organizations throughout the country. He works in the areas of governance, physician–hospital alignment strategies, credentialing, privileging, peer review, performance improvement and patient safety, medical staff development planning, strategic planning, and physician performance and behavior management. He also has expertise in how physicians and management can work together in new ways to solve quality, safety, operational, and financial challenges through the creation of population health programs and clinically integrated networks.

Dr. Burroughs serves on the national faculty of the American College of Healthcare Executives (ACHE) and the American Association for Physician Leadership (AAPL), where he has been consistently rated as a top speaker and educator. In 2017, Burroughs and Richard Priore ScD, FACHE, introduced a new national program for ACHE titled Monetizing Quality in a Pay-for-Value World. In 2016, Burroughs; John Byrnes, MD; and Priore were awarded a national development grant by ACHE to develop a 12-hour program to address C-suite collaboration with physicians and the link between quality, safety, and service outcomes and financial performance. In 2014, he and Dr. David Nash were awarded another grant by ACHE for a program to address population health and the disruptive innovative business models necessary to support it. He developed a two-day advanced physician leadership program for AAPL, which was introduced 2016. Burroughs is the author or coauthor of the following books: *Redesign the Medical Staff Model* (Health Administration Press 2015; honored with the 2016 James A. Hamilton Award for outstanding healthcare management book), *The Complete Guide to FPPE* (HCPro 2012), *Medical Staff Leadership Essentials* (HCPro 2011), *Engage and Align the Medical Staff and Hospital Management* (HCPro 2010), *A Practical Guide to Managing Disruptive and Impaired Physicians* (HCPro 2010), *The Top 40 Medical Staff Policies and Procedures,* fourth edition (HCPro 2010), *Emergency Department On-Call Strategies* (Greeley Medical Staff Institute 2009), and *Peer Review Best Practices: Case Studies and Lessons Learned* (HCPro 2008).

Dr. Burroughs is a former senior consultant and director of education services for the Greeley Company, where he was rated as one of its top healthcare consultants and educators. He is also a past medical staff president and past president of the New Hampshire chapter of the American College of Emergency Physicians, and he served as an emergency department medical director. As a member of the governing board of Memorial Hospital in New Hampshire, he chaired the ethics, succession planning, and bylaws committees and sat on the joint conference, strategic planning, and medical executive committees. He previously served as a member of the clinical faculty of Dartmouth Medical School, where his research interests included introducing EMT defibrillation and automatic defibrillation to the field.

Dr. Burroughs's passion for the outdoors has led him to serve as a physician on mountaineering expeditions, and he has reached the summits of over 5,000 peaks throughout North America, South America, Europe, Africa, and Asia. He is the coeditor of the twenty-sixth edition of the *White Mountain Guide* and the first edition of the *Southern New Hampshire Trail Guide.* He was the first person to hike and log all maintained trails in the state of New Hampshire—more than 2,000 miles.

Dr. Burroughs received his bachelor's degree at Johns Hopkins University, his medical degree from Case Western Reserve University, and a healthcare master of business administration, with honors, at the Isenberg School of Management. He is a certified healthcare and physician executive; a Fellow of ACHE, where he was recently honored with a service award; and a fellow of the AAPL.

About the Contributors

Tom Atchison, EdD, is an international healthcare consultant specializing in leading sustainable change, physician leadership development, and improving organizational performance. He has authored four books and several articles on healthcare leadership. He has a doctorate human resources development from Loyola University in Chicago.

Mary A. Baker, CPMSM, CPCS, is president of Medical Staff Plus Consulting, LLC. She has more than 35 years of domestic and international healthcare experience. She works with medical staff leaders and medical staff services professionals in areas such as credentialing, privileging, accreditation readiness, and more. She received a master's degree in healthcare administration from Central Michigan University in 2000 and a doctorate in healthcare administration from the University of Phoenix in 2008. She is also a certified provider-credentialing specialist and a certified professional medical services manager.

Kathleen Bartholomew, RN, BS, MN, is an international speaker, author, and healthcare culture expert. She has authored *Ending Nurse-to-Nurse Hostility: Why Nurses Eat Their Young and Each Other,* (HCPro 2006) and *Speak Your Truth: Proven Strategies to Improve Nurse-Physician Communication* (HCPro 2005), and she has coauthored *The Dauntless Nurse: Communication Confidence Builder* (CreateSpace 2016). From the front line to the boardroom,

Kathleen works with leaders to maximize power and synergy in their organizations and to create a truly patient-centric culture.

Steve Berger, FACHE, FHFMA, CPA, is president of Berger Healthcare Executive Training and Consulting (HETC LLC) and has previously been a hospital financial executive, ACHE lecturer, and software entrepreneur. He has also written four peer-reviewed books, including *The Power of Clinical and Financial Metrics* (Health Administration Press 2005).

Brian Betner, Esq., is a shareholder at Hall, Render, Killian, Heath & Lyman, PC, where he focuses his practice on the representation of health systems, hospitals, and other healthcare providers in a broad range of regulatory, operational, and strategic matters. He graduated from the Indiana University Robert H. McKinney School of Law and completed the health law concentration with honors; he received the Outstanding Health Law Student Award and was the executive articles editor of the *Indiana Health Law Review*. Brian proudly served in the US Navy prior to law school.

Carl Couch, MD, MMM, is an accomplished family physician and physician executive in Dallas, Texas. He formed and led Baylor Healthcare System's employed physician group for 13 years; led major system quality improvement initiatives as vice president of quality; and formed and led Baylor Scott & White's accountable care organization, comprising more than 5,000 physicians, 50 hospitals, and almost 400,000 patients. He is a recognized expert in revenue cycle management, clinical quality improvement, strategy, and leading physicians.

Dan Grauman, MBA, CPA/ABV, is a managing director and CEO at Veralon. He has more than 35 years of experience with clients, including health systems, hospitals, physician–hospital organizations, clinically integrated networks, and health plans. His work is focused on mergers and affiliations, clinically integrated networks, value-based payment, and valuation. He has published numerous articles in national publications such as *hfm* and *Becker's Hospital Review*, and he speaks nationally on healthcare trends. Dan has been accredited in business valuation by the American Institute of Certified Public Accountants.

Michael Greer is a healthcare lawyer in the Indianapolis office of Hall, Render, Killian, Heath & Lyman, PC, and focuses his practice in the area of antitrust law. He has extensive experience in counseling health systems, hospitals, and physicians on the antitrust requirements of mergers, acquisitions, joint ventures, and provider networks. In this capacity, he frequently obtains clearance from the Federal Trade Commission and the Department of Justice under the premerger reporting requirements of the Hart-Scott-Rodino Antitrust Improvements Act, and he defends providers in government antitrust investigations. He also counsels healthcare providers on day-to-day antitrust compliance issues related to provider networks, managed care contracting, dominant firms, and exchanges of competitively sensitive information.

Mike Harmer leads the enterprise analytics and data science work at Intermountain Healthcare in Salt Lake City, Utah. He is a frequent speaker at industry conferences and has been with Intermountain Healthcare for more than 20 years. Mike holds a master's degree and is a senior partner at ThinkTroop, a research consulting firm.

John M. Harris, MBA, is a director at Veralon. He has more than 30 years of healthcare experience; he combines consulting expertise with a hands-on management background, having founded a healthcare business and operated facilities. He has consulted for hospitals and health systems, accountable care organizations, clinically integrated networks, physician–hospital organizations, and health plans. His work focuses on strategy, mergers and acquisitions, clinical transformation, and value-based payment. John is a faculty member of ACHE, conducting numerous sessions annually, including the course Strategic Planning: Formulation to Action, and he is the editor of the recently published *Healthcare Strategic Planning* (Health Administration Press 2017), fourth edition.

Brent Heaton is the data governance manager at Intermountain Healthcare. Brent oversees the planning, development, operations, training, and implementation of the Data Governance Program Office. Brent has more than 20 years of experience in healthcare information technology, focusing primarily in data and analytics functions. Brent received his bachelor of science in mechanical engineering from the University of Utah in 1993.

Steven Johnson, PhD, has served as president and CEO of Health First, on central Florida's east coast, since 2011. Health First is an integrated delivery network focused on health, wellness, and disease prevention. He earned his undergraduate degree in psychology from the University of Puget Sound in Washington State, a master of science in human development, and a doctoral degree in psychology, both from the University of Kansas.

Naveen Maram, MD, MSHI, MPH, is a partner in care transformation at Intermountain Healthcare.

John Nance, JD, author of the acclaimed book *Why Hospitals Should Fly* (Second River Healthcare, 2008; winner of ACHE's 2009 James A. Hamilton Award), is a lieutenant colonel in the Air Force; a veteran airline captain; and a leader in patient safety for the past quarter-century, bringing the lessons of high reliability to healthcare. The author of 23 books, he is also the long-time aviation analyst for ABC News and *Good Morning America*.

Lonny Northrup is a medical informaticist for Intermountain Healthcare, primarily responsible for finding, piloting, and implementing new data and analytic solutions leading to improved clinical outcomes and cost reductions. In addition, Lonny regularly collaborates with other leading healthcare providers to validate solutions being evaluated and implemented and to share data from various solutions to accelerate results inside Intermountain and with other healthcare systems.

James E. Orlikoff is president of Orlikoff & Associates, Inc., a consulting firm specializing in healthcare governance and leadership, strategy, quality, patient safety, and organizational development. He is the national adviser on governance and leadership to the American Hospital Association and Health Forum. He was named one of the 100 most powerful people in healthcare in the inaugural list by *Modern Healthcare*.

Lee Pierce, BS, MIS, is the chief data officer at Intermountain Healthcare. Lee has more than 20 years of experience in healthcare information technology, specializing in business intelligence, data warehousing, data architecture, and business intelligence/ data governance. He has been accountable for the development of Intermountain's analytics infrastructure, data governance efforts, business intelligence development, and coordination of analytics and data science services throughout the enterprise. Lee is the immediate past chairman and incorporator of the Healthcare Data and Analytics Association, a national nonprofit organization with more than 400 member healthcare organizations.

Jake Poore is the founder, president, and CEO of Integrated Loyalty Systems, an Orlando-based company on a mission to change the face of healthcare. For more than three decades, including 18 years as a leader with the Walt Disney Company, Jake has taught organizations how to transform their culture to create a world-class employee and customer experience.

Sid Thornton, **PhD,** works in the field of healthcare data interoperability as a care transformation partner at Intermountain Healthcare and as an adjunct assistant research professor for the Department of Bioinformatics at the University of Utah. He has contributed to several state and national advisory committees, including Shared

Identity Services for Utah, Carequality, and the Care Connectivity Consortium. He leads research activities focused on identity relationship resolution and workflow automation in medical informatics.

William Vanaskie, FACHE, is a leadership consultant with more than 35 years of healthcare experience. His past positions include executive vice president and chief operating officer of Maricopa Integrated Health System, Phoenix, Arizona; executive vice president and chief operating officer for Parkland Health and Hospital System in Dallas, Texas; president and CEO of Robert Packer Hospital and executive vice president and chief operating officer for Guthrie Healthcare System, both in Pennsylvania; and president and CEO of St. Francis Regional Medical Center in Wichita, Kansas. He is a graduate of the United States Military Academy at West Point, and he holds a master's degree in engineering and construction management from the University of Colorado and a master's of business administration from Bucknell University. He currently serves on the faculty of the College of Health Solutions, Arizona State University.